# SPORT FIRST AID

## Sixth Edition

### EDITOR

**Robb S. Rehberg**
PhD, ATC, NREMT

### CONTRIBUTORS

**Michael Prybicien**
MA, LAT, ATC, CES, PES

**Ben Chianchiano**
MS, ATC, LAT, CSCS

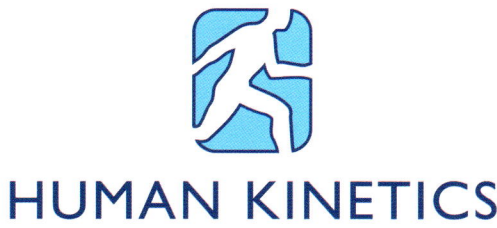

**HUMAN KINETICS**

**Library of Congress Cataloging-in-Publication Data**

Names: Rehberg, Robb S., editor. | Prybicien, Michael, other. |
   Chianchiano, Ben, other.
Title: Sport first aid / Robb S. Rehberg, PhD, ATC, NREMT, Editor, Michael
   Prybicien, Ben Chianchiano, Contributors.
Description: Sixth edition. | Champaign, IL : Human Kinetics, 2026. |
   Includes bibliographical references and index.
Identifiers: LCCN 2024033292 (print) | LCCN 2024033293 (ebook) | ISBN
   9781718216754 (paperback) | ISBN 9781718216761 (epub) | ISBN
   9781718216778 (pdf)
Subjects: LCSH: Sports injuries--Treatment. | First aid in illness and
   injury.
Classification: LCC RD97 .F525 2026  (print) | LCC RD97  (ebook) | DDC
   617.1/027--dc23/eng/20240718
LC record available at https://lccn.loc.gov/2024033292
LC ebook record available at https://lccn.loc.gov/2024033293

ISBN: 978-1-7182-1675-4 (print)

Copyright © 2026, 2014, 2008, 2004, 1997, 1992 by Human Kinetics, Inc.

This publication is written and published to provide accurate and authoritative information relevant to the subject matter presented. It is published and sold with the understanding that the author and publisher are not engaged in rendering legal, medical, or other professional services by reason of their authorship or publication of this work. If medical or other expert assistance is required, the services of a competent professional person should be sought.

The web addresses cited in this text were current as of August 2023, unless otherwise noted.

**Senior Developmental Editor:** Laura Pulliam; **Managing Editor:** Hannah Werner; **Copyeditor:** Joanna Hatzopoulos Portman; **Indexer:** Nan N. Badgett; **Permissions Manager:** Laurel Mitchell; **Senior Graphic Designer:** Sean Roosevelt; **Cover Designer:** Keri Evans; **Cover Design Specialist:** Susan Rothermel Allen; **Photographs (cover):** Harry How/Getty Images and Stu Forster - The FA/The FA via Getty Images; **Photographs (interior):** © Human Kinetics, unless otherwise noted; **Photo Asset Manager:** Laura Fitch; **Photo Production Specialist:** Amy M. Rose; **Photo Production Manager:** Jason Allen; **Senior Art Manager:** Kelly Hendren; **Illustrations:** © Human Kinetics, unless otherwise noted; **Printer:** Versa Press

We thank Liberty Office Suites in Pine Brook, New Jersey, for assistance in providing the location for the photo shoot for this book.

Printed in the United States of America     10  9  8  7  6  5  4  3  2

The paper in this book is certified under a sustainable forestry program.

**Human Kinetics**
1607 N. Market Street
Champaign, IL 61820
USA

*United States and International*
Website: **US.HumanKinetics.com**
Email: info@hkusa.com
Phone: 1-800-747-4457

*Canada*
Website: **Canada.HumanKinetics.com**
Email: info@hkcanada.com

Human Kinetics' authorized representative for product safety in the EU is Mare Nostrum Group B.V., Mauritskade 21D, 1091 GC Amsterdam, The Netherlands.
Email: gpsr@mare-nostrum.co.uk                                    E8862

This book is dedicated to the thousands of youth and high school coaches who have a positive impact on the lives of their athletes each day. Few people realize all that is required to meet the expectations of that role. More than ever, coaches are met with challenges that extend far beyond the Xs and Os of their sport. It is our hope that this book will help each coach be more prepared to manage one of the more serious of their many responsibilities and, in doing so, make their job a bit less challenging.

# CONTENTS

# PREFACE

Being a successful coach requires more than just knowing the skills and strategies of the sport. It includes being able to teach techniques and tactics, lead and motivate athletes, and manage a plethora of responsibilities. One of those duties is to be a competent first responder who is able to address athletes' injuries and illnesses.

Only about one-third of high schools in the United States have the full-time services of an athletic trainer, and one-third have no athletic trainer services at all. Even in the programs fortunate enough to have full-time athletic trainer services, only very rarely is an on-site professional present at all practices and competitions. Athletic trainers are even less likely to be available for club teams. Therefore, because sport injuries are inevitable in both practices and games, it is essential that coaches know how to fulfill their role as first responder.

This sixth edition of *Sport First Aid* is designed to prepare coaches for that role. Because coaches have many other matters to tend to, we have streamlined this book to include only those first aid topics and procedures coaches should know, and we have prioritized the information that is most important to know and most likely to be used. *Sport First Aid* also serves as the text for a course offered by Human Kinetics Coach Education.

Human Kinetics recruited us to author the book and course content to be as current and relevant as possible, while ensuring its presentation is instructionally effective for the coaching community. We have worked with coaches throughout the course of our careers and have created instructional materials and courses to help coaches understand and fulfill their injury prevention and sport first aid responsibilities. Those experiences and many years of study and work in the field have informed our decisions regarding what content would be presented in this book.

The first few chapters provide a basic background to get started, just as you would do for a new athlete entering your program. In this case, this introductory material leads you through learning your role on the athletic health care team, familiarizing yourself with the game plan for sport first aid, and getting up to speed on anatomy and sport injury lingo you need to know. We are not expecting you to absorb all of this information in your initial read-through, just as you would not expect your rookie athletes to grasp everything in their first week or two of the preseason. But after you have made your way through the entire book, with quick refreshers every now and then, repeated exposure will give you a good handle on the essentials.

The next three chapters teach first aid fundamentals, starting with step-by-step instructions on what to do when medical emergencies occur. Next are tutorials on how to assess the status of an injured or ill athlete and first aid measures to take in responding to such scenarios. This section concludes with guidance on whether to move an injured or ill athlete and, when it is appropriate, how to do it properly.

The remainder of the book covers the full spectrum of injuries and illnesses your athletes may suffer, with an emphasis on those ailments that are most common. In each of those chapters you will find concise and understandable explanations of the condition, including the causes or mechanisms, how it might be prevented, the signs and symptoms, and a description and illustrations (when helpful) of the proper first aid to be applied. Again, all of this is a lot to consume and is certainly too much for you to master from your first reading. However, simply gaining a basic awareness of what to look for and how to respond is a good start. Then you can refer back to these chapters time and again—perhaps giving more attention to those chapters that cover injuries and illnesses you have found to be more common in your sport—until you have the knowledge needed to be an effective first aid provider.

This book is not intended to make you a medical expert. However, the text, along with the course that accompanies it, should prepare you to competently serve your first responder role. By reading and studying this book, and referring back to the material for refreshers, you will be better prepared to provide basic care for athletes' injuries and illnesses.

# ACKNOWLEDGMENTS

In the fall of 1991, I was a new athletic trainer working at a high school in New Jersey. As the first full-time athletic trainer at that school, I wore many hats in addition to providing care for student-athletes, and one of those jobs included educating the coaching staff on first aid. Although I had taught first aid before, I knew somehow the content needed to address the unique needs of coaches. "How can I make this relevant for the coaches?" was a recurring question in my mind, until one day when my athletic director handed me a piece of mail he had received about a brand-new book: *Sport First Aid*, by Melinda J. Flegel. I instantly knew this book was exactly what I needed, and it didn't disappoint! Melinda, thank you for your dedication to educating coaches on a topic that is more important than any game strategy.

*Sport First Aid* was groundbreaking at the time, and Melinda's comprehensive yet easy-to-use book gave me exactly what I needed to teach our coaches what they needed to know. Since that time, the book has been used to educate generations of coaches on how to prevent, recognize, and respond to sport-related injuries and illnesses. Who knew that over 30 years and five editions later, the challenge to continue and attempt to improve upon that effort would be passed on to me and my colleagues to create the sixth edition!

Much like a championship season, creating a winning book like this takes teamwork. Thanks to Ted Miller, the "captain" of this project, for approaching me with the idea, for convincing me it was a good one, and for having the perseverance, patience, and vision to see it through to completion. Thanks also to Laura Pulliam and the entire team at Human Kinetics. You have been a wonderful partner throughout this project.

Special thanks to Mike Prybicien and Ben Chianchiano, my coauthors and driving force behind this project. Young athletes will be safer on the field, court, mat, and ice because of your countless hours researching, writing, editing, rearranging, and rewriting. Thank you for taking this journey with me. I could not be more proud to have you as colleagues and friends, and now coauthors. Equal thanks to Jennifer Prybicien and Sarina Lavooy-Chianchiano for your support and patience as Mike and Ben worked tirelessly on this project. I appreciate you sharing your husbands with us!

Finally, thanks to my wife, Joelle, and my children, Anna and Joey, for their unending love and support. None of what I do professionally would be possible without your unconditional love and support.

*Robb S. Rehberg*

# INTRODUCTION

January 2, 2023, was a Monday when most of us were trying to get back into the work routine after the holiday break. That night, millions of *Monday Night Football* viewers—and many more millions who later saw replays of the game's defining event—were provided a vivid example of why prepared and capable first aid responders at sport competitions, practices, and training sessions are so essential.

With a little more than 6 minutes remaining in the first quarter of the game between the Buffalo Bills and Cincinnati Bengals, Cincinnati wide receiver Tee Higgins caught a pass near midfield and lowered his right shoulder before ramming into the head and chest of Buffalo defensive back Damar Hamlin. Hamlin was able to wrestle Higgins to the ground with him. However, after Hamlin got up and appeared to adjust his face mask, he fell backward to the turf.

The Bills' medical staff rushed onto the field and, after quickly determining that Hamlin was suffering a cardiac arrest, immediately executed its league-approved emergency plan. Athletic trainers and physicians quickly administered CPR and defibrillation, which experts later said were crucial for not only the resumption of Hamlin's cardiac function but also his subsequent neurological function and recovery. Amazingly, through effective and diligent rehabilitation and training, Hamlin returned to the field to play the following season in five regular season games and two playoff games, mostly on special teams.

Only a very small percentage of sport first aid scenarios are as dire, dramatic, or public as Damar Hamlin's. However, that in no way minimizes the need to provide all athletes prompt and effective attention when they are suddenly injured or ill. And because many interscholastic or club sports programs still do not have medical professionals such as an athletic trainer on site at every training session, practice, or competition, it is you, the coach, who must fill the vital role of capable first aid provider until further help arrives.

It is a daunting task—one most coaches feel very uneasy about fulfilling. If you share the same uneasiness, that's good, because it means you are taking the responsibility seriously. Now let me offer assurance that you can fulfill this first aid duty.

I have had the unique opportunity to gain a 360-degree view on this issue. Through my experience as a youth and high school coach, as an athletic trainer, as a chief of emergency medical services, as a professor of athletic training and sports medicine, and now as senior medical advisor and director of game day medical operations for the National Football League, I can say that preparedness and appropriate immediate care matter, as in Damar Hamlin's case. In fact, appropriate immediate care is the most important factor in an emergency.

Much of my professional career has been devoted to helping others learn and apply first aid protocols in the athletic setting. I have helped educate parents coaching their kids' youth sports teams for the first time, veteran high school coaches who had gone many years with no training, and aspiring students who will someday be the next generation of athletic trainers and physicians. So I know what is and is not important for you to know and be able to do as a coach who works with young athletes.

*Sport First Aid* embodies that practical perspective. Its intent is not to try to make you a medical professional. Rather, the aim of the book is simply to help you provide immediate care until further help is available. My coauthors and I have made the material easy to read and grasp and have emphasized the injuries and illnesses that you are most likely to have to deal with in your role as first aid responder.

Medical emergencies in sports are rarely as serious as a heart attack, but all illnesses and injuries incurred by athletes warrant a serious, quick, and effective response. *Sport First Aid* and its corresponding course will help ensure you are prepared to provide just that.

# PART I
# BASICS OF SPORT FIRST AID

# YOUR ROLE ON THE ATHLETIC HEALTH CARE TEAM

**IN THIS CHAPTER, YOU WILL LEARN THE FOLLOWING:**

- The four-part approach of the athletic health care plan
- What the athletic health care team is and who is part of it
- How to define the respective roles of each member of the athletic health care team
- What your role is on the athletic health care team
- The types of health care providers you might work with and your role in working with them
- What emergency medical personnel, athletic trainers, and physical therapists do and your role in working with them
- The need for good communication among all members of the athletic health care team

Building a winning athletic health care team is vital to the success of any athletic organization. In fact, it is similar to assembling a successful athletic team. Members of both types of teams must understand their individual roles (assigned tasks), cooperate with others on the team to prepare for various challenging situations, and practice their own positions within the team. Without these components, it is difficult to function as an effective athletic health care team and to successfully provide first aid. Each member of the athletic health care team must ensure proper injury evaluation and subsequent care. Improper evaluation and care can cause further injury, delay the athlete's recovery, or decrease the athlete's athletic performance; in some cases, it can even cause catastrophic injury or long-term harm to the athlete.

To ensure successful role delineation, team members must understand the four-part approach of the athletic health care team. These four parts are essential for ensuring safe and successful participation in sports:

1. *Injury prevention*—Recognizing how an injury happens in order to appropriately plan and attempt to avoid the occurrence of the injury. This goal should be a primary focus for everyone involved in athletics.

2. *Injury recognition and initial first aid care*—Recognizing that when an injury occurs, the immediate care provided is essential.

3. *Injury assessment and initial treatment*—Determining the extent of the injury and what follow-up care is needed.

4. *Follow-up care*—Understanding the importance of making the correct referrals to those involved on your athletic health care team.

Protecting the health and safety of an athlete requires the participation of many different team members. These team members may include the following:

Coach

Athlete

Parent or guardian

Athletic trainer

Physicians such as primary care or specialty care physicians, physician assistants, or nurse practitioners (refer to state laws as they may vary on who can provide a diagnosis and medically clear an athlete)

Physical therapist

Dentist or oral surgeon

Optometrist

Emergency medical services such as emergency medical technicians (EMTs) or paramedics

Strength and conditioning coach

Equipment manager

The following sections explain each person's role in ensuring the health and safety of the athlete.

## Coach's Role

The coach plays a central role in protecting the health and safety of an athlete. Every coach must understand the importance of excellent communication. Coaches (head and assistant) need to communicate with all parties (athletes, parents or guardians, other coaches and staff, and various members of the athletic health care team) involved in sport safety. Coaches should establish and monitor rules, policies, and procedures with athletes, parents or guardians, and athletic health care team members alike. For teams with multiple coaches, the head coach should assume the majority of the responsibilities. Assistant coaches should stand by to assist the head coach.

Coaches are responsible for knowing and understanding the rules of their specific sport as set forth by the governing body of the sport.

Coaches must also know and understand the sport safety policies, protocols, and guidelines at their school or organization. Established policies, protocols, and guidelines guide the coach in working to ensure injury prevention, recognition, assessment, first aid, treatment, rehabilitation, and safe return to play. Examples include preparticipation physical examinations, emergency action plans, procedures for cardiac emergencies or concussion, education for injury prevention, guidelines for hydration, and procedures for extreme weather (heat, cold, or lightning).

The primary role of coaches is to minimize injury for athletes who are under their supervision. Therefore, as a coach, you are likely to be involved in each leg of the athletic health care relay—prevention, recognition and first aid care, assessment and treatment, and rehabilitation. Your role is defined by

- certain rules of the legal system and rules of your school administration,
- expectations of parents or guardians, and
- interactions with other athletic health care team members.

Minimizing the risk of injury to athletes encompasses a variety of coaching duties. As a coach, you should perform the following duties to safely train your athletes:

1. Properly plan each activity.
   - Teach the skills of the sport using the correct progression.
   - Consider each athlete's developmental level and current physical condition. Evaluate your athletes' physical capacities and skill levels with preseason fitness tests, and develop practice plans accordingly.
   - Keep written records of fitness test results and practice plans. Don't deviate from your plans without good cause.

2. Provide proper instruction.
   - Make sure that athletes are in proper condition to participate.
   - Teach athletes the rules and the correct skills and strategies of the sport. For example, in American football, teach athletes that tackling with the head (spearing) is illegal and potentially dangerous.

- Teach athletes the sport skills and conditioning exercises in a progression so that they are adequately prepared to handle more difficult skills or exercises.

- Stay current about more effective and safer ways of performing the techniques used in the sport.

- Provide competent and responsible assistants. If you have coaching assistants, make sure that they are knowledgeable in the skills and strategies of the sport and that they behave in a mature and responsible manner.

3. Warn of inherent risks.

- Provide parents or guardians and athletes with both oral and written statements of the inherent health risks of their particular sport.

- Warn athletes about potentially harmful conditions, such as playing conditions, dangerous or faulty equipment, and the like.

4. Provide a safe physical environment.

- Monitor current environmental conditions, such as windchill, temperature, humidity, and severe weather warnings.

- Periodically inspect the playing areas, the locker room, the weight room, and the dugout for hazards.

- Remove all hazards.

- Prevent improper or unsupervised use of facilities.

5. Provide adequate and proper equipment.

- Make sure athletes are using equipment that provides the maximum amount of protection against injury.

- Inspect equipment regularly.

- Teach athletes how to fit, use, and inspect their equipment.

6. Match your athletes appropriately.

- Match the athletes according to size, physical maturity, skill level, and experience.

- Do not pit physically immature or novice athletes against those who are in top condition and are highly skilled.

7. Evaluate athletes for injury or incapacity.

- Require all athletes to participate in preseason physical exams, health screenings, and sport ability screenings to detect potential health problems and monitor performance.

- If an athlete is unable to compete without pain or loss of function (e.g., inability to walk, run, jump, or throw without restriction), withhold that athlete from practice and competition.

8. Supervise each activity closely.

- Do not allow athletes to practice difficult or potentially dangerous skills without proper supervision.

- Forbid rough or boisterous play (e.g., wrestling around) during the activity.

- Do not allow athletes to use sport facilities without supervision.

9. Provide appropriate emergency assistance.

- Learn sport first aid as well as cardiopulmonary resuscitation (CPR) and use of an automated external defibrillator (AED). You can take a course through organizations such as the American Red Cross or the American Heart Association.

- Take action when needed. As a coach, you are responsible for ensuring athletes under your supervision receive immediate care if they become ill or injured. If no medical personnel are present when an injury or illness occurs, you are responsible for providing emergency care.

- Use only the skills that you are trained to administer, and provide the specific standard of care that you are trained to provide through sport first aid, CPR, and other sports medicine courses.

- For athletes who are minors, obtain a signed consent form from their parents or guardians before the season begins. For injured or ill adult athletes, specifically ask if they want help. If they are unresponsive, consent is usually implied. If they refuse help and you believe they need medical care, send for emergency medical assistance or obtain assistance from a health care provider, such as an athletic trainer, if available.

---

**SAFETY MEASURE**

**When to Return to Play**

Athletes with any of the following conditions should not return to play until they have been evaluated by the appropriate health care professional:

- Inability to bear full weight with walking, jogging, or running
- Loss of function (upper or lower extremity)
- Any signs or symptoms from a head injury
- Fever
- Dehydration
- Any heat- or cold-related issue
- Any pain-related issue

---

As a coach, you should become familiar with each of the nine duties described in this section. The first eight deal mainly with preventive measures. This book is primarily designed to help you handle duty number 9.

## Athlete's Role

Sports begin and end with the athlete. Athletes must understand the role they play in managing their own safety. Following rules, understanding guidelines and procedures, and advocating for their own well-being are cornerstones to the athletes' own safety. Their safety starts with following their school's or organization's preparticipation process.

Organizations should establish an education process for athletes, such as online education programs, informational pamphlets, or live or virtual lectures. These programs ensure that athletes are aware of signs and symptoms of foreseeable injuries or conditions and that they understand the importance of reporting these signs and symptoms to their parents or guardians, coaches, athletic trainers, or other pertinent staff members.

## Parent's or Guardian's Role

Parents or guardians can assist the athletic health care team by ensuring that their child completes the school's or organization's preparticipation sport screening. They should educate themselves as a means of assisting their child in safe participation in sports, thereby allowing for better performance and reduction of injury.

To ensure continuity of communication, parents or guardians should be encouraged to participate in their child's safety. Parents or guardians should establish an open line of communication with their child, and they should watch for the signs and symptoms of injury and illness. This awareness is an important factor in protecting the long- and short-term athletic goals of the child. When parents or guardians support the decisions of sports medicine health care professionals in terms of play restrictions, limitations, and return to play, they help set their children up for success.

To help parents or guardians actively participate in athletes' safety, the coach or athletic health care team must communicate openly with them; they should keep parents or guardians informed of injury or illness situations arising with their child. In addition, the athletic health care team should expect to answer a variety of questions from parents or guardians, such as the following:

What documents do I need to complete before practice starts?

What protective equipment do I need to provide my athlete?

What is the best way to contact you in the event of an emergency?

What exactly is my child's injury?

Can my child continue to play with this injury without making it worse?

Does my child need to see a doctor?

Is there anything I need to buy to be able to help my child compete (e.g., brace, pads, mouth guard)?

If my child is unable to play now, when is it safe to return to the sport?

Who determines when it is safe for my child to return to the sport?

Is there any return to play progression my child needs to follow?

How can this injury be prevented next time?

In summary, the role of parents and guardians on the athletic health care team entails actively staying informed about and involved in their child's safety. Coaches facilitate this role by communicating with them.

# Roles of Other Members of the Athletic Health Care Team

While the head coach plays a central role on the athletic health care team, some peripheral team members have crucial supporting roles in ensuring the health and safety of athletes. This section describes these members, their roles, and the head coach's role in interacting with them.

## Athletic Trainer

In many situations, the athletic trainer is the leader of the athletic health care team. The athletic trainer is most likely the first contact for the athlete with a medical concern. Oftentimes, the athletic trainer has already developed a rapport and relationship with the athletes. An athletic trainer (AT) is a health care professional trained in the prevention, emergency care, clinical diagnosis, therapeutic intervention, and rehabilitation of injuries and medical conditions. ATs collaborate with physicians to provide health care to the physically active. They observe for mechanisms of injury, and they can evaluate and treat injuries. Employing an AT helps to quickly determine an injury, decreases liability, and helps to rehabilitate the athlete after an injury. Having an AT on staff can facilitate a shorter recovery time for the athlete while also allowing the coaches to concentrate on coaching. An AT's ability to provide the proper physical medicine and rehabilitation techniques will provide the athlete with the environment that is most conducive to promoting healing and return to play. The AT can help to create demand-specific rehabilitation programs for athletes in a variety of sports and different positions within the sport.

Of course, prevention is the first domain for any AT. ATs are trained to prevent injury in various ways, including the following:

- Ensure proper fitting of equipment, padding, and bracing
- Ensure preventive and postinjury taping and strapping
- Assist with the administrative processes of medical and conditioning screening
- Perform field and facility inspections
- Monitor environmental factors
- Assist athletes on proper nutrition and hydration recommendations

Other functions of the AT may include the following:

- Athlete and coach education
- Injury assessment and documentation
- Emergency care
- Coordination of care
- Planning and training for emergencies during games and practices
- Communication with parents or guardians
- Injury rehabilitation
- Decisions for return to play

When an athlete has been injured, the coach's role is to work closely with the AT to provide information on how the injury occurred as well as to support the AT's decisions regarding the athlete's care, ability to participate, and compliance in a rehabilitation plan.

## Physician

Physicians play an important role on the athletic health care team. They can evaluate and diagnose illnesses and injuries, prescribe appropriate care, and also prescribe treatment and rehabilitation for illness and injury. Physicians on the athletic health care team should

- have a doctor of medicine (MD) or doctor of osteopathic medicine (DO) degree and be licensed in the state where they are practicing;
- possess fundamental knowledge of providing emergency care at sport events;
- be trained in CPR and AED; and
- have a working knowledge of trauma, musculoskeletal injury, and medical conditions affecting athletes.

In addition to the team physician, an injured or ill athlete may need to see other physicians for more specialized care. While the athlete's parents or legal guardians (or the athlete's insurance plan) may ultimately dictate the next step, the team physician can help you determine which type of physician the injured or ill athlete should see (e.g., a family practitioner, a pediatrician, an orthopedist, or a podiatrist). Types of physicians that may be involved in an athlete's care include the following:

- *Family practice and internal medicine physicians*—Specialize in general medicine.
- *Pediatricians*—Specialize in providing medical care to children from infants to teenagers.
- *Orthopedists*—Specialize in the diagnosis and treatment (which may include surgery) of injuries to the bones, ligaments, tendons, muscles, and joints.
- *Neurologists*—Specialize in the treatment of injuries to the nervous system and brain.
- *Physiatrists*—Specialize in physical medicine, including diagnosis, treatment, and rehabilitation.
- *Podiatrists*—Specialize in the medical care of foot and ankle problems.
- *Ophthalmologists*—Specialize in medicine related to proper management of eye-related issues.
- *Physician assistant*—A physician assistant (PA) is a licensed medical professional who holds an advanced degree and is able to provide direct patient care. The specific duties of a PA are determined by their supervising physician and state law, but they provide many of the same services as a primary care physician.
- *Nurse practitioner*—A nurse practitioner (NP) is a health care professional who offers a wide range of acute, primary, and specialty care services, either alone or alongside a doctor.

Once the team physician or other specialty physician has examined an athlete, the coach should support the physician's recommendations, including restrictions on sport participation. If a parent or legal guardian is not satisfied with the physician's diagnosis and treatment, seeking a second opinion may be warranted. However, it is unethical for a parent, guardian, or coach to send an injured or ill athlete to numerous physicians (often referred to as "doctor shopping") in an attempt to get permission for the athlete to resume activity.

After the team physician or other specialty physician has evaluated an injured or ill athlete, the coach, along with the parents or guardians, should urge the athlete to obtain a referral from the physician and seek follow-up care with an AT (if one is not available through the school or organization) or physical therapist at a local sports medicine clinic, physical therapy clinic, or hospital physical therapy department. (The physical therapist's role is discussed in the next section.)

## Physical Therapist

Physical therapists (PTs) are health professionals who rehabilitate individuals experiencing disease or injury. They are trained to handle a wide variety of medical problems, including cerebral palsy, strokes, heart problems, paraplegia, burns, and athletic injuries. Some PTs specialize in the evaluation, care, and rehabilitation of sport injuries.

These professionals are trained to analyze strength, joint motion, flexibility, coordination, and other physical attributes, and then instruct the athlete in an individualized rehabilitation program. They are also trained in administering modalities such as whirlpools, massage, ultrasound, and muscle stimulation as well as therapies such as joint mobilization. These modalities and therapies are important to help ease pain, decrease swelling, promote tissue healing, and restore function for a safe return to sport participation.

When an athlete has been injured, the coach's, athlete's, and parent's or guardian's roles in working with a PT are the same as working with an AT. The coach, the athlete, and the parent or guardian should provide information on how the injury occurred and support the PT's decisions regarding the athlete's care, ability to participate, and compliance in a rehabilitation plan.

## Dentist or Oral Surgeon

Both dentists and oral surgeons are medically trained to evaluate and treat conditions and injuries of the mouth, jaw, and teeth. Oral surgeons have completed a hospital surgical residency program for further training in the surgical treatment of conditions affecting the mouth, teeth and jaw, and portions of the face.

Dentists and oral surgeons can provide assistance and recommendations to athletes on mouth guards and other equipment to protect the face and mouth. When an athlete participates in a contact sport, the coach and the parent or guardian should encourage the athlete to wear an appropriate protective mouthpiece or a face protector.

## Optometrist

Although they are not medical doctors, doctors of optometry (optometrists) receive specialized training and certification in diagnosing vision problems and eye disease. They are also trained to prescribe eyeglasses, contact lenses, and drugs to treat eye disorders. When an athlete participates in a contact sport, the coach and the parent or guardian should encourage the athlete to use appropriate protective eyewear or a face protector.

## Emergency Medical Technician (EMT) and Paramedic

Emergency medical technicians (EMTs) and paramedics are trained to provide emergency medical care for a variety of situations and conditions. They are also experts in immobilizing serious injuries and providing rapid response and transportation to the appropriate emergency medical facility.

Use the following guidelines for situations when emergency medical services are needed:

- Communicate with the athletic health care team in advance, and practice emergency scenarios together.
- Have emergency contact information ready, such as parent or guardian information, medical allergies and conditions, and other pertinent information, to give to EMTs and paramedics.
- Be ready to assist in crowd control. Some people who are not needed in the situation may hinder the emergency response. It is very important that only the necessary personnel be involved in the situation.
- Have an area designated for quick access to and from your facility.
- Document the injury, event, and any first aid performed prior to the emergency team's arrival.

EMTs and paramedics are unique in that they are members of the athletic health care team who do not already know your athletes. Therefore, clear communication about your athletes' health is crucial.

## Strength and Conditioning Coach

The strength and conditioning coach can perform fitness assessments and develop and supervise the proper strength and conditioning needs of the athletes. Quality strength and conditioning coaches may have certifications from accredited organizations such as the National Strength and Conditioning Association (NSCA) or the American College of Sports Medicine (ACSM). The strength and conditioning coach works with athletes, coaches, and parents or guardians with a focus on these three goals: improve athletic performance; reduce athletic injuries; and teach lifelong fitness and movement skills (strengthen, stretch). The head coach should insist that athletes attend fitness assessments and participate in all conditioning workouts with the strength and conditioning coach.

## Equipment Manager

Some schools or organizations may assign someone to the role of equipment manager. This person should be tasked with the fitting, inspection, cleaning, maintenance, and storage of equipment. In cases when standards are in place for equipment, the equipment manager must know the standards and abide by the regulations for the equipment. For example, the equipment manager is expected to know standards for various types of helmets and adhere to rules regarding their shelf life.

In working with the equipment manager, the coach's role is to assist as needed with equipment fitting and maintenance and to enforce athletes' proper use of equipment. The coach should also help watch for equipment wear and tear. Athletes and parents or guardians can also pay attention to these details when equipment is taken home.

The importance of the athletic health care team can't be understated. Team members must all understand their roles and work within those roles. Team members should feel confident in their own abilities and in the abilities of the other team members. Organization and communication are essential components of the success of the athletic health care team. Table 1.1 summarizes the goals and common roles of each member of the athletic health care team.

**Table 1.1** Athletic Health Care Team Goals and Roles

| | GOALS OF THE ATHLETIC HEALTH CARE TEAM | | | |
|---|---|---|---|---|
| | **Injury prevention** | **Injury recognition and initial first aid care** | **Injury assessment and initial treatment** | **Follow-up care** |
| **Coach** | • Ensure athlete receives preseason screening and physical exam.<br>• Ensure athlete participates in conditioning programs.<br>• Ensure athlete wears appropriate protective equipment.<br>• Enforce safety rules. | • Watch for injuries and illnesses.<br>• Act as first responder in providing first aid assessment and care.<br>• Recommend athlete's injury or illness be thoroughly evaluated and properly treated. | • Act as first responder in providing first aid care. | • Encourage athlete to exactly follow rehabilitation and conditioning instructions.<br>• Don't allow athlete to participate until given clearance. |
| **Athlete** | • Receive preseason screening and physical exam.<br>• Participate in conditioning programs.<br>• Wear appropriate protective equipment.<br>• Abide by safety rules. | • Inform parent or guardian, coach, or athletic trainer of illness or injury.<br>• Receive injury or illness assessment by physician, athletic trainer, or physical therapist. | • Receive first aid care or physician treatment. | • Perform rehabilitation and conditioning exercises exactly as instructed.<br>• Return to activities only after given clearance. |
| **Parent or guardian** | • Ensure athlete receives preseason screening and physical exam.<br>• Ensure athlete participates in conditioning programs.<br>• Ensure athlete wears appropriate protective equipment. | • Watch for injuries and illnesses.<br>• Ensure athlete's injury or illness is thoroughly evaluated and properly treated. | • Ensure athlete receives appropriate first aid or physician treatment. | • Encourage athlete to exactly follow rehabilitation and conditioning instructions.<br>• Don't allow athlete to participate until given clearance. |
| **Athletic trainer** | • Provide preseason fitness and injury risk assessment screening.<br>• Assist with scheduling and conducting preseason physical exams.<br>• Recommend or develop conditioning programs.<br>• Inspect condition of equipment and playing areas.<br>• Recommend replacing or refurbishing faulty equipment or playing areas.<br>• Ensure proper equipment fitting for each athlete.<br>• Recommend preventive bracing or taping as needed. | • Watch for injuries and illnesses.<br>• Provide emergency medical care.<br>• Assist EMTs or paramedics in preparing an athlete for transportation to a medical facility.<br>• Recommend physician diagnosis as needed. | • Provide injury treatments (such as ultrasound) as prescribed by a physician. | • Assess athlete's symptoms and ability to function.<br>• Develop individualized rehabilitation program.<br>• Maintain athlete's fitness during rehabilitation.<br>• Safely progress athlete back into full activity.<br>• Develop and fit protective braces or pads to prevent reinjury. |

| | GOALS OF THE ATHLETIC HEALTH CARE TEAM | | | |
| --- | --- | --- | --- | --- |
| | **Injury prevention** | **Injury recognition and initial first aid care** | **Injury assessment and initial treatment** | **Follow-up care** |
| **Physician** | • Conduct preseason physical exams. | • Volunteer or contract to provide on-site emergency medical assistance at sport events.<br>• Evaluate athlete by conducting or ordering appropriate diagnostic tests. | • Prescribe appropriate treatment.<br>• Refer injured athlete to athletic trainer or physical therapist for rehabilitation. | • May recommend or prescribe specific rehabilitation exercises.<br>• May provide final clearance for return to full participation. |
| **Physical therapist** | • Provide preseason fitness and injury risk assessment screening.<br>• Recommend preventive bracing or taping as needed. | • Watch for injuries and illnesses.<br>• Act as first responder in providing first aid assessment and care.<br>• Recommend physician diagnosis as needed. | • Provide injury treatments (such as ultrasound) as prescribed by a physician. | • Assess athlete's symptoms and ability to function.<br>• Develop individualized rehabilitation program.<br>• Maintain athlete's fitness during rehabilitation.<br>• Safely progress athlete back into full activity.<br>• Develop and fit protective braces or pads to prevent reinjury. |
| **Dentist or oral surgeon** | • Recommend and fit mouth guards. | • Evaluate dental injuries. | • Treat dental injuries. | • Provide final clearance for return to full activity after dental injury. |
| **Optometrist** | • Recommend and fit appropriate protective eyewear. | N/A | N/A | • Assist with follow-up care of eye injuries when needed. |
| **Emergency medical technician and paramedic** | N/A | • Volunteer or contract to provide on-site emergency medical assessment, care, and transportation at sport events. | • Provide advanced emergency medical care. | • Transport via ambulance as needed. |

*(continued)*

**Table 1.1** Athletic Health Care Team Goals and Roles *(continued)*

| | GOALS OF THE ATHLETIC HEALTH CARE TEAM | | | |
|---|---|---|---|---|
| | **Injury prevention** | **Injury recognition and initial first aid care** | **Injury assessment and initial treatment** | **Follow-up care** |
| **Strength and conditioning coach** | • Provide preseason fitness screening.<br>• Develop and supervise conditioning programs. | • Watch for injuries and illnesses.<br>• Act as first responder in providing first aid assessment and care.<br>• Recommend athlete's injury or illness be thoroughly evaluated and properly treated.<br>• Do not allow athlete to participate until given clearance. | • Act as first responder in providing first aid care. | • Encourage athlete to exactly follow rehabilitation and conditioning instructions. |
| **Equipment manager** | • Inspect condition of equipment.<br>• Replace or oversee refurbishing of faulty equipment.<br>• Ensure proper equipment fitting for each athlete. | N/A | N/A | • Check equipment for damage or other issues. |

## Chapter 1 Recap

❏ Are you ready to provide information regarding how an injury occurred? Do you support the decisions of the athletic health care team and encourage athletes during rehabilitation?

❏ Have you become acquainted with the emergency personnel, physicians, athletic trainers, and physical therapists in your area? Do you have a list of various types of local physicians to refer athletes to?

❏ Have you developed a working relationship with a local physician? (The physician may be used as a resource and may conduct team physicals or preseason screenings.)

# GAME PLAN
# FOR SPORT FIRST AID

---

**IN THIS CHAPTER, YOU WILL LEARN THE FOLLOWING:**

- How to become and stay educated about sport first aid
- What health records you should keep for each athlete
- How to prepare a sport first aid kit and what to include in it
- How to prepare for cardiac and environmental emergencies
- What to look for when checking facilities and equipment for safety
- Why you should incorporate preseason physical exams, fitness screenings, and conditioning programs into your game plan
- How to develop an emergency action plan (EAP)

---

To prepare your team for competition, you plan practices, develop playing strategies, and train your athletes. This pregame planning process is essential to your team's success. The same is true in sport first aid; to handle injuries effectively, you must plan for them. You don't want to be caught unprepared for a critical health situation involving blood loss, unresponsiveness, or breathing difficulties. This chapter shows you how to prepare for urgent situations by enhancing and maintaining your education, gathering athletes' health records, stocking your first aid kit, incorporating physical screenings and conditioning into your overall program, and developing emergency plans.

## Your Sport First Aid Education

HK Coach Education strongly recommends that you supplement what you learn from this book (and from the Sport First Aid course) with certification in cardiopulmonary resuscitation (CPR) and automated external defibrillator (AED) use. You can obtain certification through the American Red Cross or the American Heart Association. These programs are recognized nationally as standards for providing first aid care. Upon achieving certification, you will be expected to provide the standard of care taught in the certification program.

Many youth and interscholastic sport organizations may also require additional education in the following areas:

- Concussions
- Heat illness, hydration, and environmental factors
- Cardiac emergencies

## Keeping Current

The field of sports medicine is constantly improving. Therefore, you need to keep current on the latest developments in sport first aid. The sport first aid techniques used in the future will be different from and better than the methods advocated now. Following are ways to keep up with these changes:

- Read current sports medicine books, and take appropriate online education courses to maintain certifications and learn the newest techniques.
- Keep your first aid training and CPR certification current. Most CPR certifications only last for two years.
- Attend sports medicine and sport first aid seminars and clinics. The Sport First Aid course will be updated as advances in this area warrant, so stay current by attending the course every few years.

## Recognizing Limitations

Even if you educate yourself extensively in sport first aid, do not attempt the duties of a physician, athletic trainer, or any other licensed athletic health care provider. Recognize your limitations, and provide only the care that you are qualified to provide. You can cause many years of damage to an athlete by overstepping the limits of your training. In addition, if you act irresponsibly and harm an athlete, you may end up the target of a lawsuit. If medical personnel are present, give them complete control to handle any illnesses or injuries. You can assist them if requested.

# Keeping Athletes' Health Records

Like most coaches, you probably keep statistical records of your athletes' performances. To become familiar with each athlete's health information, collect the following information:

- Consent form
- Health history form
- Emergency information card

## Consent Form

Remember, you cannot give first aid care to a minor unless you have consent. Before the season, you must have parents or legal guardians complete and return an explicitly worded consent form for their children. A consent form informs the athlete and the parent or guardian of the inherent risks of sport, and it requests permission from the parent or guardian to treat the child for an emergency illness or injury. A sample consent form is shown in figure 2.1.

## Health History Form

To train your athletes safely, it is essential that you know of any health conditions that could affect their participation in sports. Diabetes, asthma, epilepsy, heart murmurs, and skin conditions are among these conditions. If a health care provider clears an athlete with a health condition for participation, you should have a record indicating the athlete's health concerns and any related medications they need to take. To collect this kind of information, issue a health history form such as the one shown in figure 2.2.

## Emergency Information Card

In the event of an emergency, you must be able to contact the athlete's health care provider, parent or guardian (if the athlete is a minor), and a secondary contact. An emergency information card (see figure 2.3) indicates names and numbers of emergency contacts as well as medical insurance information. It should also alert you to information about preexisting medical conditions that may influence the treatment of an athlete. You must have a completed card from each athlete before the season begins. When the team practices or competes away from your school or other organization, you should take copies of the team's cards with you.

A person's health history and injury status are confidential pieces of information. Therefore, respect each athlete's privacy by keeping this information in a secure location. In addition, do not speak publicly (e.g., to fans, other athletes, media) about an athlete's condition unless you have written permission from the athlete (or their parent or guardian if a minor).

# Checking Facilities and Equipment

Although preparation and care of the playing area may be the responsibility of a groundskeeper or janitor, you are responsible for checking its safety. Litter, slippery floors, broken goals, worn playing surfaces, and the like can lead to injury. Check for hazards, and have them fixed before the season begins. Figure 2.4 provides a sample facilities inspection checklist. Use this sample to develop a checklist specific to your facilities.

Check sports equipment before every season begins. Inspect sticks, rackets, bats, gymnastics apparatus, protective helmets and pads, and other equipment for damage. Be sure that goalposts, net standards, landing pits, and gymnastics apparatus are well padded and secured. This could be the job of the equipment manager if your school or organization has one.

You will also need to prepare equipment and supplies for handling injuries. A first aid kit and ice cooler must be available on the sidelines at every practice and competition. When stocking your first aid kit, include only the items necessary for administering basic sport first aid. Omit all medicines, including over-the-counter (such as aspirin, pain medications, or decongestants) and prescription drugs. The exception to this is if a student has a prescribed medication and you have written clearance that you can administer it if needed (e.g., insulin, EpiPen, asthma medication). Best practice with regard to medication is if over-the-counter medication is needed, written clearance from the doctor, parent, or guardian should be provided if the student is a minor (under 18 years old) before administering medication. With any medication questions or concerns, it is important to check with your state and local laws, rules, and regulations. Omit items that may cause allergic reactions, such as solutions made with iodine and gloves made of latex. Be aware of latex allergies, as many first aid products may contain latex, such as tapes and wraps.

# Stocking the First Aid Kit

A well-stocked first aid kit includes the following items:

Antibacterial soap or wipes

Arm sling

Athletic tape—one-and-a-half inch

Bandage scissors

Bandage strips—assorted sizes

Blood spill kit

Cell phone

Contact lens case

Cotton swabs

CPR mouth barrier or pocket mask

Elastic wraps—three inch, four inch, and six inch

Emergency blanket

Examination gloves—latex free

Eye patch

First aid cream or antibacterial ointment

Foam rubber—one-eighth inch, one-fourth inch, and one-half inch

Hand sanitizer

Insect sting kit

Instant chemical cold packs or bags (to hold ice for ice packs)

List of emergency phone numbers

Medical release consent forms

Mirror

Moleskin

Nail clippers

Oral thermometer (to determine if an athlete has a fever due to illness)

Penlight

Petroleum jelly

Plastic bags for crushed ice

Prewrap—underwrap for tape (for taping)

Rectal thermometer (for use in cases of suspected heat illness)

Rescue blanket

Safety glasses—for first aiders

Safety pins

Saline solution for eyes

Sterile gauze pads—three-inch and four-inch squares (preferably nonstick)

Sterile gauze rolls

Sunscreen—sun protection factor (SPF) 30 or greater

Tape adherent and tape remover

Tongue depressors

Tooth-saver kit

Triangular bandages

Tweezers

## Preparing Athletes to Perform

Athletes who are in poor physical condition are more prone to injury. To ensure that athletes are ready for practice and competition, establish these routines:

- Preseason physical exam
- Preseason screening
- Preseason conditioning
- Proper warm-up and cool-down
- Use of protective equipment, bracing, and taping
- Correct skill instruction
- Sound nutritional guidance
- Ban on rough or boisterous play

### Preseason Physical Exam

The first step in preparing an athlete for participation in sports is to require a preseason physical exam. For this exam, the athlete's health care provider conducts a general health examination as well as circulatory, respiratory, neurological, orthopedic, vision, and hearing tests. The exam also includes blood and urine analyses. The health care provider should note and consider any preexisting or potential health conditions when deciding if the athlete has medical clearance for participation.

All athletes must turn in their physical exam forms before the season begins. Familiarize yourself with the records of athletes who have specific conditions that could affect their participation, such as asthma, diabetes, severe allergies, and epilepsy. Keep all forms in a secure file for future reference.

### Preseason Screening

During the preseason screening, the coach can identify players who are most qualified for specific positions, as well as those who may be developed to play the position. This includes identifying athletes who need additional development and conditioning.

Although the physical exam detects specific health problems, it does not provide insight about an athlete's fitness. A preseason screening can provide this information. Preseason screen-

## Limiting or Disqualifying Medical Conditions

The examining health care provider may discover a condition that limits an athlete's participation or disqualifies them from competition. Common disqualifying or limiting conditions may include the following:

- Uncontrolled diabetes
- Uncontrolled asthma
- Heart conditions
- Uncontrolled high blood pressure
- Epilepsy
- Previous head injury
- Previous spinal injury
- Chronic orthopedic problem (e.g., unstable knees, ankles, or shoulders)

In the past, individuals with the sickle-cell trait were often disqualified from athletic participation because it was believed that carrying the trait put them at particular risk for sudden death. However, in a large-scale study of military recruits, Casa and colleagues (2012) showed that the risk of sudden death was actually higher in those without the sickle-cell trait than in those with the sickle-cell trait. This finding does not mean that carrying the sickle-cell trait is without risk in sports; it means that this condition should not disqualify athletes from participation in sports.

ings should be conducted in the off-season by a specially trained health professional, such as an athletic trainer, or by a fitness professional, such as a certified strength and conditioning coach. Depending on the sport, each athlete should be evaluated for the following:

- *Strength* in the muscle groups most often used in the particular sport (e.g., a football player's neck strength or a basketball player's ankle strength)

- *Flexibility* or tightness in the major muscle groups and tendons (hamstrings, quadriceps, shoulder muscles, calf muscles, and Achilles tendons)

- *Endurance* in muscles that undergo repetitive or sustained contraction

- *Cardiovascular endurance* (especially for endurance athletes such as cross country runners, track athletes, triathletes, and cyclists)

- *Body composition* or percent body fat (especially important for wrestlers, gymnasts, and track athletes who severely restrict their diets to control their weight)

- *Coordination in the upper and lower body* to determine if an athlete's muscles fire quickly enough to protect a joint from injury (e.g., a timed one-leg balance test to see how long they can stand on one leg without wobbling or putting the other foot down)

These tests pinpoint potential fitness problems that can lead to injury. Coaches or athletic trainers should teach athletes conditioning exercises to help them improve these problems before the season.

## Preseason Conditioning

Get athletes in shape by starting them on a conditioning program at least 6 weeks before the season. Conditioning exercises should focus on muscle strength, cardiovascular endurance, flexibility, power, and speed needed for the sport.

To improve strength, consider these basic guidelines: Athletes need to perform at least 2 sets of 6 to 8 repetitions of each exercise, 3 days a week. Postpubescent athletes should lift at least 70 percent of their maximum weight to gain strength. Although well-supervised resistance

training has been proven safe for prepubescent athletes, you can avoid weightlifting-related injuries by emphasizing activities that require these athletes to support their own body weight (e.g., push-ups). Training 3 days a week for at least 20 continuous minutes is necessary to improve cardiovascular endurance. To improve flexibility, athletes should perform stretching exercises at least 5 days a week.

For more information on training and conditioning in the preseason, consult *Successful Coaching* (Martens and Vealey 2024).

## Proper Warm-Up and Cool-Down

Be sure that your athletes warm up before workouts, practices, and competitions. *Warming up* doesn't mean going out 5 minutes before practice and hitting or throwing a few balls. A proper warm-up is an exercise routine that prepares the body for vigorous physical activity. Athletes should warm up at least 15 minutes prior to activity using this sequence:

1. *General warm-up.* Athletes jog or bike at a low intensity for 5 to 10 minutes. The intensity of the general warm-up should cause a slight increase in the heart and breathing rates. It should also cause the athlete to break into a light sweat. The general warm-up helps to prepare the heart, lungs, muscles, and tendons for vigorous activity. Ultimately, it helps to prevent injury and to improve performance.

2. *Light exercises.* After a general warm-up, athletes continue to warm up specific areas with exercises such as push-ups, jumping jacks, abdominal crunches, lunges, or carioca (cross-over run).

3. *Sport-specific drills.* These drills allow athletes to practice the skills of their particular sport. For example, sport-specific softball drills include batting and throwing. In tennis and racquetball drills, athletes practice serves as well as backhand and forehand shots.

At the end of each practice, workout, or competition, athletes should gradually cool their bodies down. In other words, they should slowly reduce the intensity of their activity until their heart and breathing rates drop to near normal resting levels. Suddenly stopping exercise inhibits recovery from activity and can lead to problems such as fainting. Cool-down activities may include walking or light jogging for 5 to 10 minutes.

Athletes should conclude the cool-down with stretching. The muscles are very warm after activity, so they will stretch more easily and maintain the stretched position longer. Therefore, the cool-down period is a prime time for athletes to achieve long-term improvements in their flexibility. In general, muscles need to be stretched for a total of 2 to 3 minutes a day to obtain lasting improvements in length. Athletes should stretch each muscle group (appropriate to their sport) in 15- to 30-second repetitions, for a total of 2 to 3 minutes.

## Protective Equipment, Bracing, and Taping

As a coach, you should become an expert on how to properly fit and use your sport's protective equipment and instruct athletes how to correctly fit and wear it. Conduct surprise inspections to ensure that athletes adequately maintain and fit their equipment. Proper fit is especially important in contact sports such as American football, where helmets must be specially fitted and the athletes are required to wear all of their protective pads. To minimize the risk of broken equipment, conduct routine inspections and have shoulder pads and helmets refurbished and retested on a regular basis. An equipment manager would be ideal for this role if available.

Two important and often neglected pieces of equipment are mouth guards and safety glasses or goggles. Mouth guards help prevent sport-related dental injuries in a variety of sports. If any chance of eye injury exists in a sport, particularly in a contact or racket sport, athletes should use protective eyewear.

Some coaches think that bracing and taping can help athletes prevent injuries. For example, a coach might require football players to wear knee braces to prevent knee injuries or basketball players to tape their ankles to prevent ankle sprains. The use of taping and bracing is common in rehabilitation of athletic injuries. However, its use for injury prevention in non-injured athletes is questionable (see sidebar To Brace or Not to Brace?).

## Correct Skill Instruction

Many athletes become injured because they use unsafe technique. Since the technique of spear tackling was banned in football, the number of head and neck injuries among football players decreased. Baseball or softball players who dive headfirst into a base instead of sliding feet first are prone to tooth, head, and neck injuries. Many tennis players experience tennis elbow because they use incorrect backhand techniques.

You can help prevent these and other injuries by teaching your athletes safe and proper skills. Also, keep an eye out for athletes who use potentially harmful techniques. Warn them of the injuries they could suffer, and reinstruct them in the use of appropriate skills.

## Sound Nutritional Guidance

Encourage your athletes to eat balanced meals according to the MyPlate guidelines (see figure

## To Brace or Not to Brace?

Are protective bracing and taping all they're cracked up to be? They are certainly not substitutes for good technique and training. Strength, flexibility, endurance, and power are the keys to preventing injury; bracing and taping are of secondary importance. With the exception of some types of ankle braces, evidence that bracing or taping prevents injuries has not been conclusive. It is difficult to prove whether a decrease in injuries can be attributed to wearing a protective brace. Ultimately, the athlete (and parent or guardian if a minor) needs to decide on the use of preventive bracing and taping. Consulting an AT or appropriate health care provider about the benefits of taping and bracing can help you understand the right decision. Some states may require a note from a health care provider that justifies the need for the use of a brace or splint in order for the athlete to participate with it.

2.5). You can help athletes and their parents determine nutrient needs by recommending that they go to the MyPlate website (www.myplate.gov). Athletes can use tools from this website to help them determine their nutrient needs based on their size, gender, age, and activity level.

Also encourage athletes to drink plenty of fluids to maintain adequate hydration. For more details about recognizing and providing adequate hydration, see chapter 11.

### Eating on the Road

With planning and organization, an adequate high-carbohydrate, moderate-protein, low-fat (20% to 25% of total calories) diet can be obtained on the road. If budgets allow, bring along dried fruits, juices, low-fat granola bars, and other snacks that offer healthy alternatives to those offered in vending machines. Many restaurants honor special requests for teams, such as pasta bars, low-fat sandwich options, and fresh fruits and vegetables. In addition to paying attention to appropriate portions for adequate nutrition, encourage athletes to consume juices and skim milk products instead of soft drinks; baked, broiled, or boiled meats instead of fried meats; and plenty of carbohydrate-rich foods such as potatoes, rice, pasta, breads, bagels, fruits, and vegetables. Digestion takes between 2 and 5 hours depending on what is eaten, so plan meals to allow adequate time for digestion before a competition.

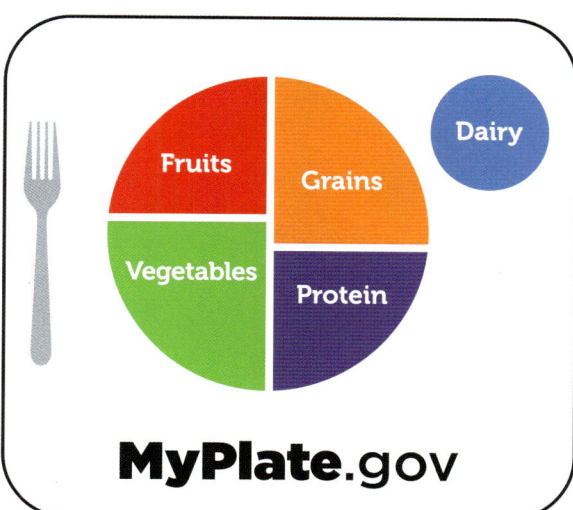

**Figure 2.5**   MyPlate.
U.S. Department of Agriculture.

An adequate diet for an athlete is like fuel for an automobile; it is energy for performance. To better inform your athletes about the quality of fuel in their diets, and to learn more about sports drinks and other nutritional issues, read *Nancy Clark's Sports Nutrition Guidebook, Sixth Edition* (Clark 2020).

### Eating for Performance

The following pregame meal guidelines can help prevent upset stomach during competition:

- Eat at least 3 hours before practices, workouts, and competitions.
- Avoid foods that are high in fat, such as french fries, potato chips, and peanut butter.
- Avoid foods that are high in fiber, such as lettuce, beans, cabbage, spinach, and nuts.
- Avoid foods that are high in sugar, such as candy bars, cakes, doughnuts, and honey.
- Eat plenty of high-carbohydrate foods that are easily digested, such as pasta, breads, low-fiber cereals, fruit juices, potatoes, and bananas.
- Eat foods that are familiar; the pregame meal is no time to try new foods.

## Ban on Horseplay

Although joking around can be harmless, rough or boisterous play such as wrestling, pushing, and hitting can lead to unintended injuries. Establish a *no horseplay* rule at the start of the season, and enforce it at all times.

# Developing an Emergency Action Plan (EAP)

Emergency medical situations may arise at any time during an activity or sport event, so the sport first aid team must be prepared. In order to provide optimal care to sports participants in an emergency or life-threatening situation, expedient action is required. Developing and implementing an emergency action plan (EAP) ensures that you are prepared to respond when a participant suddenly needs your help and that they receive the best possible care.

Effective management of emergencies requires proper planning. Preparation is the key to ensuring that appropriate resources and procedures exist. Preparation should begin well in advance of the sport season, and it should be dynamic in nature. Athletic organizations have a duty to develop an EAP that can be implemented immediately when necessary and to provide appropriate standards of emergency care to all sports participants.

Formulating an EAP specific to sports has many prerequisites, including proper education and training of individuals, development of appropriate first aid procedures for events, maintenance of appropriate medical emergency equipment and supplies, and utilization of appropriate medical emergency personnel. Through careful preparticipation physical screenings, adequate medical coverage, safe practice and training techniques, and other safety avenues, some potential emergencies may be averted. However, accidents and injuries are inherent to participation in sports, and proper preparation on the part of the sport first aid team should enable each emergency to be managed appropriately.

Developing the medical EAP must take many components into account, such as what personnel will be involved, what rules will be followed, what equipment will be available, where the arena for the contest or practice will be located, when the plan will be rehearsed, how the plan will be evaluated, and what the education processes will be for the stakeholders of the EAP. The person in charge of developing the medical EAP should ensure that all involved parties are part of the planning process. The EAP must provide detailed instructions for who will act, what actions should be taken, and how and where they will be taken.

The medical EAP should be readily available to all the members of the athletic health care team at each athletic venue. When visiting teams are coming to a venue, they, too, should be provided with a copy of the medical EAP. A separate venue-specific EAP should be developed for each venue, complete with detailed instructions and information including the address of the venue, a description of the location of emergency equipment, communication methods (cell phone, radios, landline telephones), a list of emergency telephones, a list of emergency hand signals (for use on the field), and detailed instructions for staff and emergency care personnel.

A response plan should lead the athletic health care team through conducting a thorough evaluation of an injured athlete, activating the emergency medical system (EMS), and providing effective first aid. To get started on creating your EAP, use the following guide (adapted from American Safety & Health Institute 2015):

- *Assess*—How do I evaluate the scene and the injured athlete?
- *Alert*—How do I activate the EMS?
- *Attend*—How will first aid care be provided?

## Assess

First, your plan needs to specify how you will evaluate an injured athlete. This plan should address issues such as

- what to do first when you arrive at an injured athlete's side,
- how to evaluate the safety at the scene for the injured athlete, and
- steps for evaluating responsive and unresponsive athletes.

Chapters 4 and 5 provide more detailed guidelines for evaluating injuries and illnesses.

## Alert

Next, your plan should indicate how to activate the EMS. If medical personnel are not present, how do you send for medical assistance while evaluating and providing first aid care to an athlete? To help the response go more smoothly in the event of a health emergency, you should develop a plan, before the season begins, for activating the EMS. Here's an example of an effective step-by-step approach:

1. *Delegate the responsibility of seeking medical help.* Choose a person who is calm and responsible. It can be an assistant coach, a parent, or an athlete. Make sure that this person is available during every practice and game.

2. *Make a list of emergency phone numbers.* Save a digital copy of the list in your mobile phone, and put a printed copy in your first aid kit to take to every practice and game. Include the following phone numbers:

   - Rescue unit
   - Hospital
   - Team physician (if applicable)

- Police
- Fire department

Before traveling to an away game, talk to the host coaches about emergency medical services.

3. *Take each athlete's emergency information card to every practice and game.* This information is especially important if an athlete is unresponsive and unable to tell you who you should contact or to give you that person's phone number.

4. *Give an emergency response card to the contact person calling for emergency assistance.* It will prompt the caller to provide critical information to the emergency care staff. It will also help calm the caller by providing everything they need to communicate to emergency personnel. Figure 2.6 provides a sample emergency response card.

5. *Complete an injury report, and keep it on file for any injury that occurs.* This form should provide the information requested in the sample shown in figure 2.7.

## Attend

Finally, your plan needs to indicate how first aid care will be provided. If medical personnel are present at the time of the injury, assist them as needed while they assume the care of the injured athlete. If medical personnel are not present, provide first aid care to the extent of your qualifications. Chapters 4, 5, and 6 cover first aid basics and the proper way to move an injured athlete. Part II discusses care of specific injuries.

# Handling Different Types of Injuries

Many injuries don't require emergency medical attention. An athlete who slightly twists an ankle or gets a minor bruise is not in serious condition. However, some noncritical injuries or illnesses can severely impair performance. Therefore, you should evaluate and monitor these injuries closely to ensure that no further complications occur.

All coaches should be aware of the most common serious emergencies for which a quick and effective response is critical, namely, cardiac and weather-related emergencies. You are advised to practice responding to these situations once per season as well as make sure all current guidelines are met, everyone on the sport first aid team knows their role, and their questions and concerns are addressed.

## Handling Minor Injuries

For minor injuries, follow these steps:

1. Assess the injury.
2. Attend to the injury (first aid).
3. Remove the athlete from participation if the athlete is in a great deal of pain or experiences loss of function (e.g., can't walk, run, jump, or throw).
4. Contact the athlete's parent or guardian (if a minor) to discuss the injury.
5. Suggest that the athlete see a health care provider to rule out a serious injury.
6. Complete an injury report form while the incident is still fresh in your mind.

## Handling Serious Injuries

If a serious injury or illness occurs, follow these steps:

1. Assess the safety of the scene and the athlete's level of responsiveness.
2. Send a contact person to alert emergency medical personnel and the athlete's parent or guardian (if a minor).
3. Send someone to wait for the rescue team, help them open doors and gates, and direct them to the injured athlete.
4. Assess the injury.
5. Attend to the injury (first aid).
6. Assist emergency medical personnel in preparing the athlete for transportation to a medical facility.
7. Appoint someone to go with the athlete (if none of the athlete's emergency contacts are present). This person should be responsible, calm, and familiar with the athlete. Assistant coaches or parents are best for this job.
8. Complete an injury report form while the incident is still fresh in your mind.

### Cardiac Emergencies

Sudden cardiac arrest is the leading cause of death in young athletes. Although the likelihood of such emergencies increases with age (spectators are more likely to need medical assistance related to heart problems), even healthy, seemingly low-risk youth can experience a cardiac event.

It is imperative that all members of the athletic health care team stay current with all appropriate national safety guidelines for sports. Staying current with these guidelines (among other important skills) will help members of the athletic health care team understand when to use an automated external defibrillator (AED) and give the athlete the best chance of a positive outcome. An AED is a medical device that analyzes heart rhythm and delivers an electrical shock (defibrillation) to help the heart reestablish an effective rhythm.

To improve likelihood of survival in sudden cardiac arrest, quickly applying an AED is of utmost importance. Although ambulances are equipped with AEDs, athletic health care team members should ensure that an AED is accessible during all athletic events and that every member knows where it is located. According to the American Heart Association, chances of survival from cardiac arrest decrease 7 to 10 percent for every minute a shock from a defibrillator is delayed for a victim with a shockable rhythm (Ibrahim 2007).

Take the time to review the EAP for your team's facility (or upon arrival at another facility), locate the AED, confirm it is operational and accessible, and visualize the steps necessary in case of an emergency. Taking these steps could save valuable time in the event of an emergency; it could even mean saving a life. Some states do require a separate cardiac EAP; refer to your local and state laws regarding this.

### Heat Illness Emergencies

Heat illness emergencies can result from training in extreme heat and humidity, which can be deadly for athletes. Heat illness emergencies consist of heat cramps, heat exhaustion, and heatstroke. They are summarized here and discussed in more detail in chapter 11.

Heat illness can occur even when you abide by your organization's rules regarding temperature and humidity limits and when you follow policies and procedures for practice limitations and restrictions. Heat illness is progressive; a person can transition from heat cramps to heatstroke very quickly. If an athlete is in the stages of heat cramps or heat exhaustion, cooling steps (see chapter 11) should be taken to help prevent them from transitioning to the much more serious condition of heatstroke. Symptoms of heatstroke include rapid heart rate, altered mental state, loss of consciousness, lack of sweating, and red skin. Heatstroke is a medical emergency; cooling an overheated athlete rapidly (within 30 minutes) can mean the difference between life and death. Using a cold-water tub or equivalent technique can help bring an athlete's body temperature to a safe level within 15 minutes.

### Cold Weather Emergencies

In addition to increasing chances of other injuries because of icy, wet, or windy conditions, cold weather can cause specific cold injuries such as hypothermia, frostnip, and frostbite. Preparing for these emergencies includes monitoring the temperature and making appropriate modifications. For more details on handling cold weather emergencies, see chapter 11.

### Lightning Emergencies

Lightning during sport events is extremely dangerous due to the exposure of the athletes on the field. The presence of lightning should be cause for immediate cessation of all outdoor activities until the storm has passed. Chapter 11 includes more detail on lightning injuries.

## Chapter 2 Recap

- ❑ Are you currently certified in CPR?
- ❑ Have all of your athletes filled out an informed consent form for emergency medical treatment, a health history form, and an emergency information card?
- ❑ Have you prepared and implemented a weather emergency plan?
- ❑ Do you have a well-stocked first aid kit?
- ❑ Do you require athletes to undergo extensive physical examinations and a preseason screening to pinpoint any potential health or fitness problems?
- ❑ Do you have a preseason conditioning plan? Do you incorporate warm-up and cool-down exercises into every practice and competition to help prevent injuries?
- ❑ Do you enforce policies that require athletes to wear protective equipment and refrain from horseplay?
- ❑ Do you teach athletes appropriate skills and correct technique and repeatedly warn them against using potentially dangerous techniques?

---

### ■ FIGURE 2.1
# INFORMED CONSENT FORM

I hereby give my permission for _____ to participate in _____ during the athletic season beginning_____. Further, I authorize the school to provide emergency treatment of any injury or illness my child may experience if qualified medical personnel consider treatment necessary and perform the treatment. This authorization is granted only if I cannot be reached and a reasonable effort has been made to do so.

Date _____ Parent or guardian _____

Address _____

Primary phone _____ Phone (other) _____

Family physician _____ Phone _____

Medical conditions (e.g., allergies or chronic illnesses) _____

_____

Other person to contact in case of emergency _____

Relationship to person _____ Phone _____

My child and I are aware that participating in _____ is a potentially hazardous activity. We assume all risks associated with participation in this sport, including falls, contact with other participants, weather effects, traffic, and other reasonable risk conditions associated with the sport. All such risks to my child are known and appreciated by my child and me.

We understand and agree to the conditions outlined on this form.

Child's signature _____ Date _____

Parent's or guardian's signature _____ Date _____

From R. Rehberg, *Sport First Aid*, 6th ed. (Champaign, IL: Human Kinetics, 2026).

■ **FIGURE 2.2**

# PREPARTICIPATION PHYSICAL EVALUATION HISTORY FORM

> This form should be placed into the athlete's medical file and should *not* be shared with schools or sports organizations. The Medical Eligibility Form is the only form that should be submitted to a school or sports organization.
>
> Disclaimer: Athletes who have a current Preparticipation Physical Evaluation (per state and local guidance) on file should not need to complete another History Form.

■ **PREPARTICIPATION PHYSICAL EVALUATION (Interim Guidance)**

## HISTORY FORM

Note: Complete and sign this form (with your parents if younger than 18) before your appointment.

Name: _____ Date of birth: _____

Date of examination: _____ Sport(s): _____

Sex assigned at birth (F, M, or intersex): _____ How do you identify your gender? (F, M, non-binary, or another gender): _____

Have you had COVID-19? (check one): ☐ Y ☐ N

Have you been immunized for COVID-19? (check one): ☐ Y ☐ N  If yes, have you had: ☐ One shot ☐ Two shots ☐ Three shots ☐ Booster date(s) _____

List past and current medical conditions. _____
_____

Have you ever had surgery? If yes, list all past surgical procedures. _____
_____

Medicines and supplements: List all current prescriptions, over-the-counter medicines, and supplements (herbal and nutritional).
_____
_____

Do you have any allergies? If yes, please list all your allergies (ie, medicines, pollens, food, stinging insects).
_____
_____

Patient Health Questionnaire Version 4 (PHQ-4)

*Over the last 2 weeks, how often have you been bothered by any of the following problems? (Circle response.)*

| | Not at all | Several days | Over half the days | Nearly every day |
|---|---|---|---|---|
| Feeling nervous, anxious, or on edge | 0 | 1 | 2 | 3 |
| Not being able to stop or control worrying | 0 | 1 | 2 | 3 |
| Little interest or pleasure in doing things | 0 | 1 | 2 | 3 |
| Feeling down, depressed, or hopeless | 0 | 1 | 2 | 3 |

(A sum of ≥3 is considered positive on either subscale [questions 1 and 2, or questions 3 and 4] for screening purposes.)

| GENERAL QUESTIONS (Explain "Yes" answers at the end of this form. Circle questions if you don't know the answer.) | Yes | No |
|---|---|---|
| 1. Do you have any concerns that you would like to discuss with your provider? | | |
| 2. Has a provider ever denied or restricted your participation in sports for any reason? | | |
| 3. Do you have any ongoing medical issues or recent illness? | | |

| HEART HEALTH QUESTIONS ABOUT YOU | Yes | No |
|---|---|---|
| 4. Have you ever passed out or nearly passed out during or after exercise? | | |
| 5. Have you ever had discomfort, pain, tightness, or pressure in your chest during exercise? | | |
| 6. Does your heart ever race, flutter in your chest, or skip beats (irregular beats) during exercise? | | |
| 7. Has a doctor ever told you that you have any heart problems? | | |
| 8. Has a doctor ever requested a test for your heart? For example, electrocardiography (ECG) or echocardiography. | | |

| HEART HEALTH QUESTIONS ABOUT YOU (CONTINUED) | Yes | No |
|---|---|---|
| 9. Do you get light-headed or feel shorter of breath than your friends during exercise? | | |
| 10. Have you ever had a seizure? | | |

| HEART HEALTH QUESTIONS ABOUT YOUR FAMILY | Unsure | Yes | No |
|---|---|---|---|
| 11. Has any family member or relative died of heart problems or had an unexpected or unexplained sudden death before age 35 years (including drowning or unexplained car crash)? | | | |
| 12. Does anyone in your family have a genetic heart problem such as hypertrophic cardio-myopathy (HCM), Marfan syndrome, arrhyth-mogenic right ventricular cardiomyopathy (ARVC), long QT syndrome (LQTS), short QT syndrome (SQTS), Brugada syndrome, or catecholaminergic polymorphic ventricular tachycardia (CPVT)? | | | |
| 13. Has anyone in your family had a pacemaker or an implanted defibrillator before age 35? | | | |

| BONE AND JOINT QUESTIONS | Yes | No |
|---|---|---|
| 14. Have you ever had a stress fracture or an injury to a bone, muscle, ligament, joint, or tendon that caused you to miss a practice or game? | | |
| 15. Do you have a bone, muscle, ligament, or joint injury that bothers you? | | |

| MEDICAL QUESTIONS | Yes | No |
|---|---|---|
| 16. Do you cough, wheeze, or have difficulty breathing during or after exercise? | | |
| 17. Are you missing a kidney, an eye, a testicle, your spleen, or any other organ? | | |
| 18. Do you have groin or testicle pain or a painful bulge or hernia in the groin area? | | |
| 19. Do you have any recurring skin rashes or rashes that come and go, including herpes or methicillin-resistant *Staphylococcus aureus* (MRSA)? | | |
| 20. Have you had a concussion or head injury that caused confusion, a prolonged headache, or memory problems? | | |
| 21. Have you ever had numbness, had tingling, had weakness in your arms or legs, or been unable to move your arms or legs after being hit or falling? | | |
| 22. Have you ever become ill while exercising in the heat? | | |
| 23. Do you or does someone in your family have sickle cell trait or disease? — Unsure | | |
| 24. Have you ever had or do you have any problems with your eyes or vision? | | |

| MEDICAL QUESTIONS (*CONTINUED*) | Yes | No |
|---|---|---|
| 25. Do you worry about your weight? | | |
| 26. Are you trying to or has anyone recommended that you gain or lose weight? | | |
| 27. Are you on a special diet or do you avoid certain types of foods or food groups? | | |
| 28. Have you ever had an eating disorder? | | |

| MENSTRUAL QUESTIONS | N/A | Yes | No |
|---|---|---|---|
| 29. Have you ever had a menstrual period? | | | |
| 30. How old were you when you had your first menstrual period? | | | |
| 31. When was your most recent menstrual period? | | | |
| 32. How many periods have you had in the past 12 months? | | | |

**Explain "Yes" answers here.**

_____
_____
_____
_____
_____
_____
_____
_____
_____
_____
_____
_____

**I hereby state that, to the best of my knowledge, my answers to the questions on this form are complete and correct.**

Signature of athlete: _____

Signature of parent or guardian: _____

Date: _____

From R. Rehberg, *Sport First Aid*, 6th ed. (Champaign, IL: Human Kinetics, 2026).

## ■ FIGURE 2.3
# EMERGENCY INFORMATION CARD

Athlete's name _____ Age _____

Address _____

Primary phone _____ Phone (other) _____

Sport _____

Emergency contacts (include names of two contacts) _____

Parent's or guardian's name _____

Address _____

Primary phone _____ Phone (other) _____

Alternate contact's name _____

Address _____

Primary phone _____ Phone (other) _____

Relationship to athlete _____

Insurance provider _____ Group/policy # _____

Physician's name _____ Phone _____

Are you allergic to any medications? _____ If so, what? _____

Do you have any allergies (e.g., bee stings or dust)? _____

Are you allergic to any foods? _____ If so, what? _____

Do you have _____ asthma, _____ diabetes, or _____ epilepsy? (Check any that apply.)

Do you take any medications? _____ If so, what? _____

Do you wear contact lenses? _____

Other _____

Signature _____ Date _____

From R. Rehberg, *Sport First Aid*, 6th ed. (Champaign, IL: Human Kinetics, 2026).

## ■ FIGURE 2.4
# FACILITIES INSPECTION CHECKLIST

Name of inspector _____ Date of inspection _____

Name and location of facility _____

_____

Circle **Y** (yes) if the facility is in good condition or **N** (no) if it needs something done to make it acceptable. In the space provided, note what needs to be done.

### Gymnasium

Y  N   Floor (water spots, buckling, loose sections)_____
Y  N   Walls (vandalism free and padded, if appropriate)_____
Y  N   Lights (all functioning)_____
Y  N   Windows (secure)_____
Y  N   Roof (adverse impact of weather)_____
Y  N   Stairs (well lighted)_____
Y  N   Bleachers (support structure sound)_____
Y  N   Exits (lights working)_____
Y  N   Basketball rims (level, securely attached)_____
Y  N   Basketball backboards (no cracks, clean)_____
Y  N   Mats (clean, properly stored, no defects)_____
Y  N   Uprights or projections (padded)_____
Y  N   Wall plugs (covered)_____
Y  N   Light switches (all functioning)_____
Y  N   Heating or cooling system (temperature control)_____
Y  N   Ducts, radiators, and pipes_____
Y  N   Thermostats_____
Y  N   Fire alarms (regularly checked)_____
Y  N   Directions posted for evacuating the gym in case of fire_____
Y  N   Fire extinguishers (regularly checked)_____
Other: _____

_____

### Locker rooms

Y  N   Floor_____
Y  N   Walls_____
Y  N   Lights_____
Y  N   Windows_____
Y  N   Roof_____
Y  N   Showers_____
Y  N   Drains_____
Y  N   Benches_____
Y  N   Lockers_____
Y  N   Exits_____
Y  N   Water fountains_____
Y  N   Toilets_____
Y  N   Athletic trainer's room_____
Other: _____

_____

*(continued)*

■ **FIGURE 2.4**
# FACILITIES INSPECTION CHECKLIST *(CONTINUED)*

## Field or outside playing area

Y  N    Stands_____

Y  N    Pitching mound_____

Y  N    Dugouts_____

Y  N    Track and fences_____

Y  N    Sidelines_____

Y  N    Sprinklers_____

Y  N    Garbage_____

Y  N    Security fences_____

Y  N    Water fountain_____

Y  N    Storage sheds_____

Y  N    Goalposts_____

Y  N    Net_____

Y  N    Net standards_____

Other:_____

## Pool area and equipment

### Pool

Y  N    Equipment in good repair_____

Y  N    Sanitary_____

Y  N    Slipperiness controlled (decks, diving board)_____

Y  N    Chemicals safely stored_____

Y  N    Regulations and safety rules posted_____

Other:_____

### Safety line

Y  N    Located at break point in the pool grade_____

Y  N    Bright-colored floats_____

Y  N    3/4-inch rope_____

### Ring buoys

Y  N    20-inch diameter_____

Y  N    50-foot rope length_____

### Guard chairs

Y  N    Unobstructed view_____

Y  N    Tall enough to see bottom of pool_____

### Lighting

Y  N    Adequate visibility_____

Y  N    No glare_____

Y  N    Penetrates to bottom of pool_____

Y  N    Exit light in good repair_____

Y  N    Halls and locker rooms meet code requirements_____

Y  N    Light switches properly grounded_____

Y  N    Emergency generator available_____

Other:_____

## Exits

Y   N   Accessible and secure_____

Y   N   Adequate size, number_____

Y   N   Self-closing doors_____

Y   N   Self-locking doors_____

Y   N   Striker plates secure_____

Y   N   No obstacles or debris_____

Y   N   Office and storage rooms locked_____

Other: _____

## Track

Y   N   Throwing circles_____

Y   N   Fences_____

Y   N   Water fountain_____

Y   N   Surface free of debris_____

Y   N   Surface free of holes and bumps_____

Other: _____

## First aid equipment

Y   N   First aid kit, inventoried and replenished regularly_____

Y   N   Stretcher, inventoried and in good repair_____

Y   N   Two blankets, inventoried and in good repair_____

Y   N   Spine board, inventoried and in good repair_____

Other: _____

Recommendations/observations_____

_____

_____

_____

_____

From R. Rehberg, *Sport First Aid*, 6th ed. (Champaign, IL: Human Kinetics, 2026).

Adapted by permission from *American Coaching Effectiveness Program Level 2 Sport Law Workbook* (Champaign, IL: Human Kinetics, 1985), 40-41; J.R. Olson, "Safety Checklists: Making Indoor Areas Hazard-Free," *Athletic Business* (1985): 36-38.

■ **FIGURE 2.6**
# EMERGENCY RESPONSE CARD

*Be prepared to give this information to the EMS dispatcher.*

1. Location_____
   Street address_____
   City or town_____ Zip code_____
   Directions (e.g., cross streets or landmarks)_____
2. Phone number from which the call is being made_____
3. Caller's name_____
4. What happened_____
   _____
   _____
5. How many persons injured_____
6. Condition of injured person(s)_____
7. Help (first aid) being given_____

*Note: Do not hang up first. Let the EMS dispatcher hang up first.*

From R. Rehberg, *Sport First Aid*, 6th ed. (Champaign, IL: Human Kinetics, 2026).

■ **FIGURE 2.7**
# INJURY REPORT

Name of athlete_____

Date_____ Time_____

Person performing initial emergency care_____

Mechanism of injury_____

Type of injury_____

Anatomical areas involved_____

First aid administered_____

Other treatment administered_____

Referral action_____

Person performing initial emergency care (signature)_____

From R. Rehberg, *Sport First Aid*, 6th ed. (Champaign, IL: Human Kinetics, 2026).

# ANATOMY AND TERMINOLOGY IN SPORT FIRST AID

**IN THIS CHAPTER, YOU WILL LEARN THE FOLLOWING:**

- Basic terminology used in human anatomy
- The roles of the musculoskeletal, neurological, digestive, respiratory and circulatory, and urinary systems
- How most injuries and illnesses occur
- What distinguishes acute and chronic injuries
- How to recognize the main types of acute and chronic injuries

In sports, winning takes precise execution of plays, stunts, or maneuvers. For example, in baseball, a 6-4-3 double play will never fly if a second baseman isn't in position to field the shortstop's toss and nail the throw to first base. The body functions in a similar way; all its systems and parts are connected, and they can directly affect one another. Athletes perform their best when the body's systems or parts are working together correctly. However, if one system or part falters, others may not work properly, leading to injury or illness.

This chapter provides an overview of the body's systems, anatomy, and common malfunctions (injuries and illnesses). As a coach, you need to know this information in order to provide appropriate first aid care to an athlete. With this knowledge, you can better recognize injuries and illnesses as well as more effectively communicate an athlete's symptoms and problems to emergency personnel, sports medicine professionals, and parents or guardians.

## Overview of Human Anatomy

Anatomy is the study of the structures of the body. Understanding basic anatomy can help you not only to properly train your athletes but also to better grasp first aid vocabulary, allowing you to communicate more effectively with your athletic health care team when an urgent situation arises.

The body is divided into several systems, each with unique organs and tissues. All are vital to supporting life and promoting top athletic performance. The following sections describe the systems of the body.

### Musculoskeletal System

The musculoskeletal system is made up of bones, joints, muscles, tendons, and other tissues.

#### Bones

The skeleton (bones) is the body's foundation. It serves to shape and support the body as well as to protect the brain, lungs, and heart. Figure 3.1 illustrates the anatomical terms for some of the bones.

### Joints

When two bones meet, they form a joint. Joints are also made up of ligaments, tendons, cartilage, and bursas (see figure 3.2). Without joints, the body would be unable to move. Primary joints include the hip, knee, ankle, shoulder, elbow, and wrist.

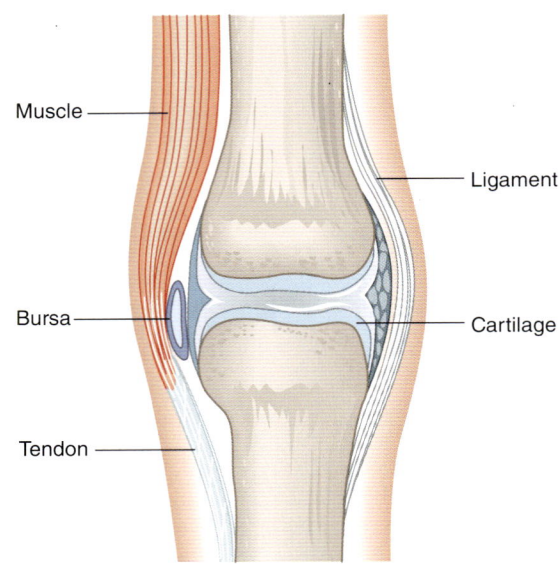

**Figure 3.2**   Joint structure.

### Ligaments

Ligaments typically attach bone to bone at joints. This function is critical to maintaining joint stability. Without ligaments, bones and joints would constantly move out of position and prevent any purposeful movement.

### Cartilage

Cartilage is a gristly type of tissue found at the end of bone. The body has several different types of cartilage. They all function primarily to absorb shock when bones hit each other and to reduce friction when bones rub together. A common example of cartilage in relation to athletic injuries is the meniscus of the knee.

### Muscles

Muscles are elastic tissues that move bones. Muscle groups that are most used (and therefore commonly injured) in sports include the trapezius, rotator cuff, quadriceps, hamstrings, and gastrocnemius (see figure 3.3). They are described as follows:

> *Trapezius*—Located over the back of the neck and shoulders and shaped like a trapezoid, the trapezius group moves the head and shoulder blade. Because they play a major role in stabilizing the head and elevating the shoulder, strong trapezius muscles are especially important in contact sports such as American football and soccer.

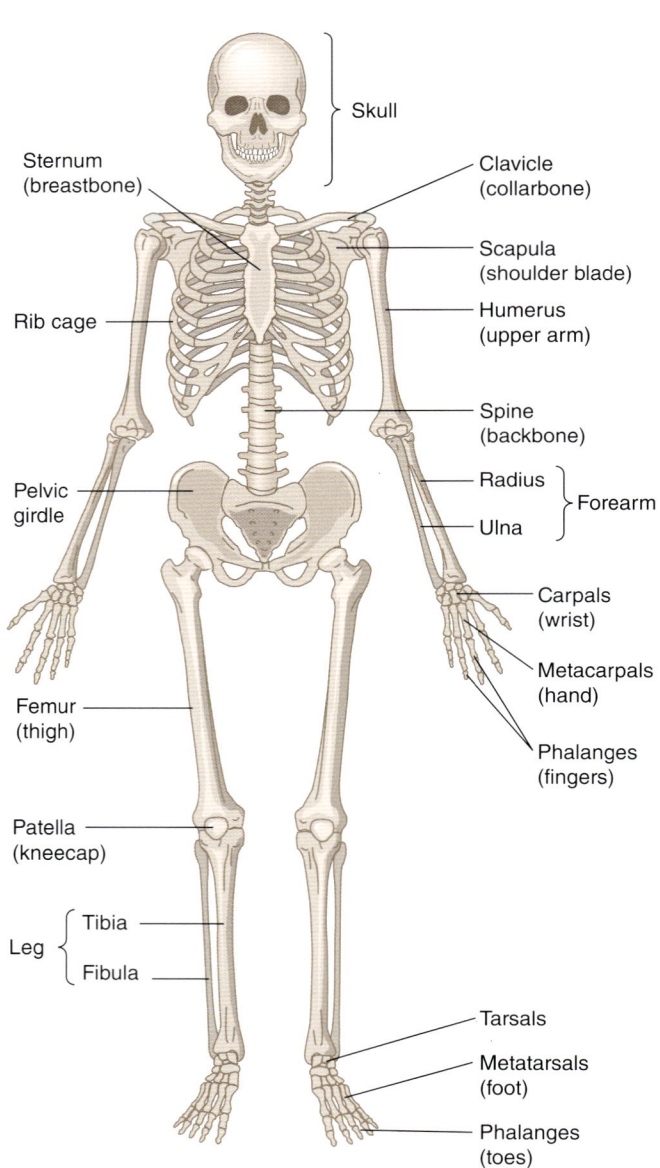

**Figure 3.1**   Bones of the human body.

*Rotator cuff*—Attaching to the shoulder blade and upper arm bone (humerus), this group of muscles is involved in throwing, swimming, and hitting (volleyball and racket sports). The rotator cuff also plays a major role in helping to hold the humerus in the shoulder socket.

*Quadriceps*—Located at the front of the thigh, these muscles straighten the knee and move the thigh forward. They help provide the power to jump and run.

*Hamstrings*—Located at the back of the thigh, these muscles bend the knee and extend the thigh backward. They help generate the force needed to propel the body forward from the landing phase of running.

*Calf*—Located on the back of the lower leg, these muscles point the foot down and also help bend the knee. They are especially active when pushing off to jump or run.

### Tendons

Tendons attach muscle to bone. They are somewhat elastic to allow for stretching or pulling by the muscles. Common tendons injured in sport (see figure 3.4) include the Achilles tendon (at the heel), patellar tendon (at the knee), biceps tendon (at the upper arm), and rotator cuff (at the shoulder). Tendons are not passive structures like ligaments. Tendon fibers are covered by several types of sheaths. One type, the synovial sheath, secretes and absorbs fluid that acts as a lubricant between tendon fibers and bundles.

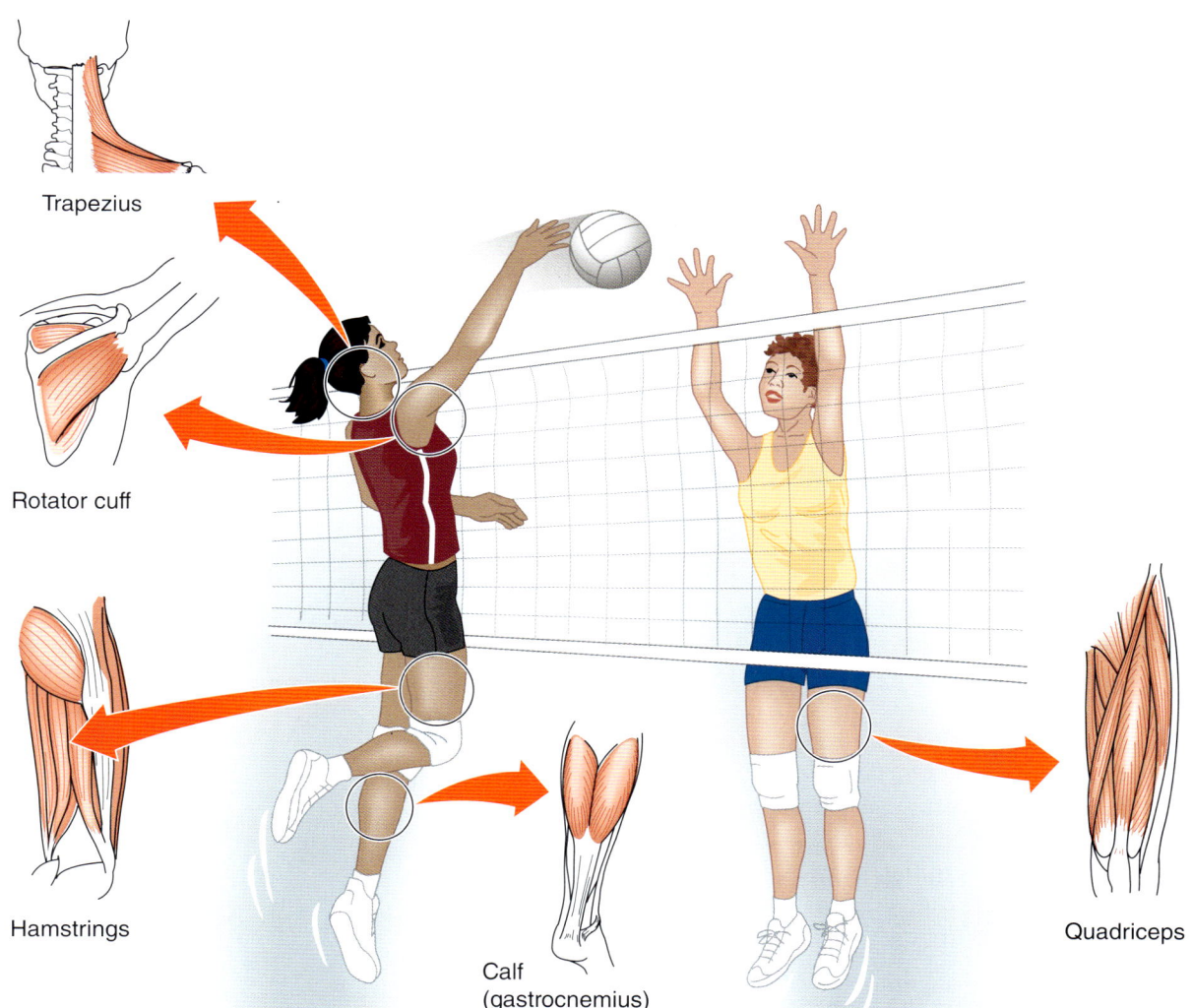

Trapezius

Rotator cuff

Hamstrings

Calf
(gastrocnemius)

Quadriceps

**Figure 3.3**   Five of the major muscle groups commonly injured in sports.

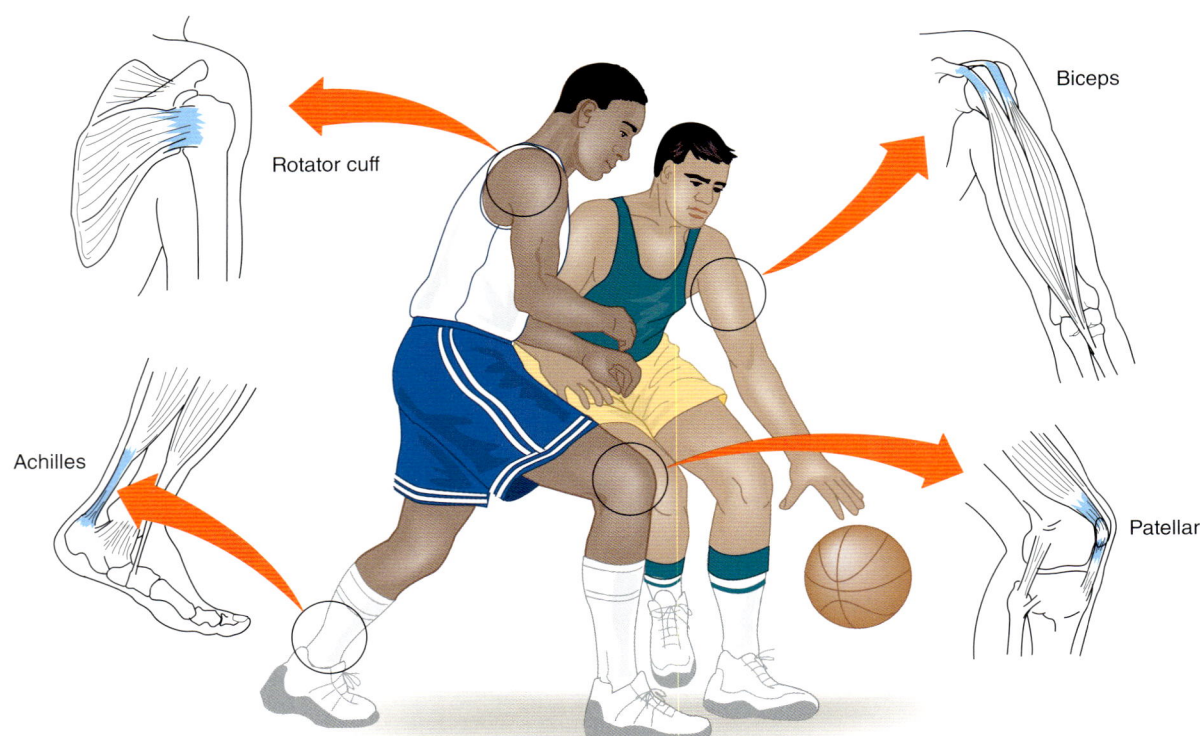

**Figure 3.4** Four tendons commonly injured in sport.

### Bursas

Bursas are small, fluid-filled sacs located between bones, muscles, tendons, and other tissues. These sacs help reduce rubbing between tissues, such as between tendons and bones. Common bursas injured in sport include the prepatellar bursa (over the knee) and the olecranon bursa (at the tip of the elbow).

## Neurological System

The neurological system is the body's control center (see figure 3.5). It is made up of the brain, the spinal cord, and a network of nerves. The brain coordinates the functioning of all systems and tissues. Digestion, breathing and heart rate, muscle contraction, and most other bodily functions depend on signals from the brain. Nerves relay these signals from the brain and also carry feedback from the tissues to the brain.

The spinal cord is the main trunk from which the nerves branch. It is protected by the spine. The vertebrae (individual bones of the spine) are held together by ligaments, and they are separated by cartilage discs (see figure 3.6).

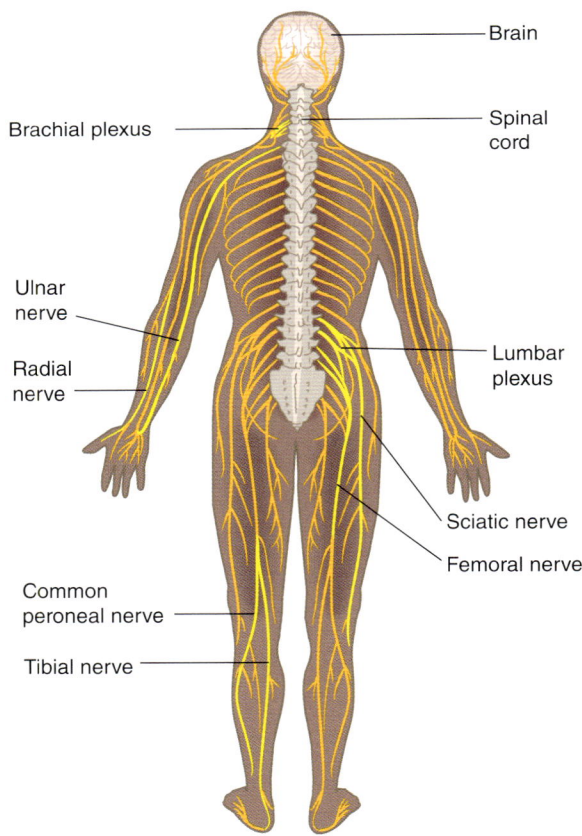

**Figure 3.5** Neurological system.

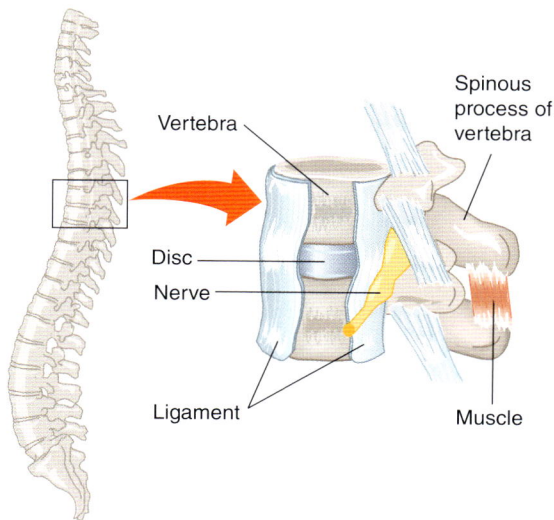

**Figure 3.6** Structures of the spine.

## Digestive System

The digestive system (see figure 3.7) is the body's energy supply center. Its organs assist in breaking down food into energy substances that fuel the muscles and other tissues. Once swallowed, food travels down a long tube (esophagus). From the esophagus, food enters the stomach, where it is partially digested. It continues on through the small and large intestines, where nutrients are further broken down and absorbed for use in the body. During this process, waste products accumulate and eventually exit from the large intestine through the rectum. The liver assists in the process by excreting a fluid (bile) that helps break down fats. The gallbladder acts as an extra reservoir for bile. The pancreas excretes fluids that aid in digestion as well as insulin, a hormone that helps regulate blood sugar levels. The appendix, which is part of the small intestine, has no known function in humans.

## Respiratory and Circulatory Systems

While the digestive system is the body's energy supplier, the circulatory and respiratory systems serve as energy releasers. These two systems work together to supply the body with the oxygen it needs to sustain life. Oxygen helps release the energy from food to fuel the tissues.

The respiratory system is the body's oxygen-transporting network. The respiratory

organs are located in the head and chest (see figure 3.8).

The circulatory system consists of the blood-transporting network shown in figure 3.9. The heart pumps the blood throughout the body via blood vessels.

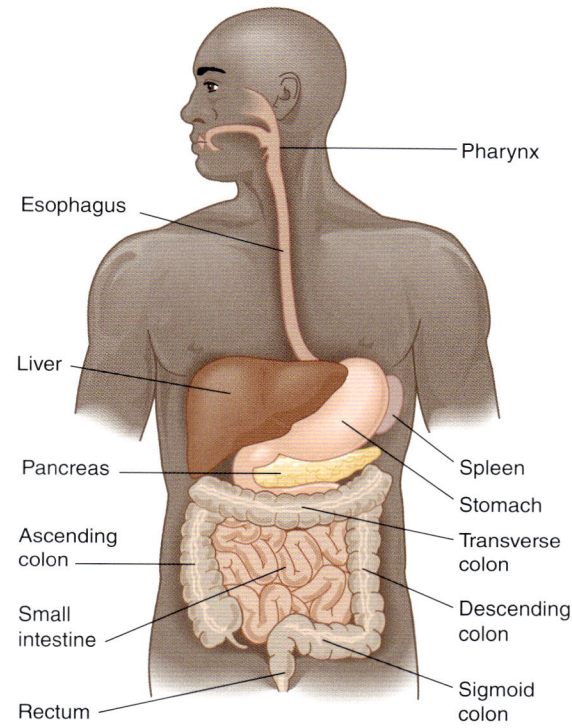

**Figure 3.7** Digestive system.

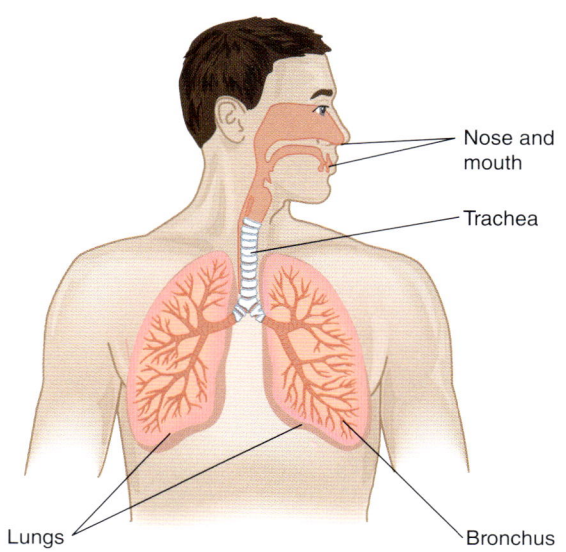

**Figure 3.8** Respiratory system.

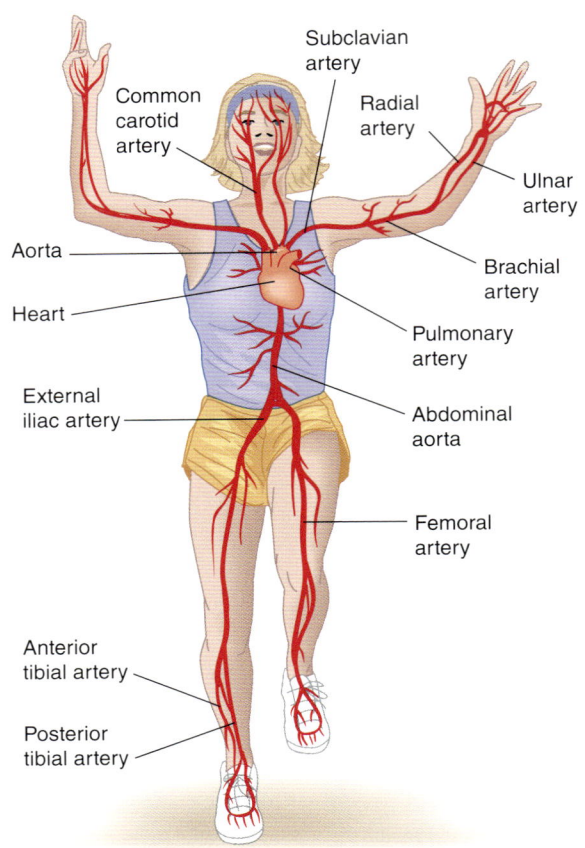

**Figure 3.9** Circulatory system.

A person breathes in oxygen-filled air through the nose, mouth, or both. This air travels down the windpipe (trachea) until it reaches the lungs. Inside the lungs, the oxygen passes through tiny sacs, called alveoli, and into thin blood vessels, called capillaries. The capillaries join together into large blood vessels, called pulmonary veins, which take the oxygen-filled blood to the heart.

The heart pumps the oxygen-filled blood through the arteries to the rest of the body. In the tissues, oxygen ($O_2$) is used to release energy, and it is broken down to a waste product called carbon dioxide ($CO_2$). The capillaries pick up the $CO_2$; this blood, called venous or low-oxygen blood, returns to the heart via the veins. The heart pumps the low-oxygen blood to the lungs, which breathe out the carbon dioxide and breathe in new supplies of oxygen.

An outline of this circulorespiratory cycle is illustrated in figure 3.10.

## Urinary System

After energy is supplied (by digestion) and then released for the body to use (by circulation and respiration), by-products result. The urinary system gets rid of these waste products from

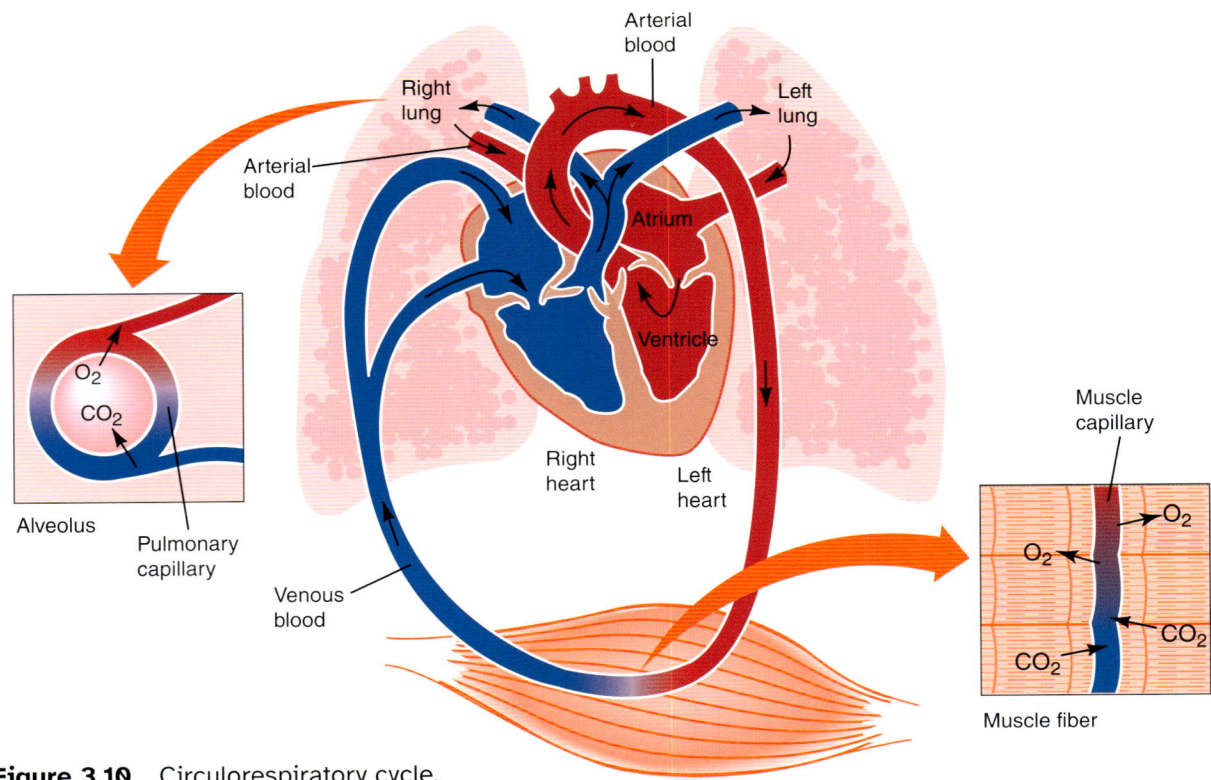

**Figure 3.10** Circulorespiratory cycle.

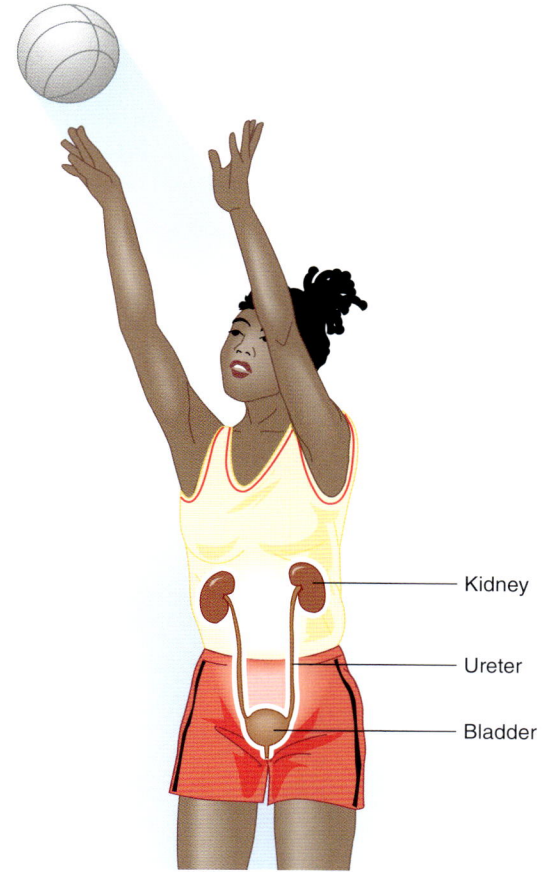

**Figure 3.11**   Urinary system.

energy breakdown. The organs shown in figure 3.11 participate in this process.

Waste products are brought to the kidneys through the blood (circulatory system). The kidneys filter out the waste products from the blood and combine them with water to make urine. Urine is released from the kidneys and travels through the ureter to the bladder. The bladder stores the urine until it is released from the body.

# Sport Injuries and Illnesses

As stated earlier in this chapter, athletes perform optimally when all of the body's systems work together correctly. Injuries and illnesses can be described as disruptions to those systems. The following section summarizes the types of injuries and illnesses you may encounter as a coach. When the classification and terminology for these injuries and illnesses become familiar to you, you will be able to recognize and respond to them more effectively.

## How Injuries and Illnesses Occur

Injuries and illnesses are often classified according to what causes them and how long it takes for them to occur.

### Causes

Injuries result from several causes (mechanisms), including compression, tension, and shearing. These injury mechanisms are defined as follows:

*Compression*—An impact injury to a specific body part that causes bleeding, superficial or deep tissue bruising, broken bones, or joint injuries. Examples of a compression mechanism include colliding with another athlete or with sports equipment, and falling on a hard surface.

*Tension*—A stretching injury that occurs when a tissue is lengthened beyond its normal limits. A tension injury can occur when using incorrect technique, landing from a jump on the wrong part of the foot, overstriding while running, having contact with another athlete that forces overstretching, or landing on an outstretched hand.

*Shearing*—A friction injury caused by two surfaces rubbing together. Contact between the skin and the ground can cause a shearing injury to the skin (e.g., when sliding into a base). Although shearing usually causes skin injuries, it can also affect other tissues, such as cartilage.

### Duration of Development

Injuries and illnesses can occur suddenly, or they can develop slowly over time. These two categories are defined as follows:

*Acute injuries and illnesses*—Occur suddenly as a result of a specific injury mechanism, such as falling or coming into contact with another athlete or equipment. Examples include broken bones, cuts, bruises, and kidney injuries.

*Chronic injuries and illnesses*—Develop over a period of several weeks or longer. Illnesses may be caused from genetic predisposition and chronic injuries may be caused by repetitive injury or trauma to the area. Examples include shin splints, tendinitis, tennis elbow, type 1 and type 2 diabetes, and epilepsy.

## Common Acute Injuries

Acute injuries occur suddenly, and they are caused by one specific injury mechanism. Common acute injuries include the following:

- Contusions
- Abrasions
- Punctures
- Cuts—incisions, lacerations, and avulsions
- Sprains
- Strains
- Cartilage tears
- Dislocations and subluxations
- Bone fractures

### Contusions

Contusions (bruises) result from a direct blow. Tissue and capillaries are damaged, and they lose fluid and blood, which causes pain, swelling, and discoloration. Superficial (skin) contusions (see figure 3.12) are minor, but deep contusions to bone or muscle can cause loss of function. If a direct blow contuses the heart, lungs, brain, or kidneys, it can cause the damaged tissue to bleed heavily, thus reducing blood flow to the organ. These types of contusions can be life-threatening. The 2021-22 National High School Sports-Related Injury Surveillance Study (Collins, Robison, and Burus 2022) reported that contusions accounted for 10.3 percent of all injuries reported in the 2021-22 school year.

### Abrasions

Abrasions occur when tissue is injured by friction or scraping. Most abrasions, such as turf burns and strawberries, injure the skin (see figure 3.13). However, the cornea (outer layer of the eye) can be abraded or scratched by dust and other objects.

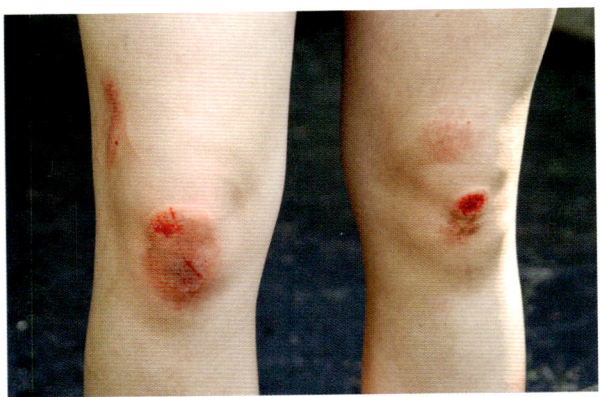

**Figure 3.13**   Abrasion.
iStockphoto.com/Judith Bicking

### Punctures

Punctures are narrow stab wounds to the skin and internal organs. In sports, they are often caused by track spikes or wood splinters (see figure 3.14). Although a superficial skin puncture may not bleed much, it is at high risk for infection because bacteria can be pushed deep into the wound. Javelins and other sharp implements used in sports can puncture inter-

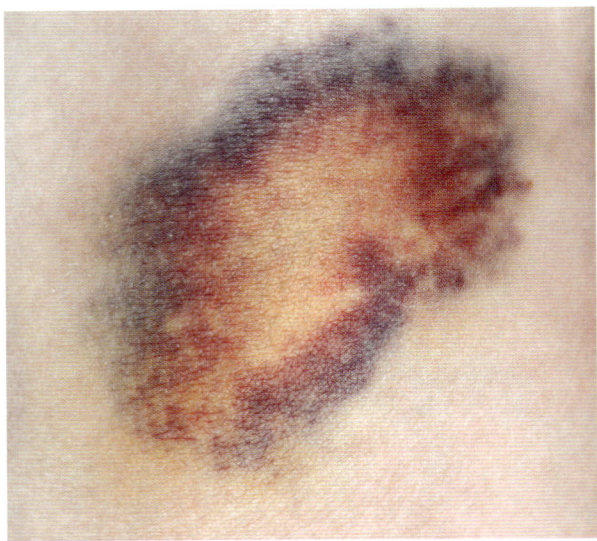

**Figure 3.12**   Contusion.
Frentusha/iStock/Getty Images

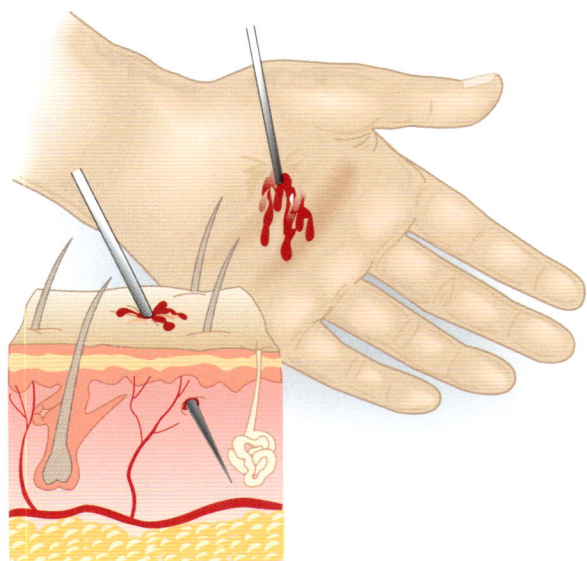

**Figure 3.14**   A puncture is a narrow stab wound.

nal organs, such as the lungs. These injuries are life-threatening, and they require prompt treatment.

### Cuts

A cut is a break or tear in the tissue. Types of cuts include lacerations, incisions, and avulsions. They are defined as follows:

*Lacerations*—Jagged, soft-tissue cuts (see figure 3.15) caused by a blow from a blunt object. Lacerations are deeper than abrasions, and they cause steady bleeding. For example, a basketball player might experience a laceration above the eye after catching an elbow to the face.

*Incisions*—Smooth cuts caused by very sharp objects, such as those made of glass or metal (see figure 3.16). These injuries usually bleed heavily and quickly. Regular, thorough inspections of facilities and equipment can help you prevent most situations where incisions could occur.

*Avulsions*—Complete tissue tears, such as tearing off the end of the earlobe (see figure 3.17). Wearing rings can sometimes cause finger avulsions; a ring can get caught in something and be forcefully pulled.

Wearing jewelry is a common risk factor for all types of cuts. Athletes can reduce the risk of cuts by removing jewelry before participating in practices and competitions.

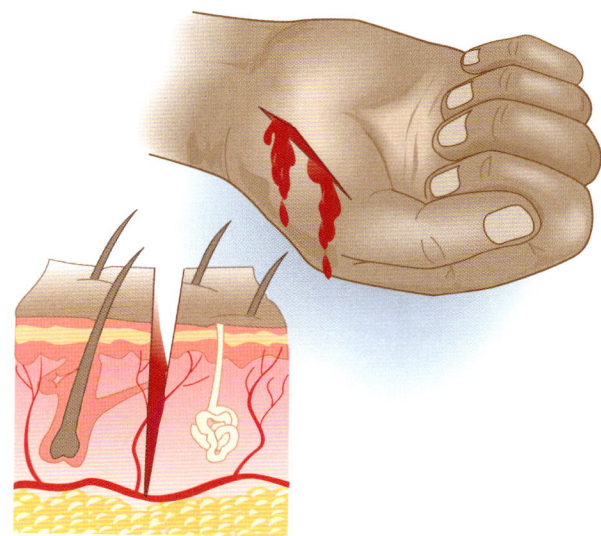

**Figure 3.16** An incision is a smooth cut that usually bleeds heavily and quickly.

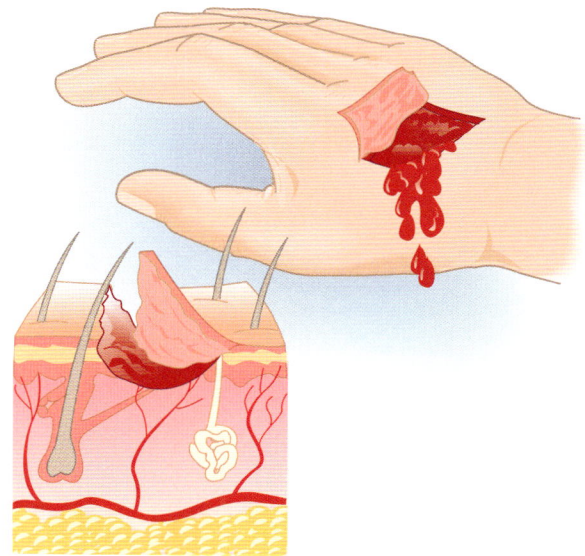

**Figure 3.17** An avulsion is a complete tissue tear.

### Sprains and Strains

In a comparison analysis of high school sport-related injuries from 2005 through 2022, sprains and strains were by far the most common type of injury reported; they accounted for 44.2 percent of injuries (Collins, Robison, and Burus 2022).

Sprains are stretching or tearing injuries to ligaments. They are classified from minor to serious as Grade I, II, or III (see figure 3.18). They are typically caused by a compression mechanism or by a torsion (twisting) mechanism.

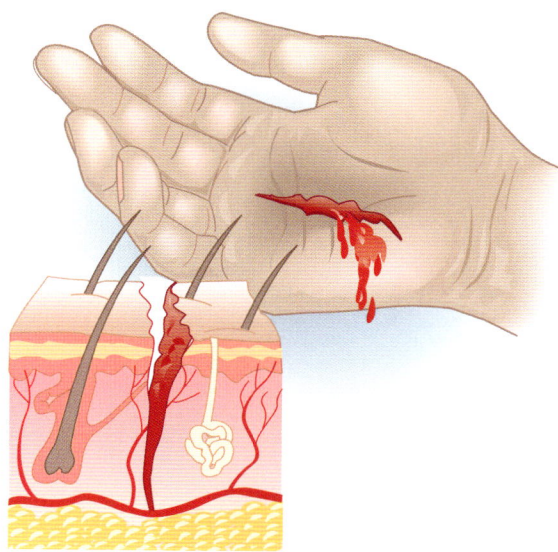

**Figure 3.15** A laceration is jagged and deep, and it causes steady bleeding.

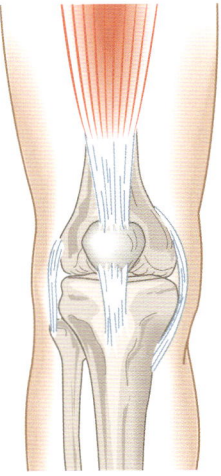

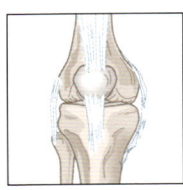

**Grade I sprain**
Ligament(s) stretched slightly
with a few fibers possibly torn

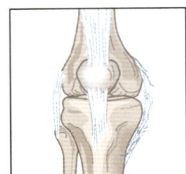

**Grade II sprain**
Ligament(s) stretched and
partially torn

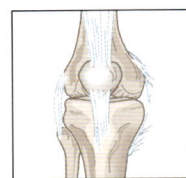

**Grade III sprain**
Ligament(s) torn completely

**Figure 3.18** Types of sprains.

In a Grade I (minor) sprain, some of the ligament fibers are stretched, and a few may be torn. A Grade I sprain results in mild pain, minimal to no swelling, and no loss of motion. A Grade II (moderate) sprain involves some ligament fiber stretching and more fiber tearing; however, portions of the ligament are still intact. A Grade II sprain causes some pain, swelling, and loss of joint function. In a Grade III (severe) sprain, a ligament tears completely. The athlete likely experiences extreme pain with any joint movement and therefore may be unable to move the joint. A Grade III sprain results in widespread swelling in the joint (particularly in ankle, elbow, finger, knee, and toe sprains).

Because ligaments support joints by holding bones together, sprains can cause serious joint instability. In addition, once stretched or torn, ligaments may not heal to be as tight as they were before the injury, leading to looseness in the joint and the possibility of numerous reinjuries (sprains). Even when ligaments heal to their original length, they can take anywhere from 6 to 12 weeks to fully heal.

Like sprains, strains are stretching or tearing injuries that occur with forceful and excessive shortening or stretching (see figure 3.19). However, strains occur in muscles and tendons.

Also like sprains, strains are classified as Grade I (minor), Grade II (moderate), and Grade III (severe). In a Grade I strain, some of the muscle or tendon fibers are stretched, but very few fibers may be torn. A Grade I strain results in mild pain, minimal to no swelling, and no loss of motion. More muscle or tendon fibers are torn in Grade II strains; however, some portions of the muscle or tendon are still intact. A Grade II strain causes some swelling, pain, loss of muscle or joint function, and possible indentation over the site of the injury. In a Grade III strain, a muscle or tendon tears completely. The athlete likely experiences extreme pain and inability to move the joint that is attached to the affected muscle or tendon. Torn muscles and tendons roll up, causing a lump.

Table 3.1 provides a breakdown of sprains and strains and their relative frequency in various youth sports.

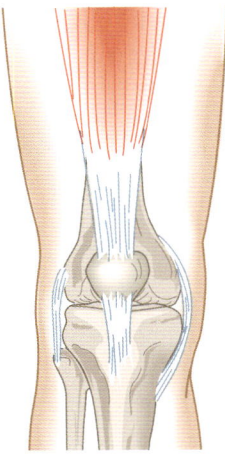

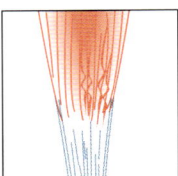

**Grade I strain**
Muscle or tendon stretched
slightly

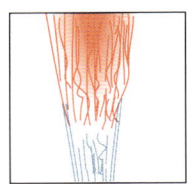

**Grade II strain**
Muscle or tendon stretched
and partially torn

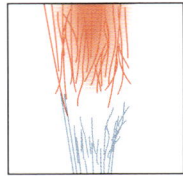

**Grade III strain**
Muscle or tendon torn completely

**Figure 3.19** Types of strains.

**Table 3.1**   Frequency of Sprains and Strains out of All Reported Types of Injury

| Sport | Percentage of game injuries | Percentage of practice injuries |
|---|---|---|
| Baseball | 41.9 | 46 |
| Soccer—boys | 34.3 | 56.7 |
| Soccer—girls | 38.5 | 55.4 |
| Wrestling | 17 | 21.3 |
| Softball—girls | 27.5 | 31.9 |
| Volleyball—girls | 55 | 43.2 |
| Football | 26.6 | 35.4 |
| Basketball—girls | 39.5 | 38.5 |
| Basketball—boys | 53.5 | 54.2 |

Data from C. Collins, H. Robison, and T. Burus, *Original Sample Summary Report. National High School Sports-Related Injury Surveillance Study, 2021-2022 School Year* (2022), https://datalyscenter.org/wp-content/uploads/2023/01/2021-22-High-School-RIO-ORIGINAL-Summary-Report.pdf.

### Cartilage Tears

Cartilage covering and between bones reduces shock and friction. If a joint's bones are twisted or compressed, they can bruise, or pinch and tear, the cartilage. Cartilage tears occur most often in the knee joint (see figure 3.20).

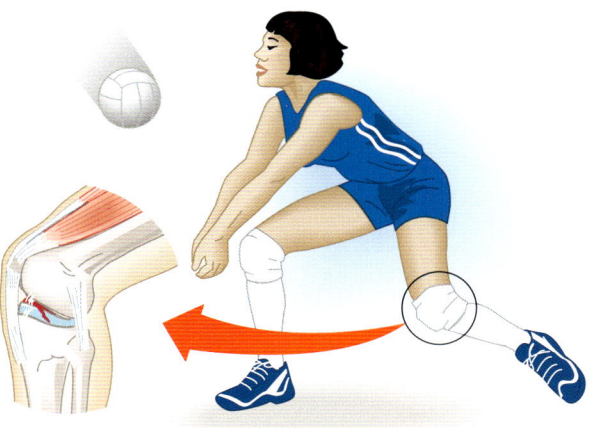

**Figure 3.20**   Cartilage tear in the knee joint.

### Dislocations and Subluxations

Sometimes when a joint is hit or twisted, the bones move out of position. In a dislocation, the bones stay out of place until a health care provider repositions them. If the bones seem to pop out of place but immediately pop back in, a subluxation has occurred. In sports, dislocations and subluxations occur most frequently at the shoulder (see figure 3.21), elbow, finger, and kneecap.

Dislocations and subluxations also injure the soft tissues around a joint. For example, ligaments are often sprained during dislocations and subluxations because they are stretched or torn when the bones move out of place. Sometimes, bones break and cartilage tears during these injuries.

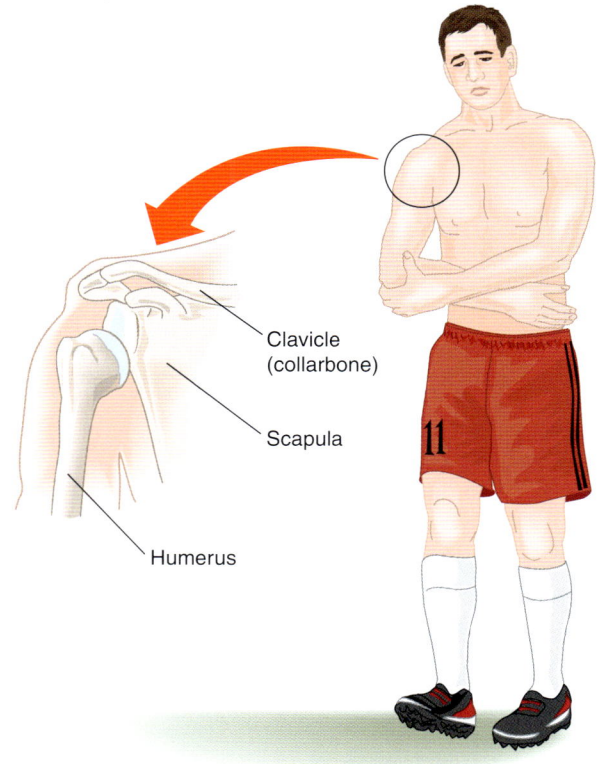

Clavicle
(collarbone)

Scapula

Humerus

**Figure 3.21**   Dislocation at the shoulder.

### Fractures

Bones that are compressed, twisted, or hit too hard can break (fracture). The two main categories of fractures are closed and open (see figure 3.22). In studies of high school sport-related injuries from the 2021-22 season, fractures accounted for 7.7 percent of sport-related injuries (Collins, Robison, and Burus 2022).

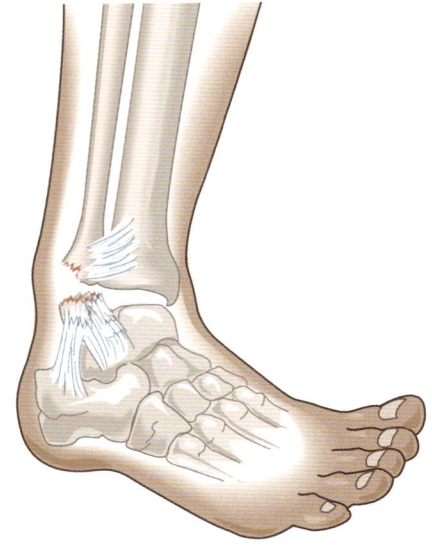

**Figure 3.23**    Avulsion fracture of the ankle.

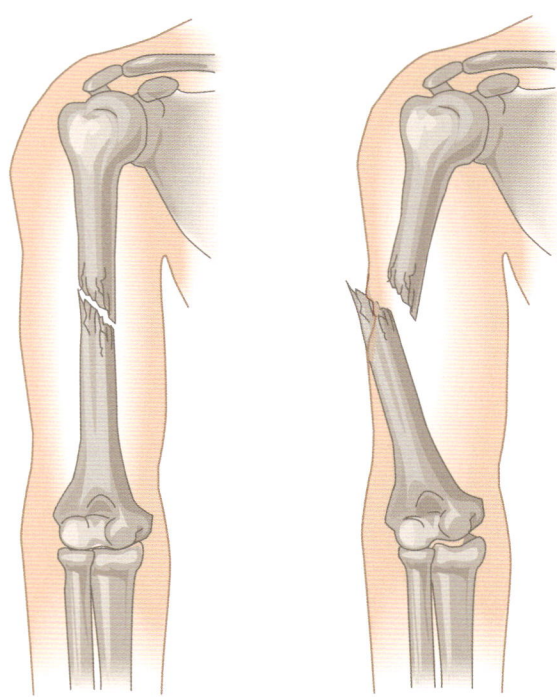

**Figure 3.22**    Closed (left) and open (right) fractures.

The most common type of fracture in sports, a closed fracture results when a bone breaks but does not protrude through the skin. Sometimes, a closed fracture causes a noticeable deformity. The two types of closed fractures prevalent in sports are avulsion and epiphyseal fractures. They are described as follows:

*Avulsion fracture*—Occurs when a sprained ligament pulls off a piece of bone. Avulsion fractures often take place in the ankle (figure 3.23) and finger.

*Epiphyseal (growth plate) fracture*—Results when the soft growth plates at the ends of bones are injured. Most often occurring in athletes before age 18, this type of fracture can affect the bone's growth. Growth plate fractures typically occur in the elbow of baseball pitchers, as shown in figure 3.24.

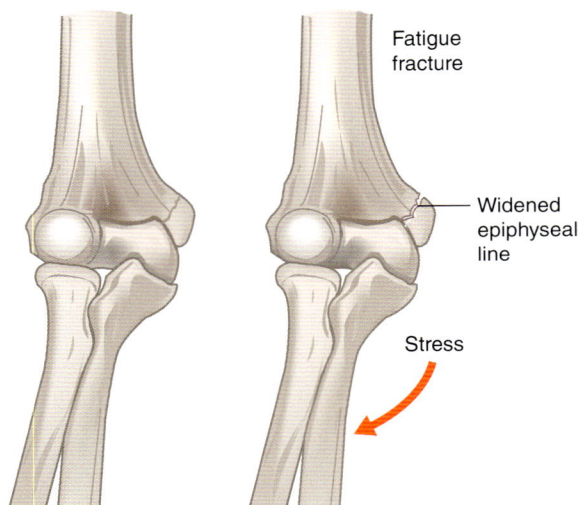

**Figure 3.24**    Epiphyseal (growth plate) fracture.

Open fractures occur when a broken bone pierces the skin. These wounds must be carefully covered with sterile gauze to help prevent infection in the exposed bone and muscle tissues. Fortunately, open fractures are rare in most sports.

## Common Chronic Injuries

Chronic injuries occur over time. They are often caused by repeated blows, overstretching, repeated friction, or overuse. Such repeated trauma can cause injuries to the muscles, tendons, bursas, and bones. These injuries typically occur in athletes who have an imbalance of muscle strength and flexibility, or in athletes who overtrain.

### Chronic Muscle Strain

If a muscle is repeatedly overworked or overstretched, a chronic strain can result. This type of injury develops over a period of weeks or months. These strains are different from acute strains because they are not caused by one specific episode (such as sprinting to first base).

### Bursitis

A bursa can become swollen and sore as a result of repeated blows or irritation. Bursitis can also be caused by tendons rubbing back and forth across the bursa. Bursitis of the elbow and kneecap (see figure 3.25) are the most common types in sports.

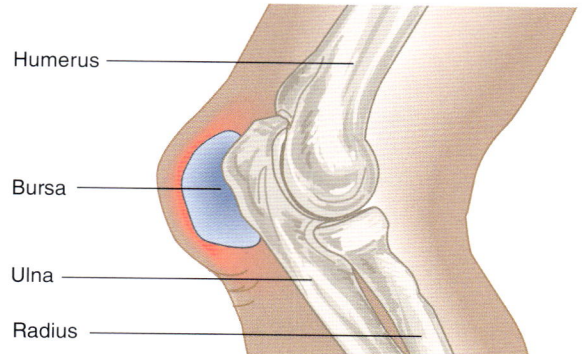

Humerus

Bursa

Ulna

Radius

**Figure 3.25**   Bursitis occurs when the bursa becomes swollen and sore.

### Tendinosis, Tenosynovitis, and Peritendinitis

Just as bursas can become irritated, repeated overstretching or overuse can cause irritation in tendons, especially if they are weak or tight. Although the various tendon injuries are all commonly known simply as tendinitis, these injuries are more accurately classified by different names based on the part of the tendon that is affected. For example, tendinosis is a condition in which microtears occur in the tendon. Tenosynovitis is an inflammation of the synovial sheath that surrounds the tendon. Peritendinitis is an inflammation or thickening of the tendon sheath (not a synovial sheath).

As with sprains and strains, tendinitis can also be classified as mild, moderate, and severe. In mild cases, symptoms include slight pain that occurs with specific skills or activities during extreme exertion. The pain subsides once the painful activity stops. Mild cases have minimal to no swelling and no loss of motion. Moderate tendinitis may cause some swelling. Pain occurs with more activities and skills, limits extreme muscle exertion, and continues up to several hours after the activity stops. In severe tendinitis, the pain intensifies; it occurs with any level of exertion, extends into daily activities, and lasts longer (sometimes more than 24 hours after activity stops). At this level, pain also limits muscle and joint function. Swelling or thickening of the tendon (particularly the Achilles or patellar tendon) becomes more prominent. Chapters 12 and 13 describe the signs and symptoms of, as well as the proper first aid care for, tendinitis at various locations on the body.

The tendons of the biceps, patella (kneecap), Achilles (heel), and rotator cuff (shoulder) are especially prone to repeated microtrauma in sports. Tendinitis of the patellar tendon and Achilles tendon (see figure 3.26) is common in athletes who experience poor muscle flexibility, muscle weakness, and overstressing through repeated running and jumping activities. The biceps and rotator cuff tendons are usually overstressed when an athlete throws with a weak and inflexible shoulder. These types of injuries can also be caused by increasing an athlete's workout or practice regimen too quickly. Generally, increasing the intensity and duration of specific exercises and workouts by 10 to 15 percent per week is considered a safe progression.

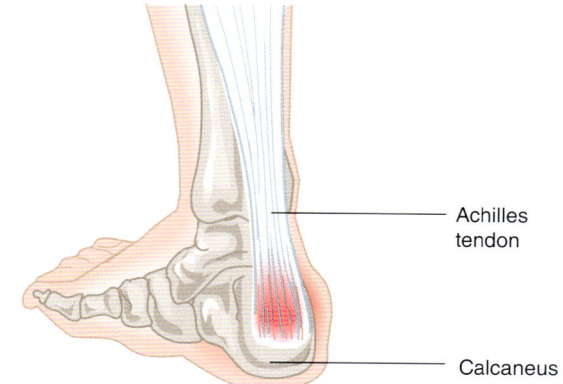

Achilles tendon

Calcaneus

**Figure 3.26**   Tendinitis results when tendons are irritated.

### *Chronic Bone Injuries*

Repeated and long-term wear and tear can cause bones to crack or grow abnormally. Two of the more prevalent types of chronic bone injuries are osteoarthritis and stress fractures.

### Osteoarthritis

Osteoarthritis is a degenerative joint disease characterized by a wearing down and inflammation of the ends of joints. It typically results from long-term wear over many years, so it is more common in postpubescent athletes. However, osteoarthritis can also develop over a shorter period as a result of one traumatic injury, such as a joint dislocation. Injuries that are ignored or left untreated in young athletes can lead to osteoarthritis in merely a few years. For example, repeated ankle or knee sprains can cause cumulative joint trauma, leading to osteoarthritis.

### Stress Fractures

Repeated stress or shock can eventually cause a bone to crack; this injury is called a stress fracture. Athletes involved in high-impact sports (e.g., running, basketball, soccer, gymnastics) and high-velocity activities (e.g., baseball pitching) are especially prone to stress fractures.

## Putting It All Together

This chapter introduced some of the injuries that you may encounter as a coach. Common injuries and their mechanisms of injury are listed in table 3.2. For an overview of what injuries affect what body parts, check out table 3.3. For more details on specific injuries, see the chapters in part II.

**Table 3.2**  Injuries and Their Mechanisms

| TYPE OF INJURY | INJURY MECHANISM | | |
|---|---|---|---|
| | Compression | Tension | Shearing |
| **Acute** | | | |
| Contusion | X | | |
| Abrasion | | | X |
| Puncture | X | | |
| Laceration | X | | X |
| Incision | X | | |
| Avulsion | X | X | X |
| Sprain | | X | X |
| Acute strain | | X | |
| Cartilage tear | X | | X |
| Dislocation and subluxation | X | X | |
| Avulsion fracture | X | | |
| Epiphyseal fracture | X | X | |
| **Chronic** | | | |
| Chronic strain | | X | |
| Bursitis | X | X | X |
| Tendinosis, tenosynovitis, and peritendinitis | | X | |
| Osteoarthritis | X | | X |
| Stress fracture | X | | |

**Table 3.3**  Examples of Injuries That Affect Specific Body Tissues

| Tissue | Injury | Type of injury |
|---|---|---|
| Bone | Closed fracture | Acute |
| | Open fracture | Acute |
| | Avulsion fracture | Acute or chronic |
| | Osteoarthritis | Chronic |
| | Stress fracture | Chronic |
| Cartilage | Tear | Acute or chronic |
| | Contusion | Acute |
| Ligament | Sprain | Acute |
| Muscle | Strain | Acute or chronic |
| Tendon | Strain | Acute |
| | Tenosynovitis | Chronic |
| | Tendinosis | Chronic |
| | Peritendinitis | Chronic |
| Bursa | Bursitis | Chronic |
| | Contusion | Acute |
| Skin | Laceration | Acute |
| | Incision | Acute |
| | Abrasion | Acute |
| | Puncture | Acute |
| | Avulsion (e.g., earlobe) | Acute |
| Eye | Puncture | Acute |
| | Abrasion (corneal) | Acute |
| Other organs (e.g., heart, kidney) | Puncture | Acute |
| | Contusion | Acute |

# Chapter 3 Recap

❑ What tissues make up a joint?

❑ Where are ligaments found? What role do they play in joint stability?

❑ What are the three mechanisms that result in most injuries?

❑ What are some common acute injuries? How do they occur?

❑ What are three types of cuts? How can you distinguish between them?

❑ What causes sprains? What tissue do they occur in?

❑ What causes strains? What tissues do they occur in?

# EMERGENCY ACTION STEPS

## INJURIES AND TECHNIQUES IN THIS CHAPTER

Imagine you are a football player. You're lining up behind your center, ready to take the snap. It's late in the fourth quarter, you're on the 30-yard line, it's fourth down, and you're down by two points. Suddenly, three hungry linebackers are staring you down from across the line. You realize your play is doomed against a blitz. You've got 7 seconds left on the play clock. What do you do? If you're able to think and react quickly, you call an audible that could save the game.

The need to recognize serious problems and react to them quickly and correctly is essential, but it is not unique to football. In sport first aid, it applies to assessing an athlete's breathing and providing basic life support. Both situations require an ability to analyze what's going on, and they both require split-second thinking and responding.

This chapter teaches you how to conduct emergency action steps to assess an injured or ill athlete. Correctly assessing an athlete can help you more accurately provide first aid care and communicate with emergency medical personnel. The chapter also guides you through potentially life-saving techniques, including proper positioning of an athlete as well as how to recognize and respond to various degrees of airway blockage.

# Emergency Action Steps

Your initial assessment of the athlete consists of these emergency action steps:

1. Assess (the scene and the athlete).
2. Alert.
3. Attend to breathing.

These steps will help you spot and care for life-threatening problems in an injured or ill athlete. Perform them quickly (in a minute or less). For a summary of these steps, see the Emergency Action Steps flowchart in the appendix.

## Assess the Scene

When an athlete goes down because of injury or illness, the first thing to consider is safety. Your immediate goal is to protect the athlete—and yourself—from harm. First, you or an assistant should instruct all other participants and bystanders to leave the athlete alone. They can cause further injury by trying to move the athlete.

Second, consider the environment. Is the athlete in danger? Consider hazards such as nearby play, crowds, downed power lines, lightning, traffic, and cold or heat exposure. If such hazards exist, you need to carefully consider how to minimize the risk of injury to yourself and evaluate if the athlete may need to be immediately moved to prevent the environment from worsening their condition. See Safety Measure: When Moving an Injured or Ill Athlete and chapter 6 for instructions on when and how to safely move an injured athlete.

Third, try to calm the athlete, and keep them from rolling around or jumping up and down, which can cause further injury. Finally, think about whether the athlete is lying in a position or wearing equipment that will prevent you from evaluating their condition or from providing first aid for a life-threatening condition. You may need to move the athlete or remove the specific equipment that is hindering the assessment or first aid care. Table 4.1 outlines positioning for various injuries and illnesses. Use it as a guide if you are presented with any of these situations.

## Assess the Athlete

As you approach the athlete, review in your mind how the injury or illness occurred. Was there a direct hit to a certain area of the body?

---

**SAFETY MEASURE**

### When Moving an Injured or Ill Athlete

In almost every case, you should let emergency medical personnel move a seriously injured athlete. Move a critically injured or ill athlete to another site only if

- the area is unsafe (e.g., because of lightning, downed electrical lines, traffic, or other runners in a road race),
- the athlete's position prevents you from providing CPR or life-saving first aid, or
- the athlete is experiencing exertional heat-related syndrome (see chapter 11).

Reposition a critically injured or ill athlete only when necessary to perform CPR, control profuse bleeding, or prevent the athlete from choking on vomit or secretions. See chapter 6 for proper techniques for moving an athlete.

---

Was a joint or body part twisted? Was the athlete stung by an insect? This information provides insight into what type of injury you're dealing with. More specific protocols are discussed in chapter 5.

Also review what you may know about the athlete's medical history. Does the athlete have a history of asthma, heart problems, kidney disorders, neurological problems, diabetes, or seizures? Has the athlete ever had this injury or condition before? This information provides additional clues to what may be wrong with the athlete, and it may help you determine what care to provide. For example, an athlete may have difficulty breathing because of an injury, or it could be due to a medical condition such as asthma. To review the steps to take in the event of an asthma attack, see the Asthma flowchart in the appendix.

When you reach the athlete, quickly determine whether they are responsive or unresponsive. Gently tap or squeeze the athlete's shoulder and ask, "Are you all right, [athlete's name]?" If an athlete is unresponsive but appears to be breathing, do not remove their helmet. If you suspect a serious injury to the head or spine, place your hands on both sides of the athlete's helmet to keep the head, neck, and spine in line.

**Table 4.1**   Positions for Ill or Injured Athletes

| Condition | Position | Rationale |
|---|---|---|
| Responsive athlete with suspected spinal injury | Manual stabilization of the head so that the head, neck, and spine do not move and are kept in line | Pain and loss of function usually accompany a spinal injury, but the absence of pain does not mean that the athlete has not been significantly injured. If you suspect an athlete could have a spinal injury, assume they do. |
| Unresponsive, uninjured athlete who is breathing but having difficulty with secretions or vomiting | Recovery position | It protects the airway by allowing fluid to drain easily from the mouth. |
| Unresponsive, injured athlete who is breathing but having difficulty with secretions or vomiting or who you must leave unattended to get help | Recovery position | It protects the airway by allowing fluid to drain easily from the mouth. |
| Unresponsive athlete who is not breathing (or you are unsure) | Flat on the back for CPR | Occasional gasps are not normal and are not capable of supplying the athlete with enough oxygen to sustain life. |
| Responsive or unresponsive athlete with signs and symptoms of shock from severe bleeding | Flat on the back | It is best to leave the athlete lying flat. If the athlete is having difficulty with secretions or vomiting, place them in the recovery position. |

# Recovery Position for a Stable Athlete

The recovery position is for an athlete who is not feeling well but has not sustained an injury. To put an athlete in the recovery position, follow these steps:

1. Kneel beside the athlete; make sure both legs are straight.
2. Bring the far arm across the chest; hold the back of the hand against the athlete's cheek that is nearest to you (figure 4.1a).
3. With your other hand, grasp the far leg just above the knee and pull it up (figure 4.1b).
4. Keeping the athlete's hand pressed against the cheek, pull on the far leg to roll the athlete toward you.
5. Adjust the upper leg so that both the hip and the knee are bent at right angles (figure 4.1c).

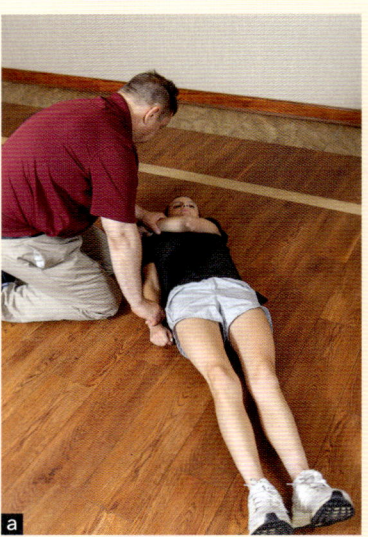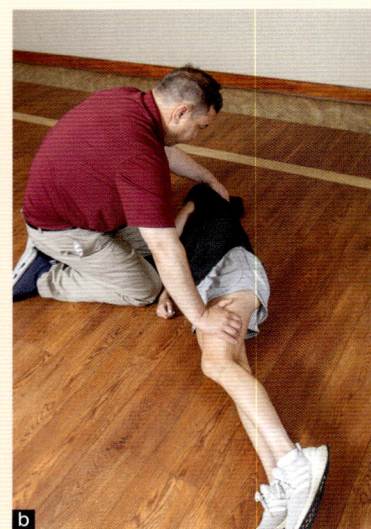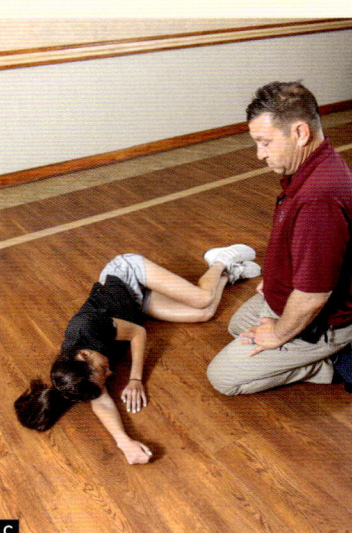

**Figure 4.1**   Recovery position: (a) bring the far arm across the athlete's chest; (b) pull up the far leg; (c) bend the hip and knee at right angles.

## Alert

If the athlete is unresponsive, or if they are responsive but are badly hurt, look or act very ill, or quickly get worse, send for emergency medical assistance (call 911) or activate your facility's emergency action plan (EAP).

## Attend to Breathing

After determining whether the athlete is responsive or unresponsive, then sending for emergency medical assistance or following your EAP, attend to the athlete's breathing.

Your objective is to see if the athlete needs CPR and to check for any other life-threatening conditions that require immediate attention, such as severe bleeding. If you don't find any conditions that are immediately life-threatening, do a more thorough physical assessment to determine the course of treatment. This assessment is described in chapter 5.

### For a Responsive Athlete

1. Identify yourself, and ask the athlete's permission to help.

2. Ensure that the athlete is fully responsive and breathing normally without making gasping, noisy, snorting, or gurgling sounds. The athlete should be able to talk and keep the airway open and clear.

3. Move the athlete only if the athlete is in an area that may cause further harm; the athlete is at risk for breathing in fluid, vomit, or blood; or you must leave the athlete alone to get help. If any of these conditions exist, you may need to move the athlete using the techniques outlined here. For a stable athlete, use the recovery position. For an injured athlete, automatically assume they may have a head or spine injury. Remember: Move an athlete only if it is necessary to protect the athlete from further harm or to provide life-saving first aid. In sports where a helmet is worn, do not remove the helmet unless it is interfering with CPR.

4. Look for and control any severe bleeding with direct pressure (see chapter 5 for more information).

5. Look for normal tissue color and body temperature. If the skin is bluish or ashen or it feels cool, it may indicate that the athlete has had reduced circulation for at least a few minutes.

6. While waiting for medical assistance, continue to monitor the athlete's alertness and make sure they are breathing normally.

7. Continue to control bleeding, monitor tissue color and temperature, and help maintain the athlete's normal body temperature.

See the Attending to a Responsive Athlete flowchart in the appendix for a summary of how to attend to a responsive athlete.

### For an Unresponsive Athlete

1. Send for emergency medical assistance, and retrieve an automated external defibrillator (AED). If other people are present, have them get the AED while you attend to the athlete.

2. Check the athlete for breathing and signs of circulation. Look to see if the athlete is moving, or if the chest rises and falls. If an unresponsive athlete is lying face down, observe if the ribs are rising and falling, indicating that the athlete is breathing. Check the athlete for no more than 10 seconds. Occasional gasps are not normal; it means they are not capable of supplying the athlete with enough oxygen to sustain life. If the athlete is not breathing or is making gasping, noisy, snorting, or gurgling sounds, you may have to move the athlete onto their back to administer CPR.

   • If you are alone and the athlete is lying face down, place the athlete's closest arm up over the head. Support the neck with your hand. Place your other hand on the athlete's hip, and roll the athlete's body toward you until the athlete is on their back. As best as you can, roll the athlete's body and head all at once to minimize injury to the spine.

   • If other people are present and the athlete is prone (on their front), use the four- or five-person rescue (described in chapter 6).

3. Begin CPR, and apply AED in accordance with CPR training. CPR uses chest compressions to help circulate blood with oxygen to the organs when the heart is not beating. Basic CPR is described as follows. However, it is not meant to take the place of certification offered through the American Red Cross, American Heart Association, National Safety Council, or other nationally recognized organizations.

### Compressions

1. Expose the athlete's chest.

2. Place the heel of one hand in the center of the chest between the nipples. Put the other hand on top of the first, and interlock your fingers (see figure 4.2a). Your fingers should be kept off the athlete's chest.

3. Position your body so that your shoulders are directly over your hands. Straighten your arms, and lock your elbows (see figure 4.2b).

4. Use your upper body weight to help compress the athlete's chest. Push forcefully straight down on the chest as outlined by your certification.

5. Release pressure and completely remove your weight at the top of each compression so the chest returns to its normal position and the heart can fill with blood.

6. Give chest compressions as outlined by your certification. Allow the athlete's chest to recoil completely. To get the most oxygenated blood to the athlete's brain and heart, minimize interruptions in chest compressions.

7. Continue chest compressions until someone with equal or higher training takes over, an AED or the EMS provider arrives, the athlete shows signs of life, or the scene becomes too dangerous or you are too exhausted to continue.

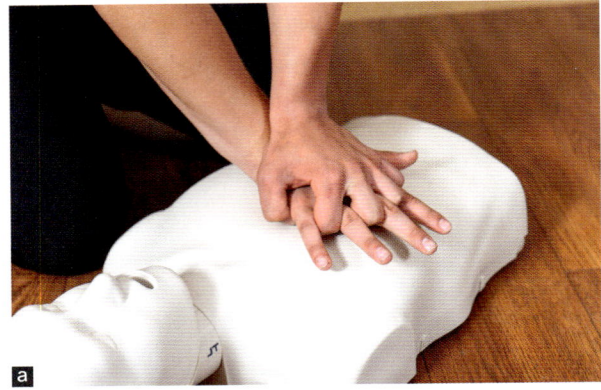

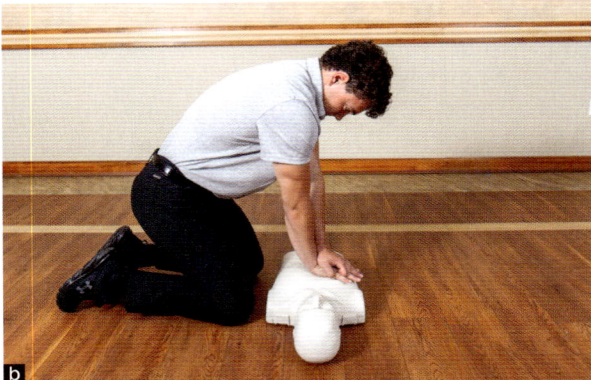

**Figure 4.2**   Position for chest compressions: *(a)* hands; *(b)* arms.

### Defibrillation

Sometimes, an athlete's heart may not be beating effectively, so blood is not effectively circulating to provide the body with oxygen. In such cases, when performing CPR, you should use an automated external defibrillator (AED) (see figure 4.3). An AED can identify two common types of heart arrhythmias. If the AED identifies these arrhythmias, it will shock the heart in an attempt to establish a normal beating rhythm. If you are alone and need to perform CPR (and the patient is an adult), then retrieve the AED and apply it as soon as possible before beginning compressions. If someone else is present, begin chest compressions and send that person to get the AED.

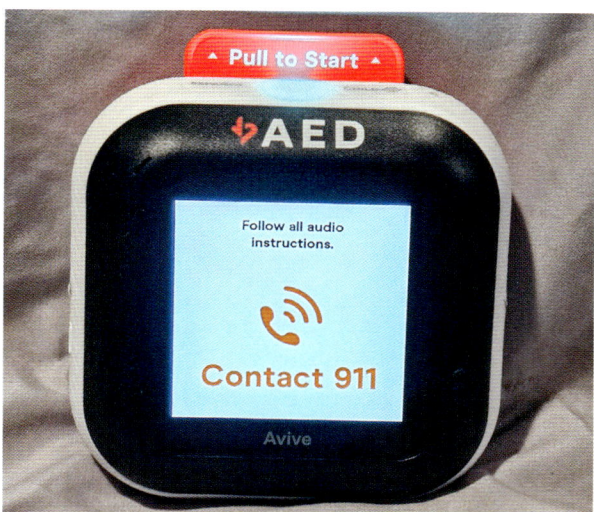

**Figure 4.3**  Automated external defibrillator (AED).

Once the AED arrives, if you are alone, do the following:

1. Turn on the AED.

2. Select and attach the adult pads if the athlete is an adult. If the athlete is a child and child pads are available, use them; if child pads are not available, use adult pads. (Note that AEDs are not used for infants.)

3. Listen to and follow the voice prompts on the AED.

4. Most AEDs will automatically begin to analyze the athlete's heart rhythm when the electrodes are fully attached. Ensure no one touches the athlete while the AED is analyzing the heart rhythm.

5. If a shock is indicated, make sure no one is touching the athlete. Stay clear of the athlete, and press the Shock button on the AED to give one shock.

6. Continue as directed by the AED until the EMS provider arrives.

If another person is available, have them open and turn on the AED while you continue CPR. Stop CPR when the pads are ready to be attached to the athlete's chest.

For a summary of these procedures, see the flowcharts Attending to an Unresponsive Athlete, CPR, and AED in the appendix.

## Airway Blockage

Airway blockage is another emergency situation that requires a quick response. In sports, an athlete's airway may become blocked due to one of the following:

- Breathing in a foreign object such as gum or food

- The tongue falling back against the throat in an unresponsive athlete

- Swelling from a direct blow or severe allergies

In these cases, the airway may have either mild or severe blockage. The first aid care that you provide depends on the kind of blockage that occurs.

This chapter deals with first aid care for airway blockage caused by a foreign object such as food, gum, or the tongue (in an unresponsive athlete). Chapter 7 addresses first aid care for airway blockage caused by swelling from severe allergic reactions. For a summary of these first aid procedures, see Airway Blockage in a Responsive Athlete and Airway Blockage in an Unresponsive Athlete in the appendix.

# MILD AIRWAY BLOCKAGE IN A RESPONSIVE ATHLETE

In mild airway blockage, the airway is partially blocked; it allows some (but not enough) air to pass through to the lungs. It is caused by a foreign object, such as gum or food, becoming lodged in the airway.

## Signs and Symptoms

- Ability to inhale, exhale, and speak
- Strong coughing or gagging as food or liquid is aspirated
- High-pitched squeaking or whistling noise (wheezing) between strong coughs

## FIRST AID

1. Ask, "Are you OK?" If the athlete says "Yes" but has trouble breathing or grasps their throat (the universal choking sign), the athlete may have a partially blocked airway.
2. Encourage the athlete to cough.
3. Monitor the athlete until (a) the object is dislodged and the athlete breathes normally, or (b) the airway becomes severely blocked (athlete is unable to cough or speak). If the latter happens, perform abdominal thrusts as described in the next section. If abdominal thrusts do not dislodge the object or if the athlete becomes unresponsive, have someone call for emergency medical assistance and begin CPR.

## Playing Status

If the object dislodges and the athlete's breathing and color in lips, skin, and nail beds return to normal, the athlete can return to activity.

# SEVERE AIRWAY BLOCKAGE IN A RESPONSIVE ATHLETE

In severe airway blockage, the airway is totally blocked, preventing air from entering the lungs. It is caused by a foreign object, such as gum or food, becoming lodged in the airway.

## Signs and Symptoms

- Grasping throat (universal choking sign)
- Inability to cough or make any sound
- Blue lips, nails, or skin

## FIRST AID

1. Ask, "Are you choking?"
2. If the athlete nods their head yes or gives the universal choking signal, then ask, "Can I help?" If the athlete nods yes or is unable to speak, cough, or cry, immediately begin abdominal thrusts.
3. If the athlete shakes their head no to "Are you choking?" send for emergency medical assistance and check for other causes of breathing difficulties (discussed in chapter 7).

## Playing Status

After receiving abdominal thrusts, even if the object dislodges and the athlete's breathing returns to normal, the athlete cannot return to play until after being evaluated by EMS providers and checked by an appropriate health care provider. Internal injuries can result from abdominal thrusts even when they are performed correctly.

## Abdominal Thrusts for Choking in a Responsive Athlete

An athlete could start choking on the sideline from attempting to eat something quickly before going back in the game. If an object is causing severe blockage, abdominal thrusts are used to force air out of the lungs to dislodge the blockage. The following steps explain abdominal thrusts:

1. Stand behind the athlete (if an adult; kneel if the athlete is a child).
2. Make a fist. Place your thumb side against the athlete's abdomen, just above the navel (see figure 4.4). If you place your fist too high, the thrusts not only will be less effective but also can break the tip of the breastbone, potentially causing internal injuries. Wrap your other hand securely around the fist.
3. Give quick inward and upward thrusts.
4. Continue the compressions until
   - the object is expelled or
   - the athlete loses responsiveness from lack of air. If this occurs, gently lower them to the ground, instruct someone to send for emergency medical assistance (call 911), and begin CPR.

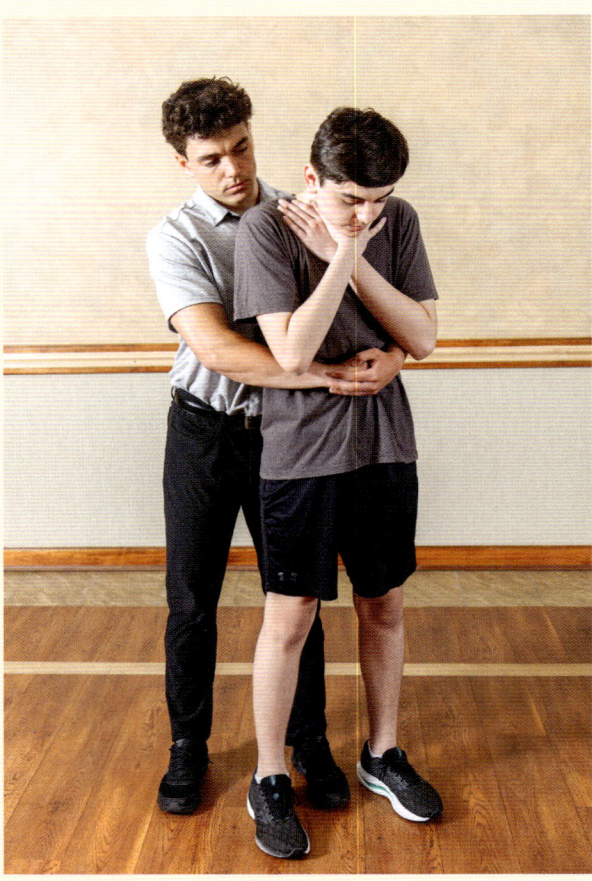

**Figure 4.4**    Hand position for abdominal thrusts.

# SEVERE AIRWAY BLOCKAGE IN AN UNRESPONSIVE ATHLETE

This situation could result from a once responsive choking athlete who becomes unresponsive or from the tongue obstructing the airway of an athlete who unresponsive. The blockage is caused by a lodged foreign object or the back of the tongue obstructing the airway.

**Signs and Symptoms**

- Unresponsive
- Not breathing

## FIRST AID

If the athlete loses responsiveness from choking, do the following:

1. If possible, protect the athlete from falling when they lose consciousness.
2. Have someone immediately send for emergency medical assistance.
3. If the athlete is not positioned on their back, move them onto their back as outlined in table 4.1.
4. If you are certain that the athlete does not have a head or neck injury, open their mouth, then remove the object if you see it. Look for signs that the tongue has slipped back and is blocking the airway. If it is, gently tilt the athlete's head back until the tongue has been cleared from the airway.
5. If the athlete still isn't breathing, continue CPR until the AED or EMS provider arrives, or until the object dislodges and the athlete shows signs of life. If the latter occurs, recheck the athlete's breathing. If the athlete is breathing (not gasping), continue to monitor breathing and monitor and care for shock as needed until the EMS provider arrives.

**Playing Status**

The athlete cannot return to activity until examined and released by a health care provider.

## Chapter 4 Recap

❑ When an athlete sustains an injury or sudden illness, what are the first steps you should take?

❑ If an athlete is unresponsive, who should be called?

❑ What are the emergency action steps, and how are they conducted?

❑ If an athlete is responsive and has mild blockage of the airway, what should you do?

❑ If an athlete is responsive and has a severe blockage of the airway, what should you do?

❑ If an athlete is unresponsive and has a blockage of the airway, what should you do?

❑ When and how do you perform abdominal thrusts for choking?

❑ When and how do you perform cardiopulmonary resuscitation (CPR)?

❑ When and how do you use an automated external defibrillator (AED)?

# ASSESSMENT IN SPORT FIRST AID

## IN THIS CHAPTER, YOU WILL LEARN THE FOLLOWING:

- How to conduct an assessment of an injured or ill athlete
- How to control profuse bleeding
- What methods you can use to minimize widespread tissue damage
- How to splint unstable injuries
- How to control slow, steady bleeding
- What to do to minimize local tissue damage

## INJURIES AND TECHNIQUES IN THIS CHAPTER

In gymnastics, flawlessly executing a difficult mount is only the beginning of a balance beam routine. Similarly, in sport first aid, the emergency action steps are only the start of assessment and care. These primary steps are pivotal skills, but they are a small portion of an entire routine. Beam specialists and sport first aid providers alike must also be able to perform more common and basic (but equally important) skills. For a gymnast, these skills may be turns and jumps on the beam. For the sport first aid provider, these skills include conducting an assessment and administering corresponding first aid techniques.

## Assessment

After you have completed the primary assessment (step 1 of the emergency action steps outlined in chapter 4) and established that the athlete is responsive and breathing, you should begin a secondary assessment to pinpoint the nature, site, and severity of an injury or illness. For an overview, consult the Secondary Assessment flowchart in the appendix. Do not begin the secondary assessment until you have ruled out a life-threatening condition. As with the emergency action steps, this assessment follows a standard pattern to ensure a thorough evaluation.

The secondary assessment has two parts: the history and the physical examination.

## History

The history step is a time to gather additional information about how the injury or illness happened. Your goal is to determine the location, mechanism, symptoms, and previous occurrences. Use the acronym SAMPLE to ensure that you cover the full history of the injured or ill athlete (National Safety Council 2016).

**S**—*Signs and symptoms*

Ask the athlete how they feel or what they feel. Look for any signs of injury, such as bleeding or deformities.

**A**—*Allergies*

Ask the athlete if they have any allergies to foods, insect bites, medications, or anything else. Look for a medical identification bracelet.

**M**—*Medications*

Ask the athlete if they are currently taking any medications (either prescribed or over-the-counter).

**P**—*Previous problems*

Ask the athlete if they have ever had this injury or illness before.

**L**—*Last food or drink*

Ask the athlete when they last consumed food or drink.

**E**—*Events*

Ask the athlete what happened that led to the situation they are in now. Ask for as many details as possible. If the athlete is unresponsive, ask bystanders what they know or saw.

## Physical Examination

The assessment of an injured or ill athlete who is responsive also includes a physical examination. This examination may detect other injuries that need first aid or additional clues to the athlete's condition.

### Inspection

Use the information from the injury history to pinpoint where you should look for obvious signs (actual physical manifestations) of an injury or illness. For example, if an athlete reports hearing and feeling a pop in the ankle, you should look for signs of an ankle injury such as a deformity or swelling. In addition, you should check for these obvious signs:

- *Bleeding*—Is it profuse or slow? Is it dark red or bright red?
- *Skin appearance*—Is the skin pale or flushed? Is it dry or sweaty? Is it blue or gray?
- *Pupils*—Compare the two pupils. Are they dilated (enlarged), constricted (small), or uneven in size? Also, use the penlight from your sport first aid kit to check whether each pupil reacts to light by constricting (see figure 5.1). If the pupils are uneven or do not react to light, the athlete may have a head injury.
- *Deformities*—Do you see any indentations or bumps? If the deformity is on one side of the body, always compare it to the opposite side.
- *Signs of sudden illness*—Is the athlete vomiting or coughing?
- *Swelling*—Do you see any puffiness around the injured area or other areas?

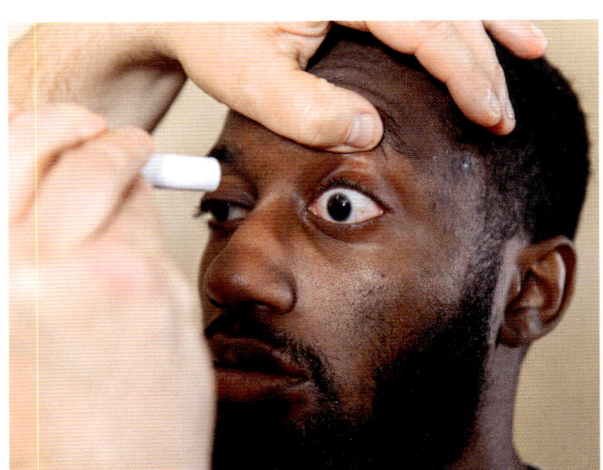

**Figure 5.1** Check whether each pupil reacts to light by constricting.

- *Discoloration*—Do you see any bruising or other marks?
- *Ability to walk, or position of lower extremity*—Does the athlete limp, or is the athlete totally unable to bear weight? If swelling exists, elevate and splint accordingly.
- *Position of an upper extremity (arm, elbow, forearm, wrist, or hand)*—Is the athlete supporting the forearm with the other hand? Is the arm held in an unusual position, such as out to the side?

For some illnesses and injuries, it's helpful to check the athlete's pulse (heart) rate to determine the regularity and strength of the heartbeat. For specific steps, see the sidebar Taking the Athlete's Pulse. If the athlete has been active, the heart rate will be faster than their resting heart rate. Table 5.1 provides normal resting heart rates for various ages. If the heart rate doesn't return to resting levels within a few minutes, or if the rate feels irregular, you should suspect a potentially life-threatening injury or illness and send for emergency medical assistance.

**Table 5.1** Normal Resting Heart Rates

| Age group (years) | Resting heart rate (beats per minute) |
|---|---|
| Children (5-12) | 60-120 |
| Adolescents (12-18) | 75-85 |
| Adults (18+) | 60-100 |

The information gathered during the inspection should help to further pinpoint the exact nature of an illness or injury. This information, combined with the palpation portion of the physical examination (discussed next), will help you determine the first aid that you will provide. In addition to previously mentioned signs and symptoms gathered during the inspection, the acronym *DOTS* is a quick and easy one for coaches. *DOTS* stands for:

**D**—*Deformities*

**O**—*Open injuries*

**T**—*Tenderness (pain)*

**S**—*Swelling*

### Palpation

Sometimes, looks can be deceiving. What appears to be an intact, fully functioning body part may in fact have severe internal damage. To get a better idea of the nature of the injury, gently touch the injured area with your fingertips. Start away from the injury; for example, if the hand is injured, start at the fingers and wrist and work your way toward the injury. Check for the following:

- *Point tenderness*—Is there an area that is extremely painful?
- *Skin temperature*—Is it hot? Cool? Sweaty? Dry?
- *Sensation*—Can the athlete feel you touching the area?
- *Deformity*—Can you feel any bumps, indentations, or differences between sides that you did not see in the inspection?

Remember that if one side of the body is injured (e.g., ribs, arm, leg), you should always compare it to the opposite side. After completing the history and physical examination, you will be better able to focus your first aid techniques on the specific injury or illness that is affecting the athlete.

Take some time to review the procedures of the secondary assessment. Upon completing the secondary assessment, you may find that you have to control external bleeding, minimize systemic tissue damage (shock), splint injuries, and minimize local tissue damage. The following section discusses these basic first aid techniques in order of priority. Remember to continue to monitor breathing even after beginning to administer first aid to the site of the injury. You must continually observe any seriously injured athlete even if their breathing is initially normal.

# Taking the Athlete's Pulse

You can take an athlete's pulse either at the wrist (radial pulse, figure 5.2*a*) or at the neck (carotid pulse, figure 5.2*b*). Because your thumb has its own pulse, you should always use your fingers to check the pulse. The carotid pulse is easier to feel than the radial pulse. However, be careful not to push too hard; you may reduce blood flow to the athlete's brain.

### Radial Pulse

1. Place the tips of your index and middle fingers just below the athlete's thumb.
2. Slide your fingertips down until you feel a bony bump.
3. Move your fingers just to the inside of the bump, toward the middle of the wrist.
4. Apply slight pressure to feel the athlete's pulse.
5. Check the pulse for no more than 10 seconds and then multiply by 6 for the number of beats per minute.

### Carotid Pulse

1. Using the hand nearest the athlete's body, place the tips of your index and middle fingers over the athlete's Adam's apple (the prominent projection of thyroid cartilage at the front of the neck).
2. Slide your fingertips back and up in the groove along the side of the neck. Use the index and middle fingers to gently apply pressure over the carotid artery.
3. Check the pulse for no more than 10 seconds and then multiply by 6 for the number of beats per minute.

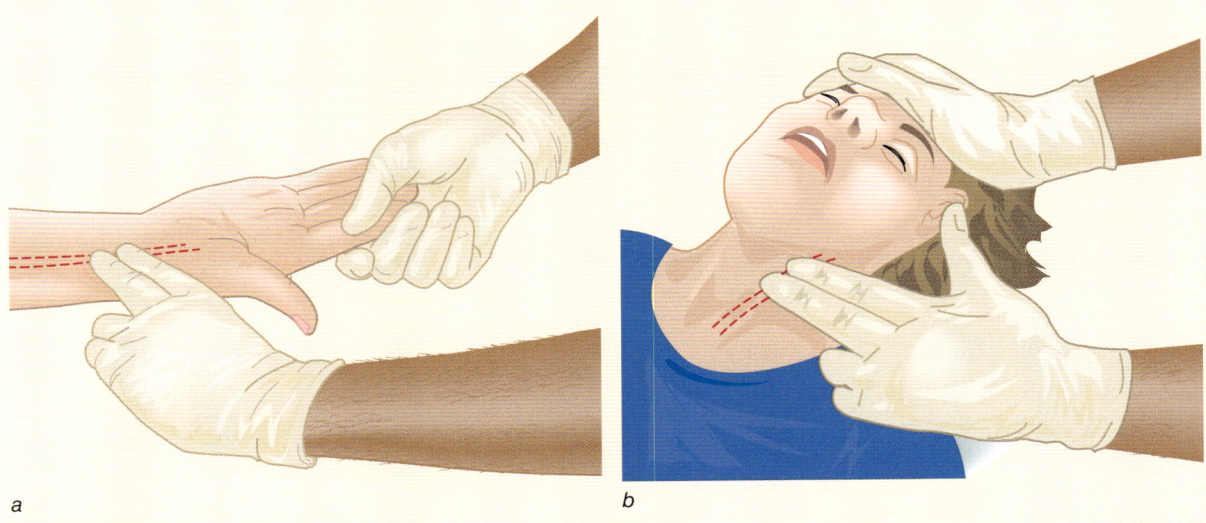

*a*                                                           *b*

**Figure 5.2**   Taking the *(a)* radial pulse and *(b)* carotid pulse.

# Universal Precautions to Protect Against Blood-Borne Pathogens

Don't let a fear of human immunodeficiency virus (HIV), hepatitis B, or other blood-borne pathogens keep you from administering first aid to injured athletes. Instead of avoiding the situation, opt to learn more about these diseases and how they can be transmitted. Contact your state athletic association for specific sport rules and policies regarding blood-borne pathogens. For example, some sports require athletes to change a bloody uniform before returning to competition.

If care of an injured athlete involves handling bloody wounds, bloody dressings or linens, body fluids, mouth guards, or bloody playing surfaces and equipment, follow these guidelines:

1. Wear disposable examination gloves (latex free, to avoid allergic reactions).
2. Wear safety glasses or a face shield if your face will be exposed to blood or body fluids.
3. Immediately wash any portion of your skin that touches blood or body fluid.
4. Bag contaminated linens or clothing, then wash them in hot water and detergent.
5. Clean contaminated floors, equipment, and other surfaces with a 1:10 solution of bleach and water. Wiping up the solution reduces its effectiveness, so you should let the surface air dry after applying the solution.
6. Remove your contaminated gloves in this manner:
   a. Without touching the bare skin, grasp either palm with the fingers of the opposite hand (see figure 5.3a).
   b. Gently pull the glove away from the palm and toward the fingers, removing the glove inside out. Hold on to the glove with the fingers of the opposite hand (see figure 5.3b).
   c. Without touching the outside of the contaminated glove, carefully slide the ungloved index and middle fingers inside the wristband of the gloved hand (see figure 5.3c).
   d. Gently pulling outward and down toward the fingers, remove the glove inside out (see figure 5.3d).

Adapted from American Safety & Health Institute.

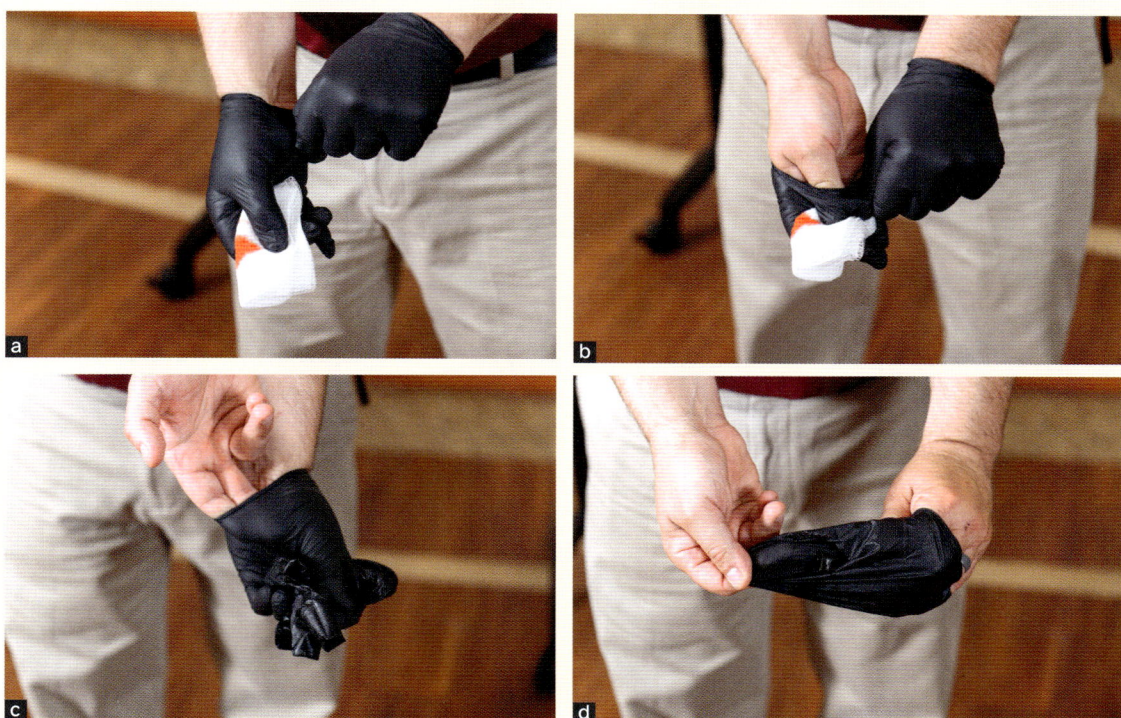

**Figure 5.3**  Proper removal of contaminated gloves.

*(continued)*

# Universal Precautions to Protect Against Blood-Borne Pathogens *(continued)*

7. Place contaminated gloves and bandages in a biohazard waste bag.

8. Wash your hands immediately after removing the examination gloves. You can use an alcohol-based hand rub; however, if your hands are visibly soiled, use soap and water.

Taking these steps all the time, regardless of who the athlete is, is called taking universal precautions. It means that you treat all human blood and most body fluids as if they were infectious for blood-borne pathogens, even if you think they aren't. In addition to taking universal precautions, also review your school district's or organization's plans for disposing of contaminated waste, handling athletes who are infected with blood-borne pathogens, reporting employee (e.g., coaches, teachers) exposure to blood-borne pathogens, and protecting employees against the transmission of blood-borne pathogens (using policies, procedures, equipment, and possibly hepatitis B vaccinations).

## Controlling Profuse Bleeding

Although it is not a common injury, profuse bleeding from an artery or vein can be life-threatening. Bleeding can also occur internally from injuries such as a bruised muscle, ruptured spleen, or bruised kidney (see chapter 9 for details on bleeding internal organs and how to care for them). The Profuse Bleeding flowchart in the appendix provides a summary of first aid techniques for this injury.

### SAFETY MEASURE

**With Bleeding Injuries**

- Do not attempt to pull out embedded objects.

- Do not remove blood-soaked bandages from a wound; doing so may cause bleeding to resume. For example, if you put gauze over an athlete's hand to stop bleeding, don't remove the gauze to see whether the wound has stopped bleeding. You'll know if it's still bleeding because blood will continue to seep through the bandages.

- Do not give aspirin to the athlete; it can cause increased bleeding.

# ARTERIAL AND VENOUS BLEEDING

Arterial and venous bleeding are profuse bleeding resulting from a cut to a limb. They are defined as follows:

- *Arterial bleeding*—Bleeding caused by a very deep incision, laceration, or puncture of an artery.
- *Venous bleeding*—Bleeding caused by a deep incision, avulsion, or puncture of a vein.

Note that once you have protected yourself from infected blood, you need to quickly determine the extent of the bleeding. A cut to a limb's artery or vein can cause profuse bleeding. The first aid steps for arterial and venous bleeding are identical. However, the causes and signs of each are slightly different.

### Signs and Symptoms

- *Arterial bleeding*—Bright red blood, or rapid or spurting bleeding
- *Venous bleeding*—Dark red blood or rapid bleeding

## FIRST AID

Specific items and techniques used to control arterial or venous bleeding include a tourniquet, wound packing, and hemostatic dressing.

### Tourniquet

A tourniquet applies intense pressure to a limb to temporarily stop blood flow (see figure 5.4). A tourniquet should be the first item used with severe, life-threatening bleeding to an extremity that cannot be controlled by other means. Tourniquets should be used in conjunction with hemostatic dressing (if available), gauze, clean cloths, and direct pressure over the wound. Tourniquets are manufactured for their specific purpose. If a tourniquet is not available, only a first aid provider trained in the use of improvised tourniquets should improvise one.

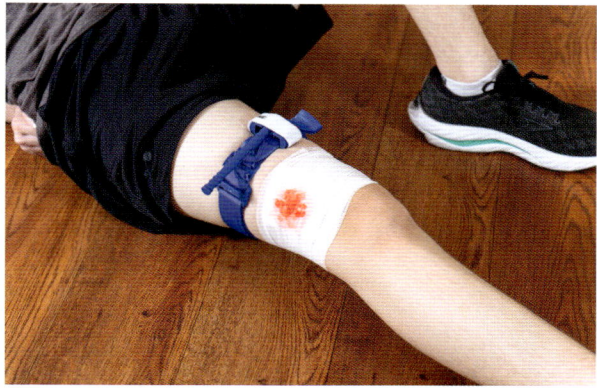

**Figure 5.4**   Tourniquet.

### Wound Packing

Wound packing is used when severe bleeding cannot be stopped by applying compression alone and when the location of the wound does not allow for the use of a tourniquet. Wound packing is placing the gauze, hemostatic dressing, or clean rags directly into the wound to control the bleeding (see figure 5.5). Wound packing can also be used in conjunction with a tourniquet on the arms and legs (if the tourniquet alone is not controlling the bleeding).

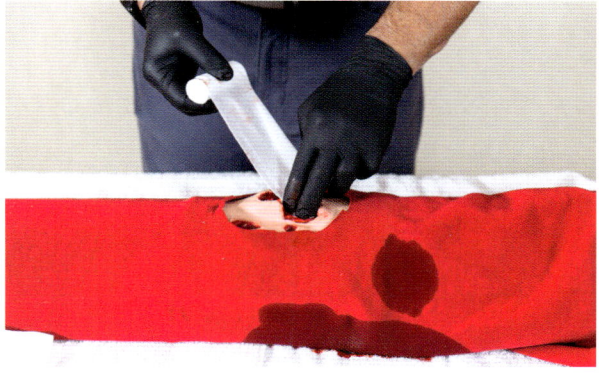

**Figure 5.5**   Wound packing.

*(continued)*

**Arterial and Venous Bleeding** *(continued)*

## Hemostatic Dressing

Hemostatic dressing is wound dressing with special properties to encourage the blood to clot faster (see figure 5.6). It is especially useful for severe bleeding where a tourniquet cannot be used. If a hemostatic dressing is available, it can be beneficial to use in life-threatening situations. When using a hemostatic dressing, direct pressure should still be used.

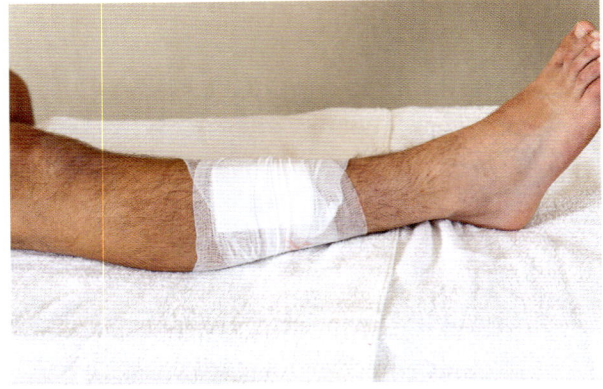

**Figure 5.6**   Hemostatic dressing.

To control arterial and venous bleeding, take the following steps depending on the location of the bleeding:

## Extremity Wound

1. Send for emergency medical assistance.
2. Put on personal protective equipment (PPE).
3. Pack the wound with hemostatic dressing (if available), gauze, or clean cloth.
4. Apply direct pressure to the wound.
5. Apply more gauze as needed.
6. If bleeding is severe and cannot be controlled, apply a tourniquet.
7. Monitor breathing and perform CPR if needed.
8. Monitor and treat for shock as needed.

## Torso, Neck, or Head Wound

1. Send for emergency medical assistance.
2. Put on PPE.
3. Pack the wound with hemostatic dressing (if available), gauze, or clean cloth.
4. Apply direct pressure to the wound.
5. Apply more gauze as needed.
6. Monitor breathing, and perform CPR as needed.
7. Monitor and treat for shock as needed.

### Playing Status

The athlete cannot return to activity until examined and released by a health care provider.

# Minimizing Systemic Tissue Damage (Shock)

Injury, illness, or dehydration can cause the body to shift into life-saving mode. The body attempts to preserve life-sustaining blood, water, and oxygen to the brain, heart, lungs, and other vital organs by diverting them from the skin, limbs, and other noncritical tissues. This condition is called shock. If not treated, shock can cause extensive and irreversible tissue damage and even death.

## SAFETY MEASURE

### When Treating for Shock

Do not give fluids to an athlete who is experiencing shock. Doing so can cause vomiting or choking.

# SHOCK

Shock is a condition in which the body diverts blood, water, and oxygen from the skin, limbs, and other noncritical tissues to the brain, heart, lungs, and other vital organs. It is caused by trauma, heat, allergic reactions, severe infection, dehydration, poisoning, low pain tolerance, or bleeding.

## Signs and Symptoms

- Weakness
- Fatigue
- Dizziness
- Nausea
- Thirst
- Anxiety
- Cool and clammy skin
- Pale or grayish skin
- Weak and rapid pulse
- Slow and shallow breathing
- Dilated pupils
- Blank stare
- Confusion
- Possible unresponsiveness
- Sweating
- Shaking or shivering
- Bluish lips and fingernails

## FIRST AID

1. Assess the scene and athlete.
2. Send for emergency medical assistance if you haven't already done so.
3. Position the athlete appropriately depending on their condition (see table 4.1).
4. Monitor breathing and provide CPR if needed.
5. Maintain normal body temperature by covering the athlete as needed.
6. Provide first aid care for bleeding and other injuries.
7. Reassure the athlete.

## Playing Status

The athlete cannot return to activity until examined and released by a health care provider.

## Splinting Unstable Injuries

Bone fractures, joint dislocations and subluxations, and Grades II and III ligament sprains should be stabilized to prevent further tissue damage. Remember that the hallmark of first aid care is to prevent further injury and to do no harm. With this goal in mind, follow these guidelines for applying splints:

1. Do not move the athlete until all unstable injuries are splinted unless the athlete is in danger of further injury, or the athlete requires repositioning for CPR or control of profuse bleeding or shock.

2. Contact emergency medical personnel, and let them splint the following:

   - Large joint dislocations (shoulder, hip, knee, kneecap, elbow, wrist, and ankle)
   - Injuries where bones create an obvious deformity
   - Compound fractures
   - Fractures of the spine, pelvis, hip, thigh, shoulder girdle, upper arm, elbow, kneecap, or shin
   - Displaced rib fractures or displaced clavicle from a severe sternoclavicular (SC) joint sprain (see chapter 12)
   - Any musculoskeletal injuries that result in loss of circulation or nerve damage signified by numbness, blue or grayish skin, cold skin, inability to move fingers or toes of the affected limb, or significant weakness of the affected limb
   - Any musculoskeletal injuries in which the athlete is also experiencing shock

3. Prevent the athlete from moving until emergency medical assistance arrives. If emergency medical assistance will arrive in 20 minutes or less, stabilize the injured limb with your hands. Place one hand above and the other below the injured area, and limit movement while you wait for emergency medical assistance.

4. If the arrival of emergency medical assistance will take longer than 20 minutes, splint the injury in the position in which you found it. However, for spine fractures, simply stabilize the head, prevent the athlete from moving, and wait for emergency medical personnel to arrive.

5. Cover the ends of exposed bones with sterile gauze.

6. Splint with rigid or bulky materials that are well padded. You don't need expensive manufactured splints. Tongue depressors, boards, cardboard, bats, magazines, blankets, and pillows can be used as splints.

7. For fractures or for severe joint sprains, immobilize the bones above and below the joint. For example, if the lower leg is broken just below the knee, immobilize the thigh and lower leg bones. For fractures that occur in the middle of a bone, stabilize the joints above and below the fracture. For instance, if the upper arm bone is broken in the middle, apply a splint and then use a sling to immobilize the elbow and shoulder.

8. Secure the splint with ties or an elastic wrap. Place the ties above and below the injury but not directly over it. Apply light, even pressure with the wrap so as not to press directly on the injury.

9. Periodically check the skin color, temperature, and sensation of the hand and fingers or foot and toes of the splinted limb. Splints that are too tight can compress nerves or arteries. If an athlete complains of numbness, if the skin appears blue or gray or feels cold, or if the nail beds appear blue, then the splint is too tight.

Figures 5.7 through 5.14 show proper splinting techniques for the upper arm, elbow, forearm and wrist, finger, thigh, kneecap, lower leg, and ankle and foot. For a summary of splinting techniques, see the Splinting flowchart in the appendix.

### SAFETY MEASURE

**When Splinting**

- Do not attempt to reposition fractured or dislocated bones. It could sever nerves and arteries as well as cause further damage to the bones, ligaments, cartilage, muscles, and tendons.
- Do not attempt to push exposed bones back under the skin.

# SPLINTING TECHNIQUES

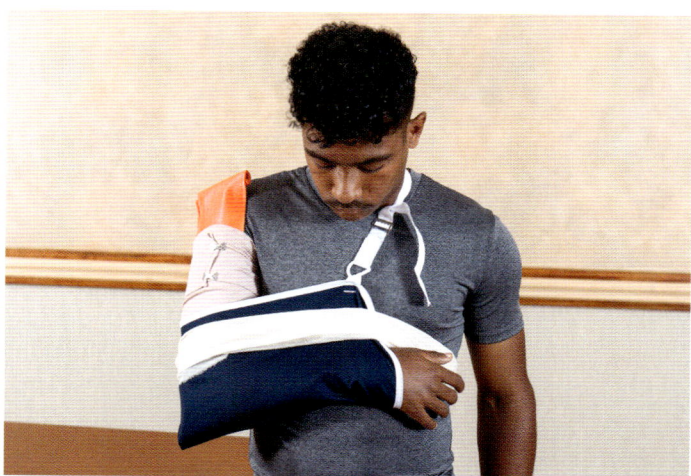

**Figure 5.7**  Proper splint for the upper arm.

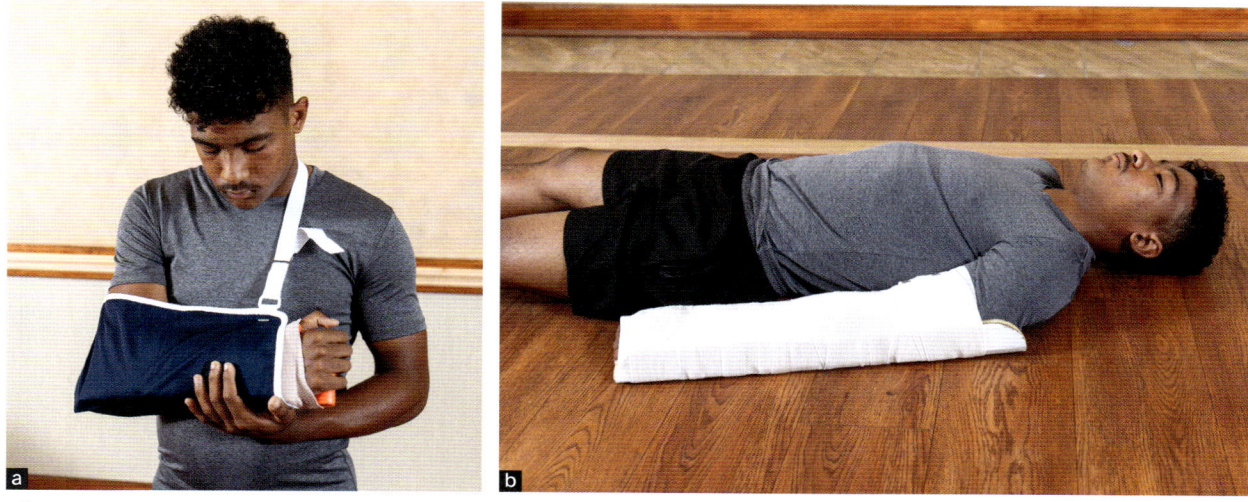

**Figure 5.8**  Proper splints for the elbow (*a, b*).

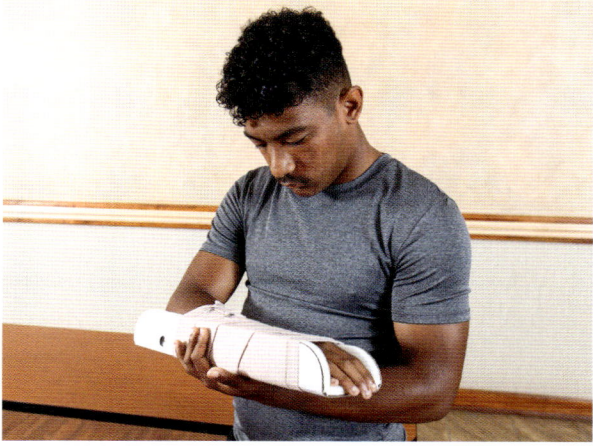

**Figure 5.9**  Proper splint for the forearm and wrist.

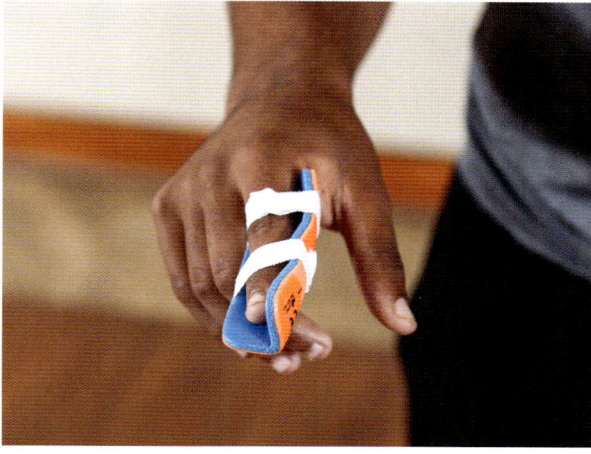

**Figure 5.10**  Proper splint for the finger.

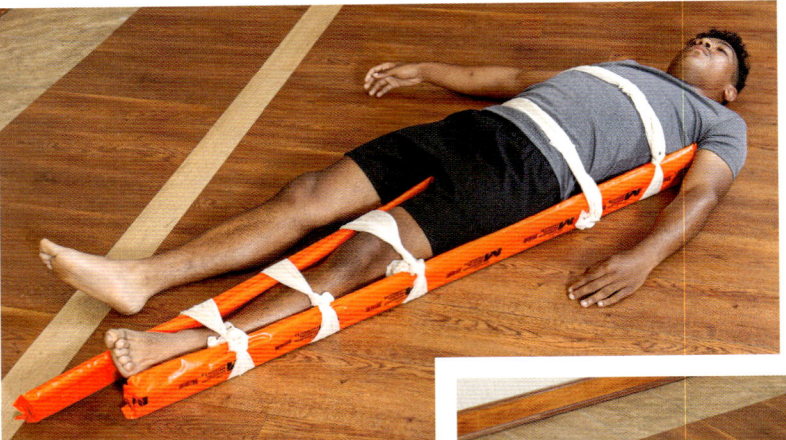

**Figure 5.11** Proper splint for the thigh.

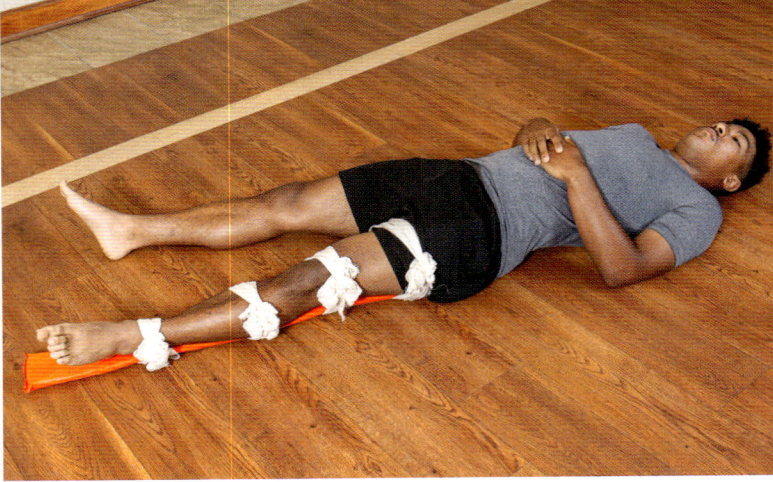

**Figure 5.12** Proper splint for the kneecap.

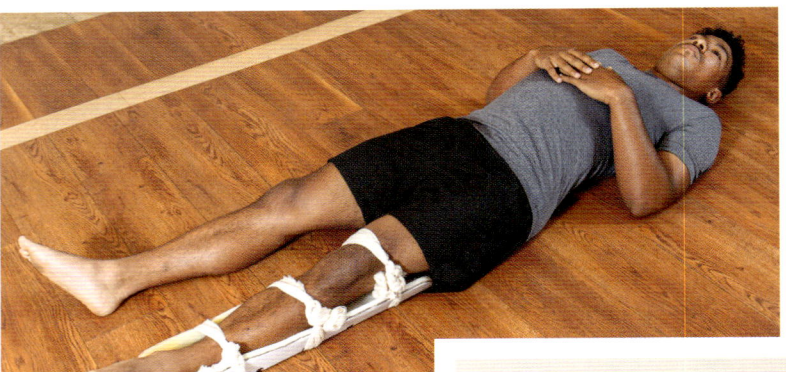

**Figure 5.13** Proper splint for the lower leg.

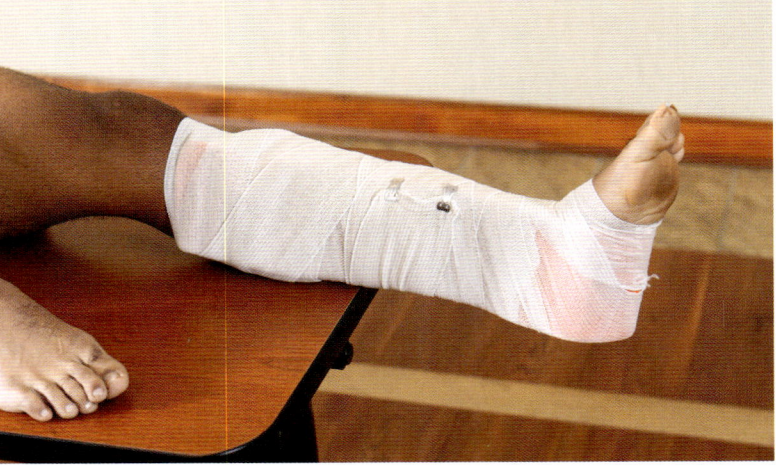

**Figure 5.14** Proper splint for the ankle and foot.

## Controlling Slow, Steady Bleeding

The following section addresses first aid for any slow, steady (capillary) bleeding of superficial wounds. For additional information and first aid procedures for abrasions and superficial lacerations, see the sections titled Face or Scalp Laceration and Eye Abrasion in chapter 14.

# CAPILLARY BLEEDING

Capillary bleeding is slow, steady bleeding from superficial wounds caused by skin abrasion or laceration.

### Signs and Symptoms

- Slow, oozing blood

## FIRST AID

1. Put on gloves and goggles or a mask as needed (if you haven't already done so) to protect yourself against blood-borne pathogens.
2. Apply sterile gauze, then firm, direct pressure over the wound with your hand.
3. Once bleeding stops, do the following:
   a. Gently clean the wound.
   b. Cover the wound with sterile gauze or a bandage.
   c. If you are unable to clean all debris from the wound, or if the wound edges gape open and do not touch (may need stitches), send the athlete to the appropriate health care provider.

### Playing Status

The athlete can return to activity if bleeding stops, and the athlete was not sent to a health care provider. The wound must be covered to protect it as well as to protect other athletes from the possible transmission of blood-borne pathogens. If the athlete is sent to a health care provider, the athlete cannot return to activity until examined and released.

# Minimizing Local Tissue Damage

If part of the body is injured, the body's local tissue reaction can cause damage to the surrounding tissues. For example, in an ankle sprain, the injured ligament bleeds and swells, and the tissues around it do as well. That reaction causes discoloration and swelling all around the ankle joint. Injury or infection to a particular area can cause the following localized tissue reactions:

- Bleeding from the injured blood vessels
- Fluid leakage from damaged tissue cells
- Swelling
- Increase in temperature
- Pain
- Loss of function (inability to use a body part)

Bleeding and fluid leakage from the damaged tissue cells can disrupt blood flow not only to the injured tissues but also to surrounding tissues. This reaction can delay healing. The best way to minimize local tissue damage is to apply the PRICE principle, which is defined as follows:

**P**—*Protection*

**R**—*Rest*

**I**—*Ice*

**C**—*Compression*

**E**—*Elevation*

Applying the PRICE principle reduces the chance of further injury to the area and minimizes swelling to help prevent further damage.

## Protection

Protect the athlete from further injury by preventing the athlete from moving and by keeping other athletes and hazards clear of the athlete.

## Rest

Rest the athlete from any activity that causes pain. If simple movements such as bending, straightening, reaching overhead, or walking are painful, *rest* means immobilizing the injured limb by splinting or preventing weight bearing with the use of crutches. The athlete cannot return to activity until examined and released by a health care provider and is able to play without pain or loss of function (e.g., no limping, no decrease or adjustments in arm movements).

If pain only occurs during strenuous workouts or sport participation, rest the athlete from the painful exercises, drills, and skills, and refer them to the appropriate health care provider.

## Ice

During the first 72 hours following an injury, ice can help minimize pain and control swelling caused by bleeding and fluid loss from the injured tissues. Ice helps control swelling after the initial injury by helping reduce blood flow (bleeding). Compression and elevation (discussed in upcoming sections) are also valuable in helping to reduce initial blood loss. Once the bleeding has stopped, these methods are needed to get rid of the swelling that has already occurred.

Ice can be applied in several ways, such as with an ice bag (see figure 5.15a), ice massage (see figure 5.15b), gel cold pack, ice whirlpool, chemical cold pack, and ice-water bucket. No matter which method is used, athletes typically experience cold, pins and needles, dull aching, and numbness sensations when ice is applied. These sensations are not unusual; they are to be expected. Table 5.2 discusses the types, applications, indications, potential downsides (cons), frequencies, and precautions of each method.

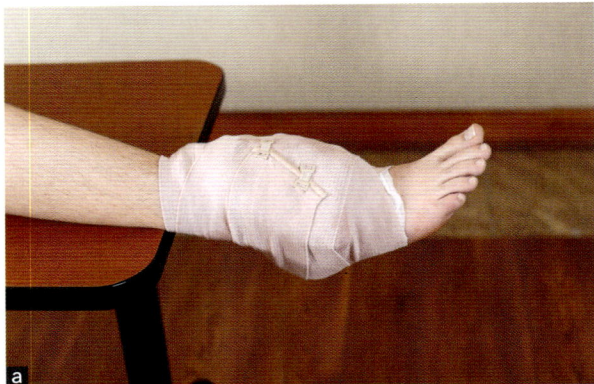

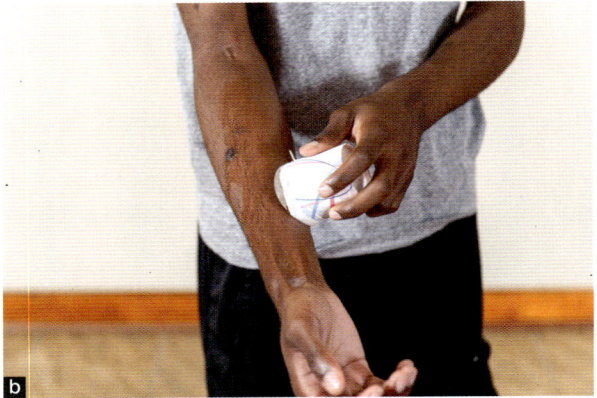

**Figure 5.15** *(a)* Ice bag and *(b)* ice massage.

**Table 5.2**  Types of Ice Application

| Type | Application | Indication | Cons | Frequency | Precautions |
|---|---|---|---|---|---|
| Ice bag | Place crushed ice (conforms the best to the body) in a plastic bag directly over injury. | Large areas, such as the back, shoulder, thigh, upper arm, chest, knee, and ankle | | • 15-20 minutes or until area feels numb<br>• Can reapply every 2 hours as needed for pain and swelling | Do not apply over open wounds or if athlete is allergic to cold. Apply a thin cloth between the skin and the ice bag. |
| Ice massage | Rub ice cube or ice frozen in a paper cup directly over injury. | Small bony areas, such as elbows, wrists, hands, and feet | | • 5-10 minutes or until area feels numb<br>• Can reapply every 2 hours as needed for pain and swelling | Do not apply over open wounds or if athlete is allergic to cold. |
| Gel cold pack | Place cooled pack over injury. | Small areas, depending on size of pack | | • 15-20 minutes or until area feels numb<br>• Can reapply every 2 hours as needed for pain and swelling | Packs have a tendency to freeze the skin, so apply a thin cloth between the skin and the pack. |
| Ice whirlpool | Submerse foot, leg, hand, or arm into icy water. | Limbs | • Typically not well tolerated<br>• Does not allow for concurrent elevation (injured area placed down into whirlpool)<br>• Inconvenient | • 10-15 minutes or until area feels numb<br>• Can repeat every 2 hours as needed for pain and swelling | Do not place athletes with open wounds in a whirlpool; it can increase risk of infection. |
| Chemical cold pack | Place cooled pack over injury. | Small areas, depending on size of pack | • May not remain cold long enough | • 15-20 minutes or until area feels numb<br>• Can reapply every 2 hours as needed for pain and swelling | Chemicals may cause skin burns if pack is punctured. Apply a thin cloth between the skin and the pack for protection. |
| Ice-water bucket | Submerse ankle, foot, wrist, or hand into icy water. | Limbs | • Typically not well tolerated<br>• Does not allow for concurrent elevation (injured area placed down into bucket)<br>• Inconvenient | • 10-15 minutes or until area feels numb<br>• Can repeat every 2 hours as needed for pain and swelling | Do not place limbs with open wounds in a bucket; it can increase risk of infection. |

## Compression

To control initial bleeding of joint or limb tissues, or to reduce residual swelling, apply an elastic wrap to an injured limb, especially the foot, ankle, knee, thigh, hand, forearm, or elbow (see figures 5.18-5.24 on page 75). Follow these steps to apply an effective compression wrap:

1. Start several inches below the injury (farthest from the heart). For example, for the forearm, start the wrap just above the wrist (figure 5.16a).

2. Wrap upward (toward the heart), in an overlapping spiral, starting with even and somewhat snug pressure, then gradually wrapping looser once above the injury (figure 5.16b).

3. Periodically check the skin color, temperature, and sensation of the injured area to make sure that the wrap isn't compressing any nerves or arteries. For example, for a forearm wrap, check the fingers and nail beds for blue or purplish tint and for coldness. Wraps that are too tight can reduce blood flow to the area and cause tissue damage.

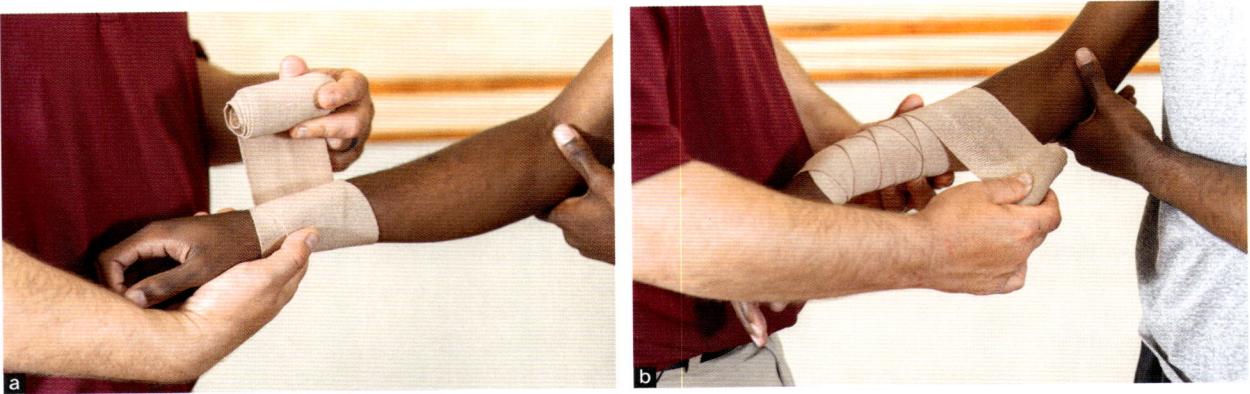

**Figure 5.16**   *(a)* Start the wrap farthest away from the heart, and *(b)* wrap in a spiral fashion with even pressure.

## SAFETY MEASURE

**When Applying Ice**

In some instances, ice can be harmful. Here are some contraindications (reasons) for which ice should not be applied:

- Do not apply ice if the athlete lacks feeling in the area.
- Do not apply ice if the athlete is allergic to cold. Allergic reactions to ice include blisters, red skin, and rashes.
- Do not ice for longer than 20 minutes; doing so can minimize the ability of the ice to restrict blood flow to the area.
- Do not apply a tight compression wrap in combination with ice; doing so may result in nerve damage.
- Do not apply ice directly over an open wound.
- Do not apply ice directly over a superficial nerve, such as the ulnar nerve (see figure 5.17a) at the elbow or the peroneal nerve (see figure 5.17b) on the outside of the knee.

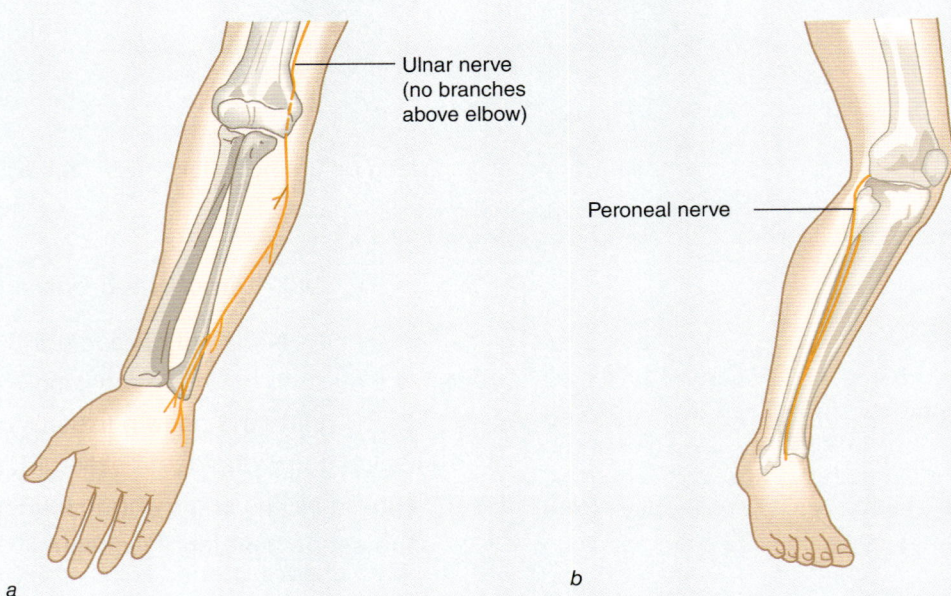

**Figure 5.17**   Do not apply ice directly over the (a) ulnar nerve or (b) peroneal nerve.

# COMPRESSION WRAPS

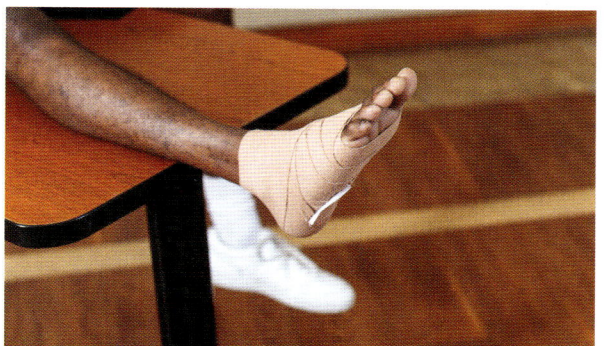

**Figure 5.18**   Foot compression wrap.

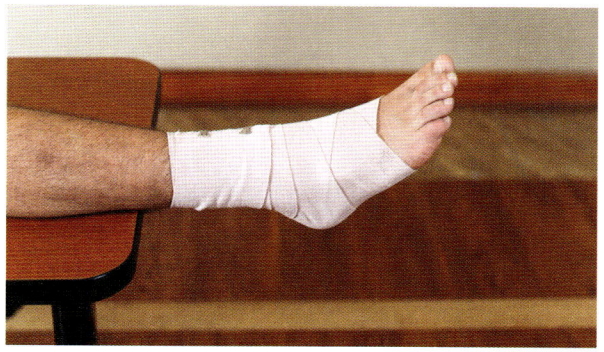

**Figure 5.19**   Ankle compression wrap.

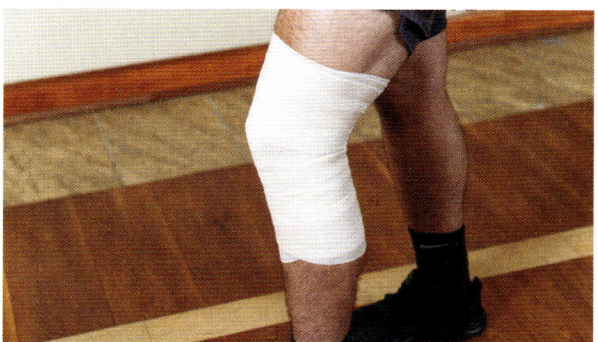

**Figure 5.20**   Knee compression wrap.

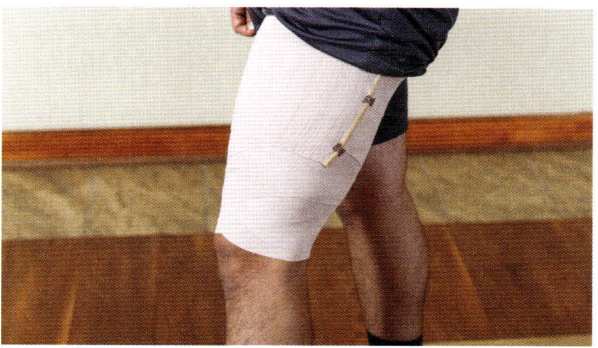

**Figure 5.21**   Thigh compression wrap.

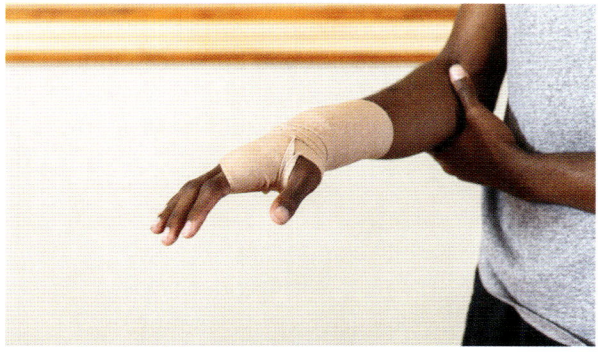

**Figure 5.22**   Hand compression wrap.

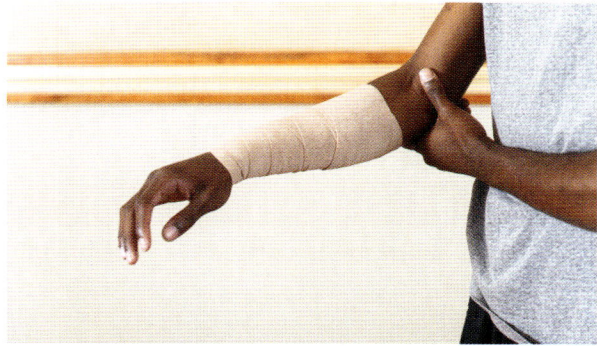

**Figure 5.23**   Forearm compression wrap.

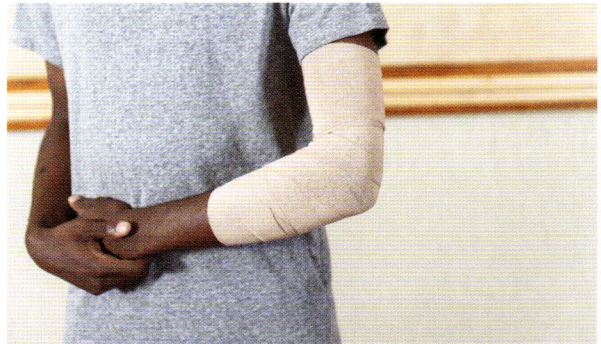

**Figure 5.24**   Elbow compression wrap.

**With Applying Heat**

If swelling from an acute injury is still present, do not apply heat. Heat causes increased blood flow to the area, so it can increase swelling. Heat therapy is generally reserved for warming up chronic muscle strains or tendinitis injuries before exercise or activity. Do not recommend or apply heat unless a medical professional prescribes it.

## Elevation

Used in combination with ice and compression, elevation can also minimize internal tissue bleeding and subsequent swelling (see figure 5.25). Elevate the injured part above the level of the heart as much as possible for the first 72 hours after the injury occurs (longer if swelling persists).

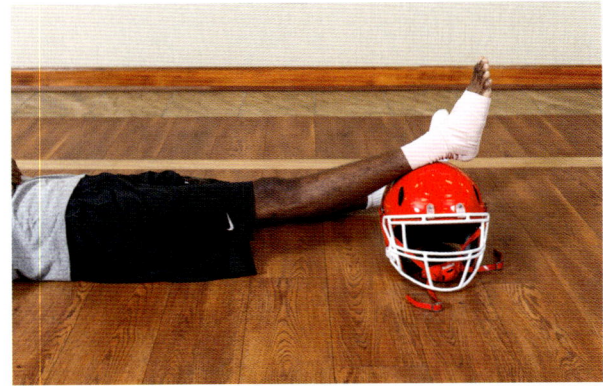

**Figure 5.25**  Elevate the injured part above heart level.

## Chapter 5 Recap

- ❑ What two criteria should be met before performing a physical examination?
- ❑ What is the difference between arterial and venous bleeding?
- ❑ How do you stop profuse bleeding?
- ❑ What are the signs and symptoms of shock?
- ❑ When is it acceptable to splint an unstable injury?
- ❑ How should a splint be applied for fractures or for severe sprains?
- ❑ What are the signs that a splint is applied too tightly?
- ❑ When can an athlete who has a wound that is bleeding slow and steady return to activity?
- ❑ What does PRICE stand for?
- ❑ What are the cons of using ice whirlpools and ice-water buckets?
- ❑ How do you correctly apply a compression wrap on the thigh?
- ❑ What is the technique for effective elevation?

# MOVING INJURED OR SICK ATHLETES

## TECHNIQUES IN THIS CHAPTER

In golf, knowing when to use a particular club for a particular situation is critical to winning. For example, a driver is used for hitting a long ball off the tee; a wedge is used to make a short, arcing shot to the green; and a putter is used for precision shots on the green. This theory also applies in sport first aid. For example, when determining when and how to move an injured or sick athlete, you must carefully select which move to do at which time in order to effectively help (and avoid further harm of) the athlete.

Perhaps the most difficult decisions in giving first aid care are when to move an athlete and when to call for emergency medical assistance. As with all first aid procedures, the basic rule for moving injured or sick athletes is to err on the side of caution. As discussed in chapter 1, your primary role as a coach is to minimize the risk of injury to athletes under your supervision. When an athlete is already injured or ill, this role includes minimizing the risk of further harm by moving.

# Moving Critically Injured Athletes

For a life-threatening or serious injury or illness, keep the athlete still while you call for emergency medical assistance to move the athlete. Critical conditions include the following:

- Breathing difficulty
- Head, neck, or back injury
- Shock
- Profuse bleeding
- Internal injuries
- Unresponsiveness
- Dislocation of a large joint (shoulder, hip, knee, kneecap, elbow, or ankle)
- Compound fracture
- Fracture of the spine, pelvis, hip, thigh, shoulder girdle, upper arm, kneecap, or shin
- Displaced fracture of the ribs or Grade III sternoclavicular joint sprain
- First-time seizure
- Serious eye injury

However, it may be necessary for you to move an athlete in these situations if (a) the athlete is in danger of further harm, or (b) it is necessary to move or reposition the athlete to provide first aid for a life-threatening condition.

## Danger of Further Harm

Following are incidents in which an athlete may need to be moved because of the potential for further harm:

- *Environmental emergencies*—Lightning, tornado, hurricane, fire, downed electrical lines, or flooding
- *Dangerous scene*—Traffic, other runners, cyclists, uncontrolled animals, or insect swarms (particularly in road races)

## Unable to Provide First Aid for Life-Threatening Conditions

Following are occasions in which repositioning an athlete is necessary to provide appropriate first aid:

- Unresponsive athlete lying on stomach or side who needs CPR
- Athlete experiencing heatstroke who must be quickly cooled with water and ice

Techniques for moving a critically injured or sick athlete include the one-person drag, the four- or five-person rescue, and the six-plus-person lift.

---

**SAFETY MEASURE**

**When Moving a Critically Injured, Unresponsive Athlete**

If an unresponsive athlete's injury was caused by a sudden and forceful movement (direct blow), compression, or twisting of the spine, assume that the athlete may have a head or spine injury. Manually stabilize the head, neck, and back, and only reposition the athlete if CPR is required.

# ONE-PERSON DRAG

The one-person drag is used to move an unresponsive athlete from a dangerous environment by yourself. The technique is as follows:

1. Squat down just beyond the athlete's head.
2. Place your hands under the athlete's armpits, and cradle the head with your forearms (see figure 6.1).
3. Partially bend your knees, while maintaining a straight back.
4. Slowly drag the athlete to a safe location.

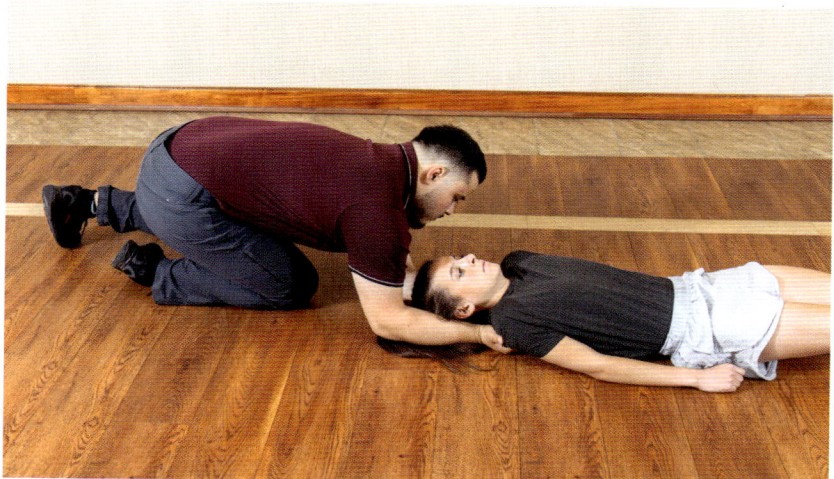

**Figure 6.1**   One-person drag.

# FOUR- OR FIVE-PERSON RESCUE

The four- or five-person rescue is used to turn over a responsive or unresponsive athlete who is lying face down, breathing normally, and must be moved or placed on a spine (back) board. This technique may also be used to roll unresponsive athletes into the recovery position to allow vomit to drain from the mouth. The technique is as follows:

1. A formally trained first aid provider goes to the athlete's head and directs the other rescuers.
2. This individual grasps the head, holding on to both sides of the head and jaw (see figure 6.2a).
3. The lead rescuer commands the other rescuers to position themselves at the shoulders, hips, and legs (see figure 6.2b).
4. A fifth rescuer (if available) places the spine board next to the athlete.
5. The lead rescuer uses the command "Ready" then "Up" to instruct everyone to roll the athlete (facing away from the board, toward the rescuers) as a unit, being sure to keep the head, neck, shoulders, trunk, hips, and legs aligned.
6. The fifth rescuer slides the board next to the athlete's back.
7. The lead rescuer, using the "Ready" and "Down" commands, instructs everyone to slowly roll the athlete onto the board as a unit (figure 6.2c).

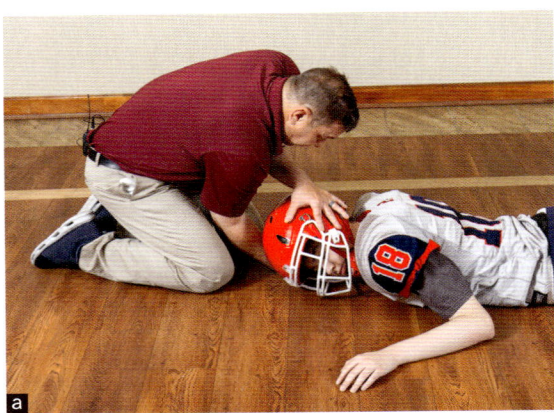
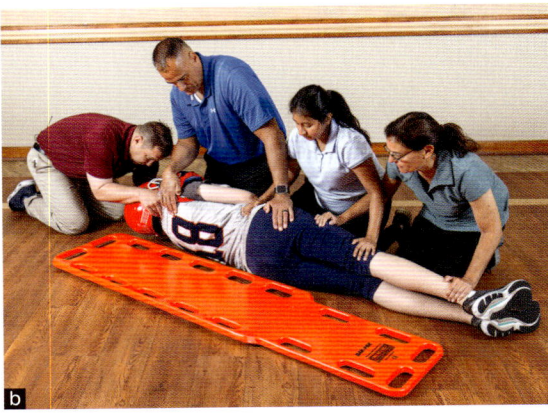
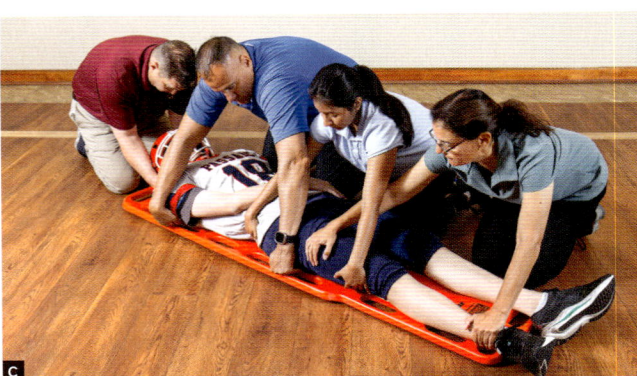

**Figure 6.2** The four-person rescue. *(a)* A trained first aid provider holds the sides of the head and jaw; *(b)* the group rolls the athlete toward the rescuers; and *(c)* the group rolls the athlete onto the board.

# SIX-PLUS-PERSON LIFT

In 2008, a study was performed to test how the six-plus-person lift compared with other methods to minimize spine movement in an injured athlete. It was concluded that the six-plus-person lift was more effective at limited spinal segment movement than other methods (Del Rossi et al. 2008). Using this technique in combination with a scoop stretcher avoids rolling the injured athlete over bulky protective equipment, which could interfere with the transfer process and bring about unwanted spinal column movements.

As described in the report, the six-plus-person lift technique requires one person to immobilize the head and neck and six more individuals (one positioned on each side of the chest, pelvis, and legs) to assist with the lift, as follows (see figure 6.3):

- Rescuer 1 provides cervical spine stabilization.
- Rescuers 2, 3, and 4 are positioned on one side at the shoulders and thorax, hips, and legs, respectively.
- Rescuers 5, 6, and 7 are positioned similarly on the other side.
- Rescuer 8 is at the athlete's feet with the spine board.

On command from rescuer 1, rescuers 2 through 7 lift the athlete approximately 6 inches (15 cm) off the ground, while rescuer 8 slides the spine board beneath the athlete. Rescuers 2 through 7 slowly lower the athlete onto the spine board. Note that this technique is to be performed only under the direction of a health care professional who has been trained in the lift (e.g., athletic trainer, EMT). This information is provided here in cases where coaches may be asked to assist.

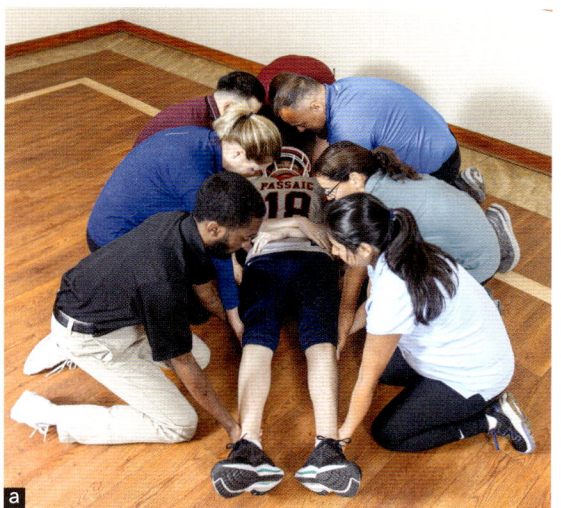 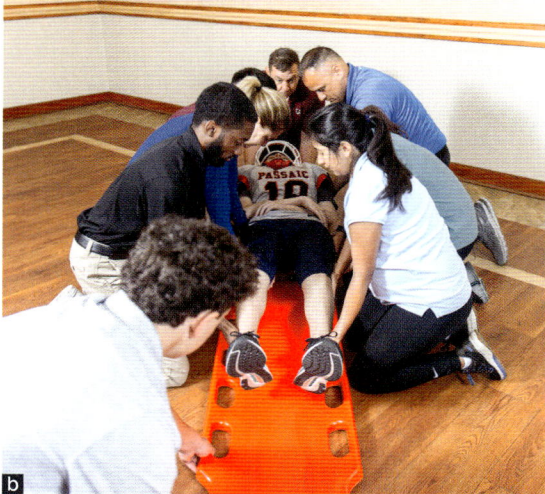

**Figure 6.3**    The six-plus-person lift. *(a)* Three people are positioned on each side of the athlete while one person stabilizes the head; and *(b)* one additional person is positioned at the feet, ready to slide the stretcher under the athlete.

## Moving Noncritically Injured Athletes

A common situation you may face is one in which an athlete has a minor or moderate injury such as a muscle pull or arm contusion. When this type of situation arises, you should use one of several types of assists: the one- or two-person walking assists or the four- or two-handed carrying assists. If you have a history of back or leg problems, or if you are considerably smaller than the athlete, do not attempt the four-handed carrying assist or the two-handed carrying assist.

Athletes who are uncritically injured can be more readily moved, but you must still exercise extreme caution. If necessary, you may move an athlete who is experiencing these conditions:

- Sprain or strain
- Solar plexus spasm
- Contusion
- Facial injury
- Closed and nondisplaced (no gross deformity) fracture of the finger, hand, wrist, forearm, ankle, or foot
- Finger dislocation

---

### SAFETY MEASURE

**When Moving Noncritically Injured Athletes**

Before moving a noncritically injured athlete, you should control profuse bleeding and immobilize or splint all unstable injuries.

---

# ONE-PERSON WALKING ASSIST

The one-person walking assist is used to walk a dazed or slightly injured athlete off the playing area by yourself. The technique is as follows:

1. Instruct the athlete to place an arm around you and hold on to your shoulder.
2. Grasp the athlete around the waist with your free hand.
3. Instruct the athlete to lean on you as needed when walking (see figure 6.4).

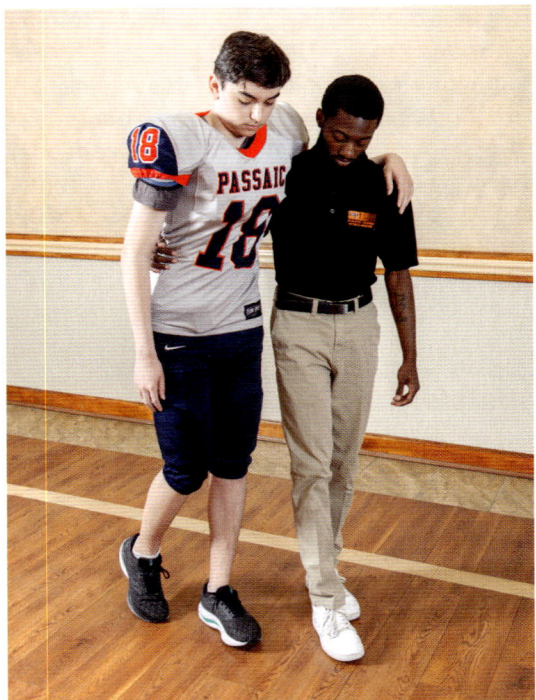

**Figure 6.4**   One-person walking assist.

# TWO-PERSON WALKING ASSIST

The two-person walking assist is used to walk a dazed or slightly injured athlete off the playing area with the help of another person. The technique is as follows:

1. Instruct the assistant to follow your directions so as not to endanger the well-being of the athlete.
2. Stand on opposite sides of the athlete.
3. Place the athlete's arms around you and your assistant, and instruct the athlete to hold on to your shoulders.
4. Hold the athlete around the waist.
5. Slowly walk to the sidelines, supporting the athlete with your arms and shoulders (see figure 6.5).

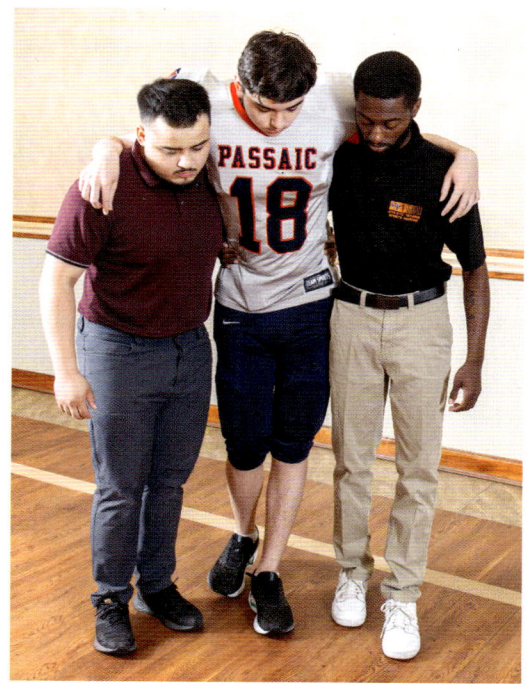

**Figure 6.5**   Two-person walking assist.

# FOUR-HANDED CARRYING ASSIST

The four-handed carrying assist is used to move (with the help of another person) a responsive and coherent athlete who is not able to walk but is able to assist you in moving them; the athlete holds on to the rescuers' shoulders. This carry is especially useful if it is too far or too difficult for the athlete to move with the two-person walking assist. The technique is as follows:

1. Instruct the assistant to follow your directions so as not to endanger the well-being of the athlete.
2. Stand behind the athlete, and face each other.
3. Grasp your right forearm with your left hand, and instruct the assistant to do the same.
4. Then grasp each other's left forearm with your right hand (see figure 6.6a).
5. Instruct the athlete to sit on your and your assistant's arms and to place their arms around your shoulders (figure 6.6b).

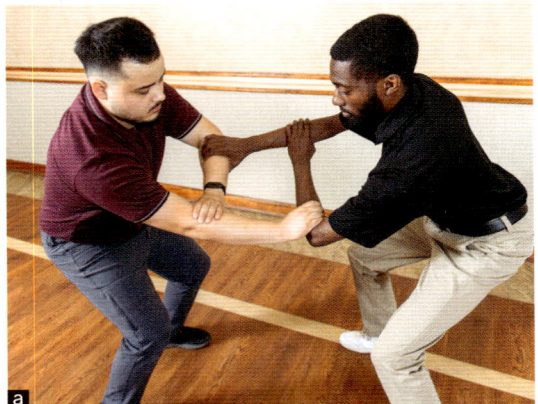

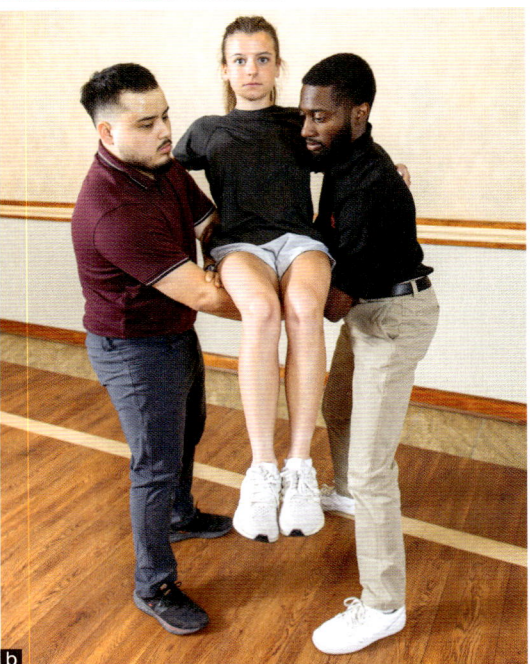

**Figure 6.6**  Four-handed carrying assist.

# TWO-HANDED CARRYING ASSIST

The two-handed carrying assist is used to move (with the help of another person) a slightly dazed athlete who is not able to walk and needs additional support from the rescuers. The technique is as follows:

1. Instruct the assistant to follow your directions so as not to endanger the well-being of the athlete.
2. Stand behind the injured athlete, facing your partner.
3. Grasp each other's forearms nearest the athlete (see figure 6.7a).
4. Instruct the athlete to sit on your and your assistant's arms and to put their arms around your shoulders.
5. Support the athlete's back with your free arms (see figure 6.7b).
6. Slowly lift the athlete by straightening your legs.

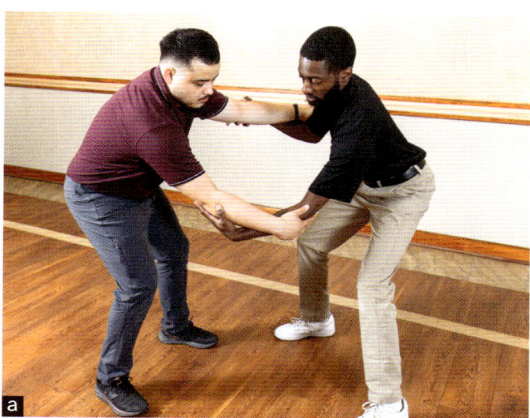

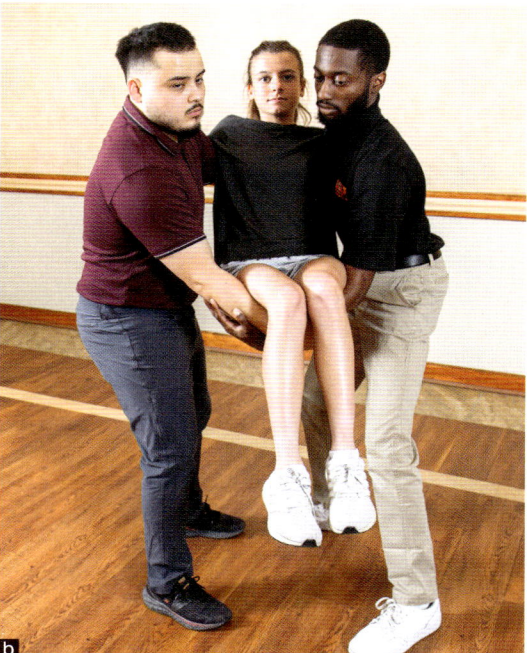

**Figure 6.7**   Two-handed carrying assist.

For a summary of guidelines for moving athletes who are ill or injured, see the Moving an Injured or Sick Athlete flowchart in the appendix. In addition, table 6.1 matches the type of transfer to use in each injury situation.

**Table 6.1** Type of Transfer to Use in Each Injury Situation

| Situation | Number of rescuers | Type of transfer |
|---|---|---|
| Moving an unresponsive athlete in danger of further injury if left in present location | 1 | 1-person drag |
| Moving an unresponsive athlete in order to assess or to provide life-saving first aid | 4 or more | 4- or 5-person rescue |
| Moving an athlete to limit spine movement and provide life-saving first aid | 6+ | 6+-person lift |
| Walking a dazed or slightly injured athlete off the playing area | 1 2 | 1-person walking assist 2-person walking assist |
| Moving a responsive and coherent athlete who is not able to walk but is able to assist in moving themselves | 2 | 4-handed carrying assist |
| Moving a slightly dazed athlete who is not able to walk and needs additional support from rescuers | 2 | 2-handed carrying assist |

## Chapter 6 Recap

❑ What injuries are considered so serious that an athlete should not be moved until emergency medical assistance arrives?

❑ Under what two conditions may you move a critically injured athlete?

❑ If you suspect an injured athlete has head, neck, or back injuries but the athlete must be moved, what guidelines must you follow?

❑ What two methods can be used to move a critically injured athlete?

❑ What two things must be done before moving an athlete with a closed, nondisplaced fracture, or a strain or sprain?

❑ What four methods can be used to move a noncritically injured athlete?

# PART II
# INJURY-SPECIFIC AID

# RESPIRATORY EMERGENCIES AND ILLNESSES

## IN THIS CHAPTER, YOU WILL LEARN THE FOLLOWING:

- How to identify the signs and symptoms of anaphylactic shock, asthma, collapsed lung, throat contusion, pneumonia or bronchitis, solar plexus spasm, and hyperventilation
- What first aid care to provide for each of these conditions
- How to prevent allergies, asthma, bronchitis, and pneumonia from progressing into life-threatening emergencies

## INJURIES AND CONDITIONS IN THIS CHAPTER

Consider this basketball scenario: You're down by one point, six seconds remain on the clock, you have no time-outs left, and your team is inbounding the ball from under your opponent's basket. You have precious little time to waste; if your team doesn't have a set play to handle the full-court press and get the ball to your best scorer, the clock will run out and your team will lose the game. This level of urgency also applies to situations involving respiratory emergencies and illnesses. If you don't have a set plan for handling them, time could run out for the affected athlete.

Various types of respiratory emergencies and illnesses can occur during activity. While choking and respiratory distress were covered in chapter 4, allergic reactions, contact injuries, sickness, and anxiety can also cause breathing problems in athletes. (See the appendix for an overview of first aid protocol for Anaphylactic Shock and Asthma.) This chapter will help you prepare to deal with these additional respiratory emergencies and illnesses.

# ANAPHYLACTIC SHOCK

Anaphylactic shock is a severe allergic reaction where the body responds with swelling of the throat, lips, or tongue. Causes include exposure to an allergy-causing substance, such as insect venom, pollen, molds, latex, certain foods (e.g., peanuts, seafood), and drugs.

## Signs and Symptoms

- Chest tightness
- Difficulty breathing
- Dizziness
- Anxiety
- Wheezing or gasping
- Swollen tongue, lips, throat, or eyes
- Bluish or grayish skin, fingernails, or lips
- Hives
- Abdominal cramping
- Nausea or vomiting
- Mental confusion

## FIRST AID

If the athlete is prone to allergic reaction, they may carry emergency medication known as epinephrine, which is administered through an auto-injector. If so, do the following:

1. Send for emergency medical assistance.
2. If the athlete is responsive, assist them in administering the medication. If they are unresponsive, you may administer it if permitted by state law. However, do so only if you have been trained to use it properly and the medication has been prescribed by the appropriate health care provider.
3. Administer the medication by following the directions on the auto-injector.
4. Put the athlete in a position for easiest breathing. If they are unresponsive but breathing, put them in the recovery position unless head or neck injury is suspected.
5. Monitor breathing, and be prepared to give CPR if needed.
6. If symptoms continue after the first dose of epinephrine has been given, and if EMS personnel are not expected to arrive within 5 to 10 minutes, administer a second dose of epinephrine, using a second auto-injector (National Safety Council 2016).

If the athlete does not have antidotal medicine, do the following:

1. Send for emergency medical assistance.
2. Put the athlete in a position for easiest breathing. If the athlete is unresponsive but breathing, put them in the recovery position.
3. Monitor breathing, and be prepared to give CPR if needed.

## Playing Status

If CPR or emergency medical personnel were necessary, the athlete cannot return to activity until examined and released by a health care provider. Athletes who recover without needing life-saving first aid or emergency medical assistance must also be examined and released by the appropriate health care provider.

## PREVENTION

- Reminders for athletes to bring auto-injectors to practice and competition
- Inspection of playing area for insect nests
- Allergy action card on file (see figure 7.4 at the end of the chapter)

# COLLAPSED LUNG

A collapsed lung occurs when air escapes from the lung into the space between the lung and chest wall (pleural space) and pressure prevents the lung from expanding normally (see figure 7.1). Causes include a direct blow to the ribs that compresses or tears the lung, spontaneous collapse of a lung that is not caused by an injury, or puncture by a sharp object (e.g., broken rib, arrow, javelin). Signs and symptoms include chest pain, bruise or open wound to the chest, sucking sound coming from a chest wound, or increased breathing rate. If you suspect a collapsed lung, send for emergency medical assistance, cover any wound with nonporous material or gauze, and provide first aid and CPR if needed.

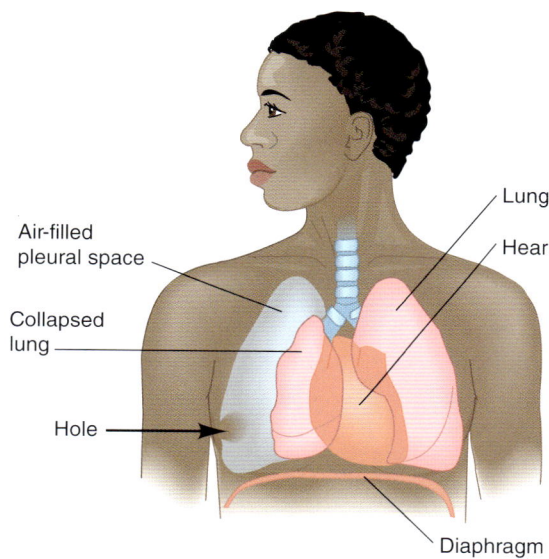

**Figure 7.1**   Collapsed lung.

# ASTHMA

Asthma is a condition in which the air passages in the lungs constrict and interfere with normal breathing (see figure 7.2). Causes include allergic reaction to dust, molds, pet dander, or other substances; exposure to cold environments such as ice-skating rinks; exposure to smoke or other inhaled substances; or adverse response to strenuous exercise.

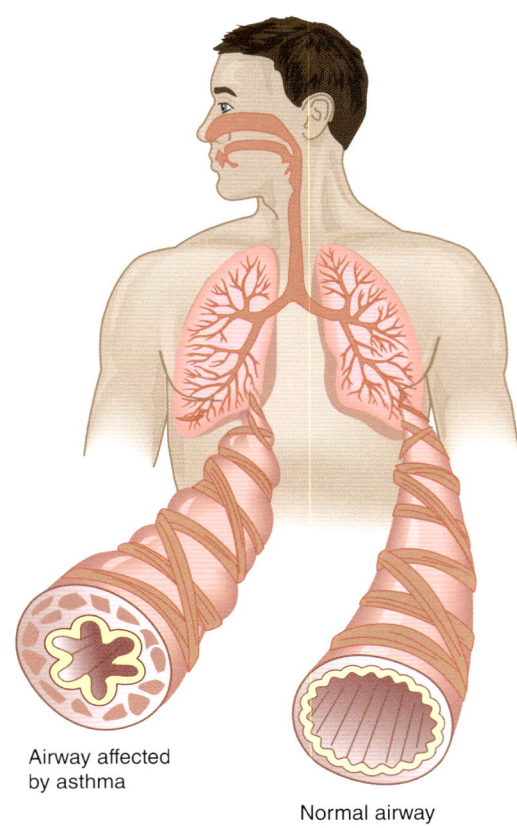

Airway affected
by asthma

Normal airway

**Figure 7.2**   Constricted breathing passages caused by asthma.

## Signs and Symptoms

- Tightness in the chest
- Shortness of breath or trouble exhaling
- Wheezing when breathing
- Increased respiratory and pulse rate
- Blue or gray fingernails, lips, or skin
- Noticeably frightened appearance

## FIRST AID

If the athlete has an asthma inhaler or other medication, do the following:

1. Send someone to retrieve the inhaler or other medication, and have the athlete use it as prescribed by their medical provider.
2. If necessary, assist the athlete in using the inhaler or taking the medication. Do so only if you are permitted by state law, it has been prescribed by a physician, and you have been trained to use it properly.
3. Monitor breathing, and provide CPR if needed. If CPR is needed, send for emergency medical assistance.
4. Monitor the athlete's skin and lip color. If either changes to blue or gray, send for emergency medical assistance.
5. If the athlete shows no signs of improvement a few minutes after administering the medication, call for emergency medical assistance.
6. If the athlete recovers within a few minutes, call the athlete's parent or guardian to take them to their health care provider.

If asthma medicine is not available or the athlete does not respond to it, do the following:

1. Send for emergency medical assistance.
2. Monitor breathing, and provide CPR if needed.
3. Place the athlete in a seated or semireclining position (45°).
4. Monitor and treat for shock as needed.
5. Reassure the athlete.

### Playing Status

If CPR or emergency medical personnel were necessary, the athlete cannot return to activity until examined and released by a health care provider. Athletes who recover without needing life-saving first aid or emergency medical assistance must also be examined and released by the appropriate health care provider.

## PREVENTION

- Monitor all athletes with asthma, and refer to the appropriate health care provider if necessary
- Adequate rest during play
- Asthma action card on file (see figure 7.4 at the end of the chapter)
- Reminders for athletes to bring medication to all practices and games

# HYPERVENTILATION

Hyperventilation is rapid breathing that creates a deficit of carbon dioxide in the bloodstream, upsetting the oxygen–carbon dioxide balance. Causes include an overexcited athlete who breathes too rapidly or a blow to the solar plexus.

## Signs and Symptoms

- Shortness of breath
- Numbness or tingling around the mouth or in the arms, hands, and feet
- Dizziness or light-headedness
- Weakness
- Chest pain
- Panic or anxious feeling
- Rapid breathing
- Increasing pulse rate
- Fainting (could result if athlete doesn't recover)

## FIRST AID

1. Speaking calmly, reassure the athlete.
2. Place the athlete in a seated or semireclining position (45°).
3. Encourage the athlete to breathe naturally.
4. Instruct the athlete to inhale slowly, hold one second, then exhale slowly through pursed lips.
5. If the athlete does not recover within a few minutes, send for emergency medical assistance, monitor breathing, and provide CPR as needed. Also, check for other injuries that could be contributing to the problem.

## Playing Status

The athlete can return to activity once breathing returns to normal. Monitor the athlete for signs of recurrence. If CPR or emergency medical personnel were necessary, the athlete cannot return to activity until examined and released by a health care provider.

## PREVENTION

- Calming strategies for anxiety
- Correct breathing technique instruction

# SOLAR PLEXUS SPASM

The solar plexus is a nervous system structure located just below the rib cage (see figure 7.3). In this condition, the diaphragm, which causes the lungs to expand with air, experiences spasms because of signals sent to it from the solar plexus. It is commonly described as having the wind knocked out of you. Causes include a direct blow to the area below the rib cage.

## Signs and Symptoms

- Inability to inhale
- Labored breathing or hyperventilation
- Pain just below the sternum (breastbone)
- Possible temporary unresponsiveness

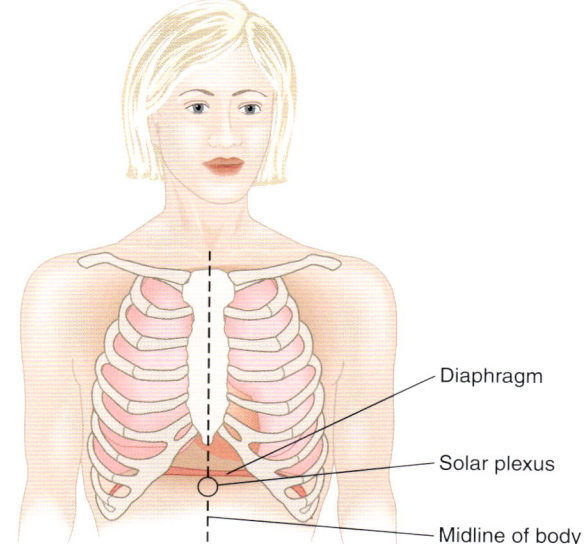

**Figure 7.3**   Location of the solar plexus; when hit hard, it can temporarily paralyze the diaphragm.

## FIRST AID

1. Speaking calmly, reassure the athlete.
2. Loosen constrictive clothing.
3. Encourage the athlete to relax.
4. Instruct the athlete to take a short breath followed by a slow, deep breath.
5. Monitor breathing, and provide CPR if needed. If CPR is needed, send for medical assistance.
6. If the athlete still has pain or does not recover in a few minutes, call for emergency medical assistance.
7. Monitor for signs and symptoms of other internal injuries; watch for shock, vomiting, or coughing up blood.

## Playing Status

The athlete can return to activity if breathing returns to normal and no deformity or pain exists in the affected area. If CPR or emergency medical personnel were necessary, the athlete cannot return to activity until examined and released by a health care provider.

## PREVENTION

- Use of appropriate protective padding in contact sports such as football and ice hockey

# PNEUMONIA OR BRONCHITIS

Pneumonia and bronchitis are inflammation, or viral or microorganism infection, of the lungs that can cause fluid or mucus to collect in the lungs. Causes include infection by a microorganism; irritation by an inhaled substance such as dust or chemicals; or chronic respiratory problems such as asthma. Signs and symptoms include shortness of breath or labored breathing, chest tightness or pain, fatigue, fever or chills, muscle aches, coughing (possibly with mucus), or wheezing during expiration. If the athlete is experiencing fever, cough, and congestion, refer them to the appropriate health care provider. The athlete cannot return to activity until examined and released by a health care provider.

# THROAT CONTUSION

A throat contusion is a bruise that may interfere with air passing to the lungs. Causes include a direct blow to the throat area (e.g., getting hit with a baseball, softball, or hockey puck, or getting hit by an elbow in basketball or football). Signs and symptoms include pain in the throat; pain and difficulty swallowing; shortness of breath or gasping for air; increased breathing rate; swelling, discoloration, or deformity in the throat area; crunchy or grating sound when touched; voice changes (may vary from hoarseness to total inability to speak); wheezing or coughing; or coughing up or spitting blood. In the event of a throat contusion, follow basic first aid. In severe situations, monitor the athlete's airway, breathing, and circulation, and perform CPR or use an AED if needed. For prevention, enforce wearing throat protectors in sports where rules mandate that they are worn.

## Chapter 7 Recap

❑ How do you manage anaphylactic shock?

❑ What should you do if an athlete has a collapsed lung caused by a hole in the chest?

❑ What can an athlete and coach do to help prevent and manage asthma attacks?

❑ What should you do if an athlete is hyperventilating?

❑ When should an athlete with bronchitis or pneumonia not participate in activity?

❑ What signs indicate when a throat contusion is potentially life-threatening?

## ■ FIGURE 7.4

# STUDENT ASTHMA/ALLERGY ACTION CARD

## SCHOOL OR CHILD CARE
## ASTHMA/ALLERGY ACTION PLAN

Asthma and Allergy Foundation of America

aafa.org

*Attach or insert ID photo*

Name:

DOB:

Parent/Guardian #1 Name:

Address:

Phone (home):                    Phone (work):

Parent/Guardian #2 Name:

Address:

Phone (home):                    Phone (work):

Emergency Contact #1 Name:

Relationship:                    Phone:

Emergency Contact #2 Name:

Relationship:                    Phone:

Physician Child Sees for Asthma/Allergies:

Phone:

Other Physician:

Phone:

### Daily Asthma Management Plan

Identify the Things That Start an Asthma/Allergy Episode
(Check each that applies to the child)

☐ Animals          ☐ Bee/insect sting   ☐ Respiratory infections

☐ Dust mites       ☐ Exercise           ☐ Change in temperature

☐ Pollens          ☐ Smoke              ☐ Strong odors

☐ Food:            ☐ Chalk dust/dust    ☐ Molds

☐ Other:

### Control of Child Care Environment
(List any environmental control measures, pre-medications, and/or dietary restrictions that the child needs to prevent an asthma/allergy episode.)

### Daily Medication Plan for Asthma/Allergy          (Emergency medicines listed on next page)

| MEDICINE | HOW MUCH | HOW OFTEN/WHEN TO USE |
|---|---|---|
|  |  |  |
|  |  |  |
|  |  |  |

### Outside Activity and Field Trips          (List medications that must accompany the child when participating in outside activities and/or field trips)

| MEDICINE | HOW MUCH | HOW OFTEN/WHEN TO USE |
|---|---|---|
|  |  |  |
|  |  |  |
|  |  |  |

*(continued)*

# ■ FIGURE 7.4
## STUDENT ASTHMA/ALLERGY ACTION CARD (CONTINUED)

### Asthma Emergency Plan

Emergency action is necessary when the child has symptoms such as:

#### Steps to Take During an Asthma Episode:

1. Assess symptoms.
2. Give emergency asthma medications as listed below.

| MEDICINE | HOW MUCH | HOW OFTEN/WHEN TO USE |
|---|---|---|
|  |  |  |
|  |  |  |
|  |  |  |

3. Check symptoms after _____ minutes. Give medicine again if symptoms have not improved.
4. Allow child to stay in school or at child care setting if:
5. Contact parent/guardian.
6. Seek emergency medical care if the child has any of the following:

Signs and symptoms of severe asthma episode

- No improvement after treatment
- Hard time breathing with:
  - Chest and neck pulled in with breathing
  - Child hunched over
  - Nose opens wide
- Trouble walking or talking
- Stops playing and cannot start activity again
- Lips, gums, or fingernails turn gray or white on darker skin or blue on lighter skin

### Allergy Emergency Plan

Child is allergic to:

#### Steps to Take During an Allergy Episode:

1. Assess symptoms.
2. Give medicine as listed below.

| MEDICINE | HOW MUCH | HOW OFTEN/WHEN TO USE |
|---|---|---|
|  |  |  |
|  |  |  |
|  |  |  |

3. Check symptoms after _____ minutes.
4. Allow child to stay in school or at child care setting if:
5. Contact parent/guardian.
6. Seek emergency medical care if the child has any of the following:

Symptoms of severe allergic reaction

- Mouth/Throat: itching and swelling of lips, tongue, mouth, throat; throat tightness; hoarseness; cough
- Skin: hives; itchy rash; swelling
- Gut: nausea; abdominal cramps; vomiting; diarrhea
- Lung*: shortness of breath; coughing; wheezing
- Heart: pulse is hard to detect; "passing out"

*If child has asthma, asthma symptoms may also need to be treated.

Severe symptoms need immediate treatment and medical help

### Special Instructions

☐ I have instructed _____ in the proper way to use their medications. It is my professional opinion that they should carry their asthma/allergy medicines by themselves.

☐ It is my professional opinion that _____ should not carry their asthma/allergy medicines by themselves.

| | | |
|---|---|---|
| Physician Signature | Date | Parent/Guardian Signature | Date | Child Care Provider's Signature | Date |

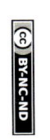

# HEAD, SPINE, AND NERVE INJURIES

Consider this scenario: You are a coach on a high school wrestling team. While a 14-year-old athlete on your team was horsing around with a teammate, the teammate picked him up and dropped him on his head. He was instantly unable to move his arms and legs. You have just arrived at his side, and you observe that he is extremely scared. Do you know your emergency action plan for a spinal injury? It is vital that you take the initial and follow-up steps on your plan; your athlete's life depends on it.

Sport participation is among the leading causes of catastrophic cervical spine injury (CSI) in the United States. Sport-related spine injury can be devastating and have long-lasting effects on athletes and their families. Providing the best care for patients with spine injuries is essential for optimizing postinjury outcomes. To ensure safe on-field management, we must develop and practice the plan to be used in the event of a serious head, neck, and possible spinal cord injury. (Courson et al. 2020).

## Head Injuries

When most people hear the term *head injuries*, they immediately think of concussions. While concussions are not the only type of head injury, they are the most common in sports. The Centers for Disease Control estimates that 5 to 10 percent of athletes will experience a concussion in any given sport season (Theye and Mueller 2004). According to the University of Pittsburgh Medical Center (UPMC), about 1.7 to 3 million sport- and recreation-related concussions occur annually; 300,000 of them are from playing football. In addition, about 50 percent of concussions go unreported (UPMC n.d.). An athlete can sustain a concussion by hitting their head on the ground or by their head hitting an object when they fall. A concussion can also occur during a player-to-player collision or when an athlete is hit in the head by an object such as a ball or bat. However, a concussion doesn't necessarily result from an obvious event such as a blow to the head; it can also result from a hit to the body that creates enough force to jolt the brain inside the skull. For this reason, it is important to always refer an athlete with signs and symptoms of a concussion to a health care professional, and remember the adage, *When in doubt, sit them out.* In other words, if you suspect a concussion has occurred, get your athlete some help rather than having them immediately return to play.

Signs of concussion vary from person to person. Athletes with concussions may experience one or more signs and symptoms. People used to use phrases such as *getting dinged* or *getting your bell rung* to describe so-called mild concussions. Today, concussions are more accurately recognized as brain injuries. Therefore, regardless of the number or severity of signs and symptoms, concussions must be taken seriously.

Concussion signs and symptoms fall within four categories: physical, cognitive, emotional, and sleep-related. Some of the signs of concussion include difficulty remembering (amnesia), behavioral changes, slowed reaction time, and loss of consciousness. Physical symptoms may include any combination of symptoms. While a headache is the one most commonly reported, lack of a headache does not rule out a concussion. Common cognitive symptoms include feel-

ing as if in a mental fog, feeling mentally slow, and trouble concentrating or staying focused, especially for an extended period. In addition, the athlete may have a delay in memory recall. Emotional symptoms can include irritability or sadness, or simply feeling more emotional than usual. Vision problems, feeling off-balance, and dizziness may also occur. An athlete may experience problems falling asleep or staying asleep as well as feel drowsy during the day. See table 8.1 for a list of concussion signs and symptoms.

Blows to the head don't just stun the brain; they can disrupt blood flow, cause electrical and chemical imbalances, and possibly injure brain cells. These changes are microscopic; more often than not, they are not visible on brain magnetic resonance imaging (MRI) scans or skull X-rays. However, they can be detected by neurological tests that assess an athlete's cognition, memory, multitasking ability, emotional functioning, and motor (movement) skills such as balance and reaction time. In addition, headaches, dizziness, nausea, and other signs and symptoms from minor hits are actually manifestations of microtrauma to the brain.

Approximately 20 percent of high school athletes playing contact sports will get a concussion in a given year (UPSM n.d.), but researchers have found that concussions are not limited to athletes in contact sports. Injury records across various sports have revealed that even noncontact sports show surprising rates of concussion. In one of the most comprehensive studies of sport-related injuries, the rate of concussion was analyzed across 20 high school sports from 2013 through 2018 (Kerr et al. 2019). Not surprisingly, the highest occurrence was found in football, which

**Table 8.1**  Concussion Signs and Symptoms

| Physical | Cognitive | Emotional | Sleep-related |
|---|---|---|---|
| Headache<br>Nausea<br>Vomiting<br>Balance problems<br>Dizziness<br>Fatigue<br>Vision problems<br>Sensitivity to light<br>Sensitivity to noise<br>Numbness or tingling<br>Feeling dazed or stunned | Feeling as if in a fog<br>Feeling mentally slow<br>Difficulty concentrating<br>Difficulty remembering<br>Confusion about recent events | Irritability<br>Sadness<br>Nervousness<br>More emotional than usual | Drowsiness<br>Hyposomnia<br>Hypersomnia<br>Poor sleep quality<br>Trouble falling asleep |

accounted for 43.8 percent of reported concussions. Other sports with significant concussion rates included girls' soccer (11.1%), wrestling (5.9%), boys' soccer (5.5%), and cheerleading (4.6%) (Kerr et al. 2019).

After experiencing a concussion, an athlete's return to activity depends on their recovery period. Although Marar and colleagues (2012) found that 40 percent of concussion symptoms (headache, dizziness, difficulty with concentration, confusion, light sensitivity, and nausea) in U.S. high school athletes resolved in 3 days or fewer, symptom resolution does not necessarily mean that the athlete is fully recovered. Recovery can take a week, a month, 6 months, or even longer. The duration does not depend on how the athlete feels or looks. An athlete who looks and feels fine can still have less obvious symptoms, such as impaired cognition, memory, multitasking ability, emotional functioning, and motor (movement) skills, which indicate that the brain has not fully recovered. If an athlete returns to participation before the brain is fully recovered, the brain can experience further injury when the athlete is mildly bumped or jarred too soon. This injury is known as second-impact syndrome, which can cause excessive and life-threatening brain swelling.

Repeated blows (even minor ones) can lead to cumulative brain damage and long-term impairment of brain function. Reports of long-term health issues in athletes after repeated blows to the head have brought concussions to the forefront of the media and to the attention of lawmakers. However, for all the hype and all of the well-intentioned laws, the challenges are still the same. How do you recognize the signs of a brain injury? More important, what can be done to prevent it? Information on causes, signs and symptoms, and first aid strategies to minimize long-term or permanent brain injury follows.

Brain injuries are commonly caused by one of two mechanisms:

1. A direct blow to the head can injure the skull or brain tissue on the side of contact (see figure 8.1a) or the brain tissue on the side opposite the contact (see figure 8.1b). For example, if an athlete's head hits a goalpost, they could experience a skull fracture at the site of contact, or they could experience a brain injury on the same side or opposite side.

2. A sudden, forceful jarring or whipping of the head, without contact, can also injure the brain. This movement can cause the brain to bounce back and forth in the skull. Some people have theorized that these jarring types of injuries may also cause fractures at the base of the skull.

Keep in mind that no minimum threshold or amount of force is required to cause a concussion. In addition, what seems like a minor blow to the head may not cause concussion symptoms in one person but could cause one or more symptoms of varying severity in another person. Like fingerprints, no two concussions are alike. The Head Injury flowchart in the appendix summarizes how to assess and provide first aid care for injuries to the head.

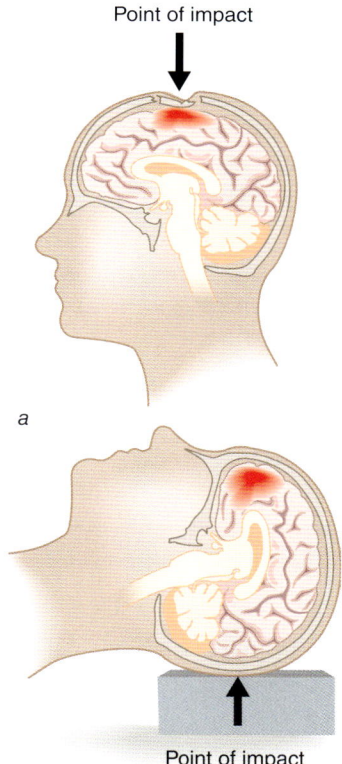

Point of impact

*a*

Point of impact

*b*

**Figure 8.1**   *(a)* Skull injury from a direct blow; *(b)* brain injury on the opposite side of a direct blow.

### SAFETY MEASURE

**No Ammonia Caps or Smelling Salts**
Using ammonia caps or smelling salts to rouse an athlete may cause them to suddenly jerk their head and worsen the condition.

# HEAD INJURY

A head injury may be caused by a direct blow to the head or by a sudden, forceful jarring or whipping of the head.

**Signs and Symptoms**

See table 8.1 for signs and symptoms of a head injury. If any signs or symptoms occur (including symptoms not listed), always refer to a health care provider.

## FIRST AID

If an athlete exhibits any of the signs or symptoms of a head injury (see table 8.1), remove them from participation immediately. Symptoms such as headache or ringing in the ears may be the early signs of a more serious injury. In these cases, do the following:

1. Continue to monitor the athlete, and send for emergency medical assistance if signs and symptoms worsen.
2. Refer the athlete to the athletic trainer (if available) for further evaluation.
3. If no athletic trainer is available, immediately contact the parent or guardian and have them take the athlete to the appropriate health care provider.
4. Give the parent or guardian a checklist of signs and symptoms to monitor (see table 8.1).

For injuries with more severe signs, such as confusion, unsteadiness, vomiting, convulsions, increasing headache, increasing irritability, unusual behavior, arm or leg weakness or numbness, neck pain with a decrease in motion, pupil abnormalities, or unconsciousness, do the following:

1. Immediately send for emergency medical assistance and your athletic trainer (if available).
2. Stabilize the head and neck until emergency medical personnel take over. If an athlete is wearing a helmet, leave it on when stabilizing the head and neck. Avoid jarring the head or neck unnecessarily, especially if the athlete is also wearing shoulder pads.
3. Monitor the athlete for breathing difficulty, and perform CPR if necessary.
4. Control any profuse bleeding, but avoid applying excess pressure over a head wound.
5. Monitor the athlete for shock, and treat as needed.
6. Immobilize any fractures or unstable injuries as long as you do not jostle the athlete, which may worsen their condition.

## Playing Status

When can an athlete return to a sport after a brain injury? This is a decision that must be made by a health care provider trained in the management of concussion. Check your state law or the regulations of the National Federation of State High School Associations (NFHS) to ensure that your athletes are receiving mandated care and supervision. The NFHS, as well as most state concussion laws, prohibit athletes from returning to activity until examined and released by a health care provider. All states now have laws in place that address sport-related concussion. Some may have additional or more strict guidelines for return to play. Additionally, many state concussion laws require school athletic programs to have a concussion policy that must be followed, so be sure you know what your athletic program's concussion policy states, and be sure to follow it.

### PREVENTION

- Concussion education for coaches, athletes, and parents or guardians (see figure 8.2)
- Athlete preseason physical exam and baseline cognitive brain testing, if affordable
- Neck strengthening exercises in preseason and in-season conditioning programs
- For sports requiring helmets, regular checks for damage and replacement if necessary, proper fit, and instruction for securing helmets
- Reminder not to use the top of the helmet as the point of contact when tackling or checking another player or lowering the head just before contacting another athlete
- Training and spotting at all times for gymnastics and cheerleading
- Encouragement for athletes to report signs of brain injury in teammates

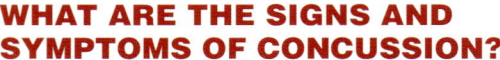

# CONCUSSION FACT SHEET FOR PARENTS

## WHAT IS A CONCUSSION?

A concussion is a type of traumatic brain injury. Concussions are caused by a bump or blow to the head. Even a "ding," "getting your bell rung," or what seems to be a mild bump or blow to the head can be serious.

You can't see a concussion. Signs and symptoms of concussion can show up right after the injury or may not appear or be noticed until days or weeks after the injury. If your child reports any symptoms of concussion, or if you notice the symptoms yourself, seek medical attention right away.

## WHAT ARE THE SIGNS AND SYMPTOMS OF CONCUSSION?

If your child has experienced a bump or blow to the head during a game or practice, look for any of the following signs of a concussion:

### SYMPTOMS REPORTED BY ATHLETE:

- Headache or "pressure" in head
- Nausea or vomiting
- Balance problems or dizziness
- Double or blurry vision
- Sensitivity to light
- Sensitivity to noise
- Feeling sluggish, hazy, foggy, or groggy
- Concentration or memory problems
- Confusion
- Just not "feeling right" or is "feeling down"

### SIGNS OBSERVED BY PARENTS/GUARDIANS:

- Appears dazed or stunned
- Is confused about assignment or position
- Forgets an instruction
- Is unsure of game, score, or opponent
- Moves clumsily
- Answers questions slowly
- Loses consciousness (even briefly)
- Shows mood, behavior, or personality changes

[ INSERT YOUR LOGO ]

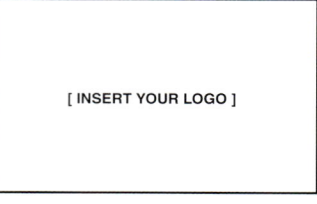

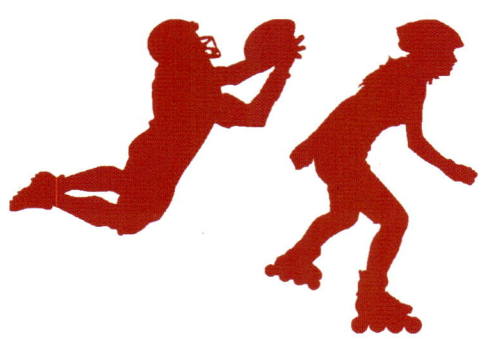

**Figure 8.2** CDC HEADS UP concussion fact sheet for parents.

Content Source: CDC's Heads Up Program. Created through a grant to the CDC Foundation from the National Operating Committee on Standards for Athletic Equipment (NOCSAE).

# Spine Injuries

A blow to the back, a swing of a club, or any sudden and forceful move can injure the spine or nerves. As discussed in chapter 3, the spine is a column of bones (vertebrae) that protect the spinal cord. The bones are held together by ligaments and muscles, and nerves branch out from between bones in the spinal column (see figure 3.6). Cartilage discs located between the vertebrae help absorb shock between the bones.

A direct blow, forceful twisting motion, compression, or forceful stretching beyond normal range of motion to any portion of the spine can cause a variety of spine injuries, including sprains, strains, contusions, fractures, and ruptured discs. Sprains, strains, and contusions are the most common sport-related back injuries. More severe spine and neck injuries, such as ruptured discs and vertebral fractures, are less common. According to Collins, Robison, and Burus (2022), cheerleading has the highest occurrence of all neck injuries (4.8%), followed by wrestling (2.9%) and football (1.5%). Injuries to the spinal cord, nerves, and cartilage can cause numbness; in more severe injuries, they can cause temporary or permanent loss of function (paralysis) in certain body parts.

As a coach, it is not important to know the type of back or spine injury an athlete has experienced. Your first aid care will be dictated by the signs and symptoms described here. Always suspect a serious head or spine injury in an unconscious athlete. Never move the athlete during the evaluation unless you are unable to check for breathing or you need to move the athlete away from a dangerous area.

## SAFETY MEASURE

### When an Athlete Is Wearing a Helmet and Shoulder Pads

If you suspect a serious spine injury, you should check for signs of circulation (breathing, coughing, or movement) and stabilize the head, neck, and spine; however, leave the helmet and pads on.

# SUSPECTED SPINE INJURY

Causes of a spine injury include a direct blow to, compression of, or torsion (twisting) of the spine. Signs and symptoms of a possible spine injury include pain over or near the spine; numbness or tingling in the extremities; responsiveness (if unresponsive or not fully alert, assume a head or neck injury); inadequate breathing; profuse bleeding; blood or fluid leaking from the mouth, nose, or ears; spine deformity; and paralysis.

If any signs or symptoms are present, assume the athlete has a spine injury and administer the appropriate first aid. Send for emergency medical assistance, and check for breathing without moving the athlete; if CPR is required, have someone hold the head still while you perform CPR. If the athlete is breathing, stabilize the head and neck until emergency medical personnel take over. (Leave an athlete's helmet on when stabilizing the head.) Avoid jarring the head or neck unnecessarily, especially if the athlete is also wearing shoulder pads. If the athlete's breathing is normal, continue to monitor breathing; perform CPR if necessary. Control any profuse bleeding, but avoid applying excess pressure over a head wound. Monitor and treat for shock if necessary. Let emergency medical personnel stabilize any other possible fractures or unstable injuries.

Playing status of an athlete with this injury should be determined only by the health care provider treating the athlete. For prevention of neck injuries, incorporate neck strengthening exercises into your preseason and in-season conditioning program. Ensure use of heads-up tackling technique in football, and always use spotters for gymnastics and cheerleading events.

## Nerve Injuries

Athletes can sometimes experience a pinched, stretched, or bruised nerve. This type of injury can occur close to the spinal column or near a joint where a nerve is located (e.g., the nerve along the inside of the elbow, often called the funny bone). In this chapter, the discussion of nerve injuries is limited to one that occurs near the cervical spine, called a burner or stinger. It is a common nerve injury for athletes, especially those in contact sports.

# BURNER OR STINGER

A burner or stinger occurs when a group of nerves (brachial plexus) coming out of the neck and running to the shoulder are overstretched. This overstretching is caused when the head is flexed (tilted forward) or extended (tilted back) and forced quickly to one side and tilted down (see figure 8.3).

## Signs and Symptoms

- Tingling or burning in the neck, shoulder, or arm
- Electrical shock sensation in the neck or shoulder
- Arm feeling dead or heavy
- Arm or hand numbness on one side (Ask the athlete to name the finger that you are touching.)
- Arm or hand weakness on one side (Have the athlete squeeze your fingers with each hand; any significant difference in the strength of the injured arm compared to the uninjured arm means that the nerve has been stretched and possibly injured.)

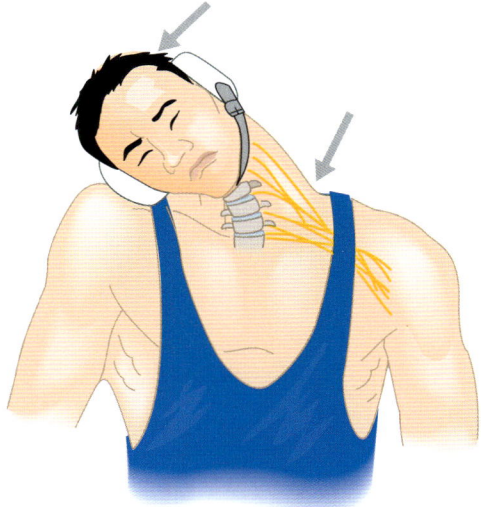

**Figure 8.3**   Mechanism of a burner or stinger injury.

## FIRST AID

If sensation and strength do not return within 5 minutes, or if tenderness or deformity of the spine exist, do the following:

1. Call your athletic trainer (if you have one), or send for emergency medical assistance.
2. Stabilize the head and spine.
3. Monitor breathing, and provide CPR if needed.
4. Monitor and treat for shock as needed.
5. Stabilize any other unstable injuries.
6. If the sensation and strength return within a few minutes, call the athlete's parent or guardian and have them take the athlete to the appropriate health care provider.

## Playing Status

Athletes exhibiting signs and symptoms of a nerve injury cannot return to activity until examined and released by a health care provider. Medical supervision is especially important with burners because they can become a recurring problem and lead to long-term nerve damage.

## PREVENTION

- Neck strengthening exercises in preseason and in-season conditioning programs
- Prevention of helmets used as a point of contact when tackling or checking
- Neck rolls recommended for all football players with prior neck injuries
- No diving into water with a depth of less than 6 feet (2 m)
- Spotters for gymnasts or cheerleaders practicing skills or routines

## Chapter 8 Recap

❑ What kind of injury should you look for if an injury is the result of a direct blow, sudden or forceful movement to the head, spinal compression, or spinal torsion?

❑ Why do you need to evaluate these injuries quickly and treat them properly?

❑ What are some signs and symptoms of a head injury?

❑ When should you refer the athlete with a suspected head injury to a health care provider?

❑ What are some signs and symptoms of a spine injury?

❑ When is it acceptable for an athlete with a burner or stinger to return to activity?

❑ What can be done to help prevent neck burners or stingers?

# INTERNAL ORGAN INJURIES

## IN THIS CHAPTER, YOU WILL LEARN THE FOLLOWING:

- How to recognize when an athlete has an internal injury, such as a ruptured spleen, bruised kidney, or testicular trauma
- How to discern whether an athlete is in an early or an advanced (and life-threatening) stage of an internal organ injury
- How to care for the injured athlete while waiting for emergency medical assistance
- What to monitor if an athlete is exhibiting minor signs of an internal injury
- What information to give the parent or guardian of an athlete who has incurred an internal organ injury

## INJURIES AND TECHNIQUES IN THIS CHAPTER

The body is often subjected to tremendous forces in sport. With pitches careening off a batter's flanks at 90 miles per hour (145 km/h), and the shoulder pads of 230-pound (104 kg) linebackers slamming into a quarterback's numbers, it's a wonder that delicate internal organs aren't injured more often. Fortunately, the body has built-in armor—the ribs and pelvis—to help deflect some of the blows to its organs. In the rare instances when one of an athlete's internal organs is injured, prompt recognition and emergency medical care are critical. These injuries may initially appear minor, but they can quickly progress into life-threatening conditions. Therefore, it is essential that medical personnel handle internal organ injuries. The most common internal injuries in sports are ruptured spleen, bruised kidney, and testicular trauma. (Collapsed lung is also considered an internal injury; it is included in chapter 7 as a respiratory emergency.) You can help minimize complications of these injuries by learning how to

1. recognize the signs and symptoms of spleen, kidney, and testicular injuries;

2. monitor the injured athlete until medical help arrives; and

3. educate the athlete and parent or guardian about the signs and symptoms of internal injuries.

A serious internal injury often takes a few hours to appear. Therefore, it is essential that an injured athlete be monitored in case their condition worsens. You should inform the athlete's parent or guardian about the injury, and provide them with information on signs and symptoms that the athlete's condition has become life-threatening. You may give them copies of the first aid protocols for the injury. Internal injury protocols are summarized in the Spleen Injury, Bruised Kidney, and Testicular Trauma flowcharts in the appendix.

## SAFETY MEASURE

### With Suspected Internal Injuries

- Do not give an athlete with suspected internal injuries food or water. If any of the digestive organs are injured, food or fluid intake can leak out into the abdominal cavity, increasing the risk of infection. If an internal injury requires surgery, food or fluid intake can increase the likelihood of vomiting and potential aspiration while under general anesthesia.

- Do not allow an athlete with possible internal injuries to leave a game or practice without being monitored by a responsible adult.

- If an athlete experiences an apparently minor blow in the area of an internal organ, inform both the athlete and the parent or guardian of the signs and symptoms of a serious internal injury before you allow the athlete to go home.

# RUPTURED SPLEEN

The spleen is an organ that acts as a reservoir of red blood cells. A ruptured spleen is a life-threatening contusion injury to the spleen that is caused by a direct blow to the left side of the body, under the stomach and lower ribs (see figure 9.1). The blow injures the spleen tissue, which can cause internal bleeding. Early signs and symptoms of a spleen injury include pain, tenderness, or an abrasion or bruise in the upper left abdominal area. Later, more advanced signs and symptoms may include pain in the left shoulder or neck, feeling faint or dizzy, rapid pulse, vomiting, rigid abdominal muscles, low blood pressure, or shortness of breath.

If you suspect a spleen injury, it is crucial that you call for medical assistance as soon as possible while you monitor breathing, vital signs, and for shock until help arrives. If more advanced signs and symptoms are not present but pain continues for more than 15 minutes, have the parent or guardian transport the athlete to a hospital emergency room (or call for medical assistance if they are not available). Before an athlete returns to play, they should be evaluated by appropriate medical personnel and obtain proper medical clearance. To help prevent a spleen injury, athletes should wear protective padding when playing. Those diagnosed with mononucleosis should not participate in sports until cleared by their health care provider; mononucleosis can cause the spleen to enlarge, making it easier to rupture.

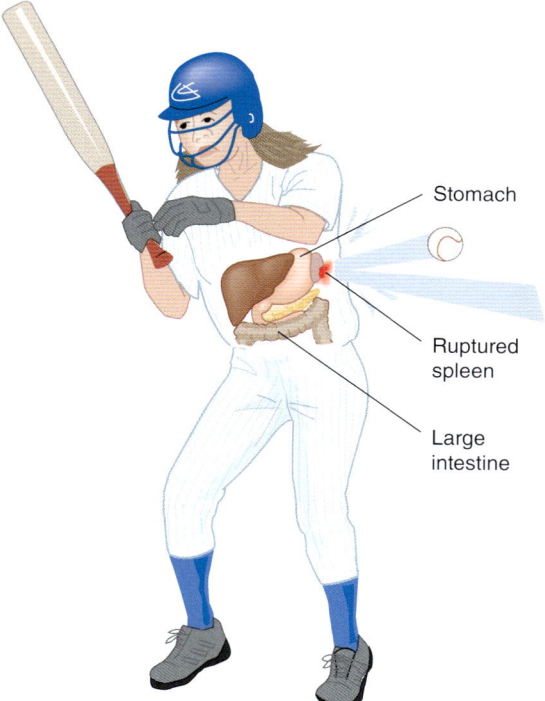

Stomach

Ruptured spleen

Large intestine

**Figure 9.1**   Location of a spleen injury.

# BRUISED KIDNEY

A bruised kidney (kidney contusion) is caused by a direct blow to either side of the mid back. Signs and symptoms of early-stage kidney contusion include pain at the site of the blow (see figure 9.2), a bruise or abrasion, and tenderness over the injured area. More advanced signs and symptoms may include pain that moves to the low back, outside thighs, or front pelvic area; feeling faint, dizziness, abdominal swelling, increased heart rate, frequent burning urination, cloudy or bloody urine, vomiting, rigid back muscles over the injury site, skin that is cool to the touch, or pale skin.

If you suspect a kidney injury, it is crucial that you call for medical assistance as soon as possible while you monitor breathing, vital signs, and for shock until help arrives. If more advanced signs and symptoms are not present but minor symptoms continue for more than 15 minutes, have a parent or guardian transport the athlete to a hospital emergency room (or call for medical assistance if they are not available). Before an athlete returns to play after a suspected or confirmed kidney injury, they should be evaluated by an appropriate medical provider and obtain proper medical clearance. To help prevent kidney injuries, athletes in contact sports should wear protective padding.

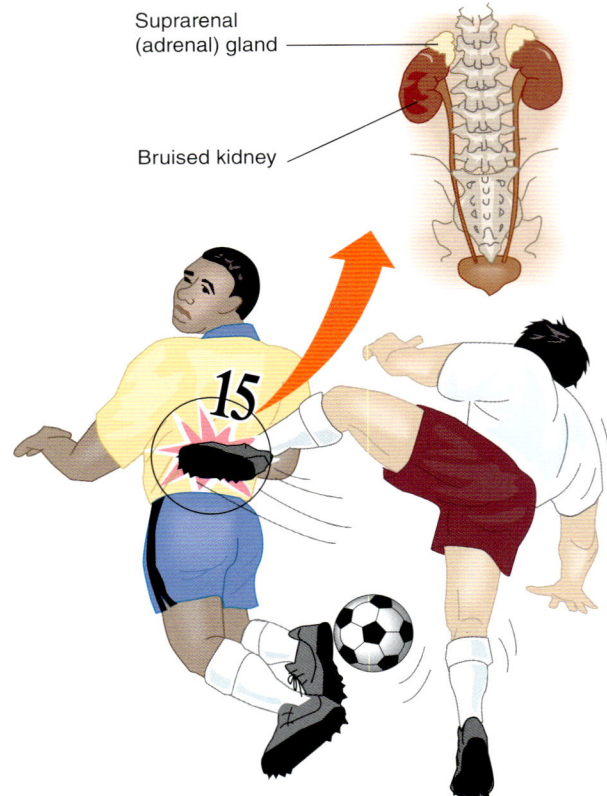

Suprarenal (adrenal) gland

Bruised kidney

**Figure 9.2**   Location of a kidney injury.

# TESTICULAR TRAUMA

Testicular trauma is caused by a direct blow to the groin area, which may cause contusion or other injuries. In severe injuries, the testicles can rupture or the testicular cord can be twisted (cutting off blood flow to the testicles, which can lead to sterility).

## Signs and Symptoms

- Pain
- Nausea
- Swelling, discoloration, and deformity
- Spasm of testicles
- Retraction of testicles
- Bloody or cloudy urine
- Vomiting

## FIRST AID

1. Assist the athlete into a comfortable position.
2. Encourage the athlete to take slow, deep breaths.
3. Apply ice to the area for 15 minutes.
4. Send the athlete to the appropriate health care provider if the pain does not stop after 20 minutes; if the testicles retract; if the athlete has bloody or cloudy urine; or if the testicles exhibit swelling, discoloration, or tenderness more than an hour after the injury occurred (Koester 2000).
5. If the athlete recovers within a few minutes, or if the testicles exhibit swelling, discoloration, or tenderness more than an hour after the injury occurred (Koester 2000), notify the athlete's parent or guardian. Explain to the athlete and parent or guardian how to identify signs and symptoms of a more severe injury (bloody or cloudy urine; retracting of testicles; or swelling, discoloration, or tenderness of testicles).

## Playing Status

The athlete cannot return to activity until the pain subsides or until examined and released by a health care provider.

## PREVENTION

- Wearing athletic supporters and protective cups in contact sports

## Chapter 9 Recap

❑ What are mild symptoms and signs of a ruptured spleen?

❑ Why should an athlete with a possible internal organ injury not be given food or fluid?

❑ What are the advanced symptoms and signs of a potentially life-threatening kidney injury?

❑ What are the signs and symptoms of a serious testicular injury?

# SUDDEN ILLNESSES

## IN THIS CHAPTER, YOU WILL LEARN THE FOLLOWING:

- How to recognize when an athlete is experiencing a diabetic emergency and how to provide first aid care if one occurs
- How to recognize the signs and symptoms of grand mal and petit mal seizures
- How to recognize adverse reactions to drugs and supplements
- How to prevent fainting and provide first aid care for it
- How to recognize the signs and symptoms of airborne diseases (influenza or COVID-19)
- How to recognize the signs and symptoms of gastroenteritis
- How to prevent airborne diseases and gastroenteritis from spreading among your athletes

## INJURIES AND CONDITIONS IN THIS CHAPTER

A botched dismount, wild pitch, dropped baton, or net serve can suddenly change the course of a competition. Likewise, an acute illness, such as a new diabetes diagnosis, can suddenly change the athlete's ability to perform.

An immediate onset of illness can happen to anyone. Too often, athletes continue to play while sick, and they attempt to hide their illness from their coach. As a coach, you should ask your athletes to be alert to, and to report, common illnesses such as the flu. It is also essential that you know about athletes' medical conditions, such as diabetes and epilepsy, and know how to respond to them in an emergency. This chapter will help you to recognize and provide first aid care for a diabetic emergency, a seizure, a drug overdose or reaction, an adverse supplement reaction, fainting, influenza and COVID-19, and gastroenteritis.

## Diabetes

Diabetes is a condition that affects the body's ability to properly produce and regulate insulin. Produced in the pancreas, insulin is a hormone that controls the uptake of sugar (glucose) by body tissues. Glucose is the primary energy source for tissues, especially the brain and kidneys. Without proper insulin levels, the tissues can receive either too much glucose (hyperglycemia) or not enough glucose (hypoglycemia). In type 1 diabetes, which often begins in childhood, the body does not produce insulin. Type 2 diabetes, which is more common, prevents the body from properly using insulin. Type 2 diabetes is becoming increasingly prevalent among children, teens, and young adults.

People with serious diabetic problems may need to take insulin injections or use an insulin pump, which delivers insulin in small amounts through a small tube inserted just under the skin. People with type 2 diabetes often take insulin pills. Because exercise and diet can affect the amount of insulin the body needs, athletes with diabetes should be closely monitored for signs of diabetic illness. An athlete who is having problems regulating diabetes is prone to either an insulin reaction or ketoacidosis. Diabetic ketoacidosis is a serious complication of diabetes when the body does not produce

enough insulin and the blood then becomes acidic as a result of the body breaking down fat too quickly (see page 118), both of which can become life-threatening.

The National Athletic Trainers' Association (NATA; Jimenez et al. 2007) recommend that athletes with type 1 diabetes undergo a medical evaluation before they start an exercise program or participate in sports in order to do the following:

- Determine whether any disease or complication may occur or be aggravated by playing a sport.
- Develop a proper plan for safe exercise and sport participation.

The NATA position statement on the management of athletes with type 1 diabetes (Jimenez et al. 2007) recommends that each athlete with diabetes have a diabetes care plan to follow while undertaking any activity in sports. The plan should include the following:

- Blood glucose monitoring, including information about the monitoring frequency and the figures that contraindicate a sport.
- Insulin therapy, including type of insulin and dose, and strategies for adjusting and correcting it according to the type of activity planned. (Athletes may either inject their insulin or use a pump device that administers their insulin.)
- Recommendations for recognizing and treating hypoglycemia, including instructions on the use of glucagon (to include in the athlete's go bag with diabetic supplies and prescriptions).
- Contact details of parents or guardians and other emergency contacts, including their health care provider.
- Identification, such as a medical alert bracelet, that indicates their condition.

This section explains appropriate first aid measures for these diabetes-related conditions. The Hypoglycemia in an Athlete With Diabetes and Hyperglycemia flowcharts in the appendix summarize first aid protocols for these conditions.

# HYPOGLYCEMIA IN AN ATHLETE WITH DIABETES

Hypoglycemia is a condition in which an athlete's blood sugar (glucose) level drops below its normal level. Although each athlete's precise target level may vary, generally, when the blood glucose level has fallen below 70 milligrams per deciliter, you need to take action to raise it to its target level. Hypoglycemia is caused by high insulin levels, which may result from medications taken to control blood glucose levels. Therefore, hypoglycemia is also called an insulin reaction or insulin shock.

## Signs and Symptoms

### Mild to Moderate

- Hunger
- Irritability
- Slight weakness
- Dilated pupils
- Trembling
- Sweating
- Strong, rapid pulse

### Severe

- Confusion
- Convulsions
- Unresponsiveness

## FIRST AID

According to the American Diabetes Association (ADA) (2023), when treating an athlete with hypoglycemia, you should take the following steps:

### Mild to Moderate

1. Remove the athlete from all activity.
2. Have the athlete test their blood glucose level. If it measures below 70 milligrams per deciliter (mg/dL), go to step 3; if it's above 70 mg/dL, see Hyperglycemia.
3. Follow the 15-15 rule: Give the athlete 15 grams of carbohydrate to raise blood glucose, and check it after 15 minutes. If it is still below 70 mg/dL, provide another serving. Many people tend to want to eat as much as they can until they feel better, which can actually cause blood glucose levels to shoot way up. Using the stepwise approach of the 15-15 rule can help prevent high blood glucose levels. One serving may be in any of the following forms:
   - Glucose tablets (see instructions on the package)

*(continued)*

**Hypoglycemia in an Athlete With Diabetes** *(continued)*

- Gel tube (see instructions on the package)
- Juice that contains at least 15 grams of carbohydrate (check label for amount)
- 1 tablespoon of sugar or honey
- Hard candies, such as jelly beans (check label for amount)

4. If the athlete does not recover, or if signs progress to severe, send for emergency medical assistance.
5. Monitor breathing, and provide CPR if needed.
6. Inform the athlete's parent or guardian. Make a note about any episodes of hypoglycemia, and have the athlete and their parent or guardian consult with their diabetic health care team for guidance on how to avoid hypoglycemia in the future.

### Severe

1. To prepare for a possible reaction, make sure the athlete always brings their emergency medication and supplies, including glucagon, to practices and competitions.
2. In cases of severe hypoglycemia, the athlete will show obvious signs and symptoms and will not be able to continue with physical activity. If they are able, please have them test their blood sugar. If they are not able to test their blood sugar, please assume a severe low and go to step 3.
3. Administer glucagon. Glucagon is used to treat someone with diabetes when their blood glucose is too low to treat using the 15-15 rule. They may be unresponsive or may be unable to swallow. Glucagon is available by prescription; it is either administered by injection, or it is puffed into the nostril. Injectable glucagon products are available in two ways: a kit with powder that must be mixed with sterile water, and a premixed solution that is ready to use. For each of your athletes with diabetes, you need to know how to administer their glucagon to treat severe hypoglycemia.
4. Send for emergency medical assistance.
5. Place an unresponsive athlete in the recovery position.
6. Monitor breathing, and provide CPR if needed.

### Playing Status

For athletes with mild to moderate hypoglycemia, consult with the athlete's health care provider for a plan. The athlete may be able to return to activity as soon as their blood glucose returns to their target level. Athletes with severe hypoglycemia cannot return to activity until examined and released by a health care provider.

### PREVENTION

- Careful monitoring of athletes during practices and competitions
- Use of predetermined hand signals for athletes who are not feeling well
- Wearing of alert bracelet, band, or necklace
- Athlete's go bag with blood glucose meter, ketone meter or ketone test strips, fruit juice or candy, protein snack, and emergency glucagon at practices and competitions
- No participation for athletes with uncontrolled diabetes

# HYPOGLYCEMIA IN AN ATHLETE WITHOUT DIABETES

Hypoglycemia can also occur in athletes who have not been diagnosed with diabetes. It is generally caused by going too long without eating.

## Signs and Symptoms

- Dizziness
- Muscle weakness
- Fatigue or exhaustion

## FIRST AID

According to Climan (2023), when you suspect that an athlete who is not previously diagnosed with diabetes has hypoglycemia, you should follow these steps:

1. For an athlete who is awake and able to swallow, encourage them to swallow some version of glucose (gel, tablets, sugar, honey, candy, or juice). If symptoms do not resolve within 10 minutes, or if they worsen, send for emergency medical assistance.
2. For a young athlete who is awake but unwilling or unable to swallow glucose, apply a teaspoon of granulated sugar and water or honey under the tongue.
3. For an athlete who is not awake or is not able to swallow, administering glucose orally is not recommended; send for emergency medical assistance immediately.

## Playing Status

The athlete can return to play when feeling well enough to do so. If they have hypoglycemia a second time during the same season, please speak to the parent and refer the athlete to the appropriate health care provider.

## PREVENTION

- Meal and snack breaks for athletes at regular intervals
- Education for athletes to recognize signs and symptoms of hypoglycemia

# HYPERGLYCEMIA

Severe or prolonged insulin deficiency can result in a high level of blood glucose (hyperglycemia). The body tries to compensate for the low insulin level by eliminating excess glucose through urine. This increased urination leads to dehydration and electrolyte imbalance. The initial drop in insulin may result from stress, extreme temperatures (too hot or too cold for the athlete), certain medications, too much or not enough food, or too much exercise for the athlete. Understanding what is typical for each athlete can give you a better idea of individual causes.

Prolonged hyperglycemia can lead to ketoacidosis. Diabetic ketoacidosis is a serious complication of diabetes when the body does not produce enough insulin and the blood then becomes acidic as a result of the body breaking down fat too quickly, both of which can become life-threatening. Early signs and symptoms of ketoacidosis may include excessive thirst, dry mouth, nausea, sweet or fruity-smelling breath, or excessive urination. If you suspect early-stage ketoacidosis, remove the athlete from all activities, and recommend that the athlete check blood glucose (if they have a monitor). Encourage the athlete to hydrate with water, or a zero-carbohydrate (zero-sugar) drink. Monitor the athlete; if signs and symptoms progress further or do not improve within a few minutes, send for medical assistance. Athletes in early-stage ketoacidosis cannot return to activity until insulin and blood glucose levels are stabilized. Consult with the athlete's health care provider to establish a plan for the athlete's return to activity.

More advanced signs and symptoms as ketoacidosis progresses may include headaches; abdominal pain; dry, red, warm skin; weak pulse; rapid pulse; heavy breathing; or vomiting. For advanced ketoacidosis, send for emergency medical assistance immediately. Place the athlete in the recovery position, and provide CPR if necessary. Athletes with severe ketoacidosis cannot return to activity until examined and released by a health care provider.

To help prevent ketoacidosis, you should carefully monitor athletes who have diabetes, and provide them with frequent fluid breaks during practices and competitions. An athlete with diabetes should wear an alert bracelet, band, or necklace. In addition, they should carry a go bag that includes a blood glucose meter, a blood ketone meter or ketone test strips, fruit juice or candy, a protein snack, and their emergency glucagon. Do not allow an athlete with uncontrolled diabetes to participate in sports.

## Seizures

A wide variety of health issues can cause seizures. Therefore, when evaluating an athlete who has just experienced a seizure, you should also look for other health problems. Please refer the reader to the athlete's health history, discussed in chapters 2 and 5. Epilepsy is the primary cause of most seizures, but other causes exist as well. The Seizure flowchart in the appendix outlines the first aid protocols for petit mal and grand mal seizures.

---

**SAFETY MEASURE**

**With Seizures**

When an athlete has a seizure, do not restrain them, try to place anything in their mouth, or try to pry their teeth apart.

---

# SEIZURE

A seizure is an episode of abnormal electrical activity within the brain. It can lead to sudden changes in an athlete's alertness, behavior, and muscle control. Causes include epilepsy, head injury, brain infection or tumor, drug abuse, respiratory arrest, high fever, heatstroke, hypoglycemia, drug reaction, or medication discontinuation.

## Petit Mal Seizures

A minor (petit mal) seizure, also known as an absence seizure, causes a person to blank out or stare into space for a few seconds. Petit mal seizures are most common in children, and they typically don't cause any long-term problems. These types of seizures are often set off by a period of hyperventilation. Although petit mal seizures are a type of epilepsy (a condition that causes seizures), not everyone who has a seizure has epilepsy. Usually, a diagnosis of epilepsy can be made after two or more seizures.

Petit mal seizures usually occur in children aged 4 to 14 (Johns Hopkins Medicine n.d.). While it is possible to have a petit mal seizure at any age, it is uncommon for this type of seizure to continue into adulthood. On any given day, a child could have 10, 50, or even 100 petit mal seizures that go unnoticed. Most children who have typical petit mal seizures are otherwise in good health. However, these seizures can get in the way of learning and affect concentration at school and during sports, so prompt treatment is important.

Petit mal seizures often occur along with other types of seizures that cause muscle jerking, twitching, and shaking, so they can be confused with other types of seizures. Doctors need to pay close attention to symptoms to make the correct diagnosis, which is important for effective and safe treatment. An athlete who experiences seizures should be advised to wear identification, such as a medical alert bracelet.

Signs and symptoms of petit mal seizures may include a dazed or inattentive manner, confusion, loss of coordination, loss of speech, or repetitive blinking or other small movements. If you suspect a petit mal seizure is occurring, rest the athlete from activity for the remainder of the day, monitor for possible progression into grand mal seizure, and inform the athlete's parent or guardian. If the seizure is caused by an injury or illness, or if it is a first occurrence, the athlete must be examined by an appropriate health care provider and cannot return to activity until released by a health care provider.

*(continued)*

**Seizure** *(continued)*

## Grand Mal Seizures

A major (grand mal) seizure, also known as a generalized tonic-clonic seizure, causes a loss of consciousness and violent muscle contractions. It's the type of response most people picture when they think about seizures. Usually, a grand mal seizure is caused by epilepsy. However, this type of seizure can be triggered by other health problems, such as extremely low blood sugar, a high fever, or a stroke.

Many people who have a grand mal seizure never have another one and don't need treatment. Someone who has recurrent seizures may need treatment with daily anti-seizure medication to control and prevent grand mal seizures. Signs and symptoms of a grand mal seizure may include the following:

- Wide-open eyes
- Stiff or rigid body
- Violently contracting muscles in spasms or convulsions that usually stop in 1 to 2 minutes
- Temporary pause in breathing, progressing to deep breathing after the seizure
- Bluish skin or lips
- Unresponsiveness, followed by gradual return to responsiveness
- Uncontrolled urination during the seizure
- Temporary confusion after the seizure

If you suspect a grand mal seizure has occurred, clear all objects away from the athlete. Protect the athlete's head with a pillow or other available soft material, and do not restrain the athlete. Do not try to place anything in the athlete's mouth, and do not try to pry their teeth apart.

After the convulsions stop, check breathing; provide CPR if needed. If the athlete does not have epilepsy, check for other possible injuries or illnesses. If the athlete has no suspected head, spine, or other injuries, place them in the recovery position. If the athlete is known to have epilepsy and recovers within a few minutes, call the parent or guardian. If the athlete has another injury or illness, is experiencing a seizure for the first time, has a prolonged epileptic seizure (more than 5 minutes), has prolonged confusion or unresponsiveness (more than 15 minutes), has difficulty breathing, or does not have epilepsy, you should send for emergency medical assistance.

If the seizure is caused by an injury or illness, or if it is a first occurrence, the athlete must be examined by an appropriate health care provider and cannot return to activity until released by a health care provider. An athlete who experiences seizures should be advised to wear identification, such as a medical alert bracelet.

# Substance Abuse

Substance abuse is another possible cause of sudden illness in an athlete. An athlete may overdose on a substance or experience an adverse reaction to it. Substances fall into the following broad categories:

- *Depressants*—These substances include alcohol, narcotics (morphine, heroin, and codeine), barbiturates (phenobarbital), gamma-hydroxybutyric acid (GHB; "liquid ecstasy," "soap," "easy lay," "Georgia home boy"), opioids, Rohypnol ("rophies," "roofies," "roach," "rope"), and ketamine ("special K," "vitamin K"). These drugs depress the central nervous system, so athletes may use them to achieve a relaxed, calm feeling. Athletes may also use GHB as a synthetic steroid for bodybuilding.

- *Stimulants*—Cocaine (crack and powdered) and amphetamines are the most common stimulants. These drugs stimulate the nervous system, and some athletes take them to feel quicker and more alert.

- *Combination drugs*—Methylenedioxy-methamphetamine (MDMA; "ecstasy," "Adam," "XTC," "hug," "beans," "love drug") includes both stimulant and hallucinogenic properties. Some effects of MDMA may include increased extroversion and sense of well-being.

As a coach, you should learn to recognize the signs and symptoms of possible overdose from or adverse reactions to these drugs. Moreover, you should educate and counsel your athletes about the dangers of drug use so that you won't have to take the following first aid measures. There are many great resources and educational programs beyond this book that you can utilize to assist you in the education of your athletes.

# DEPRESSANT OVERDOSE OR REACTION

A depressant overdose or reaction is a dangerous and possibly life-threatening response to taking a depressant (reaction) or taking an excessive amount of a depressant (overdose).

**Signs and Symptoms**

- Relaxed feeling, or appearance of intoxication
- Fatigue
- Depression (ketamine/opioids)
- Pale, cold, and clammy skin
- Constricted pupils that may not respond to light
- Rapid and weak pulse
- Possible unresponsiveness
- Shallow breathing that may stop
- Choking or gurgling sounds

After long-term use of depressants or opioids, a person may experience coma, seizures, anterograde amnesia (decreased ability to remember events experienced while taking the drug), hallucinations or delirium, or impaired motor function.

## FIRST AID

1. Rest the athlete from all activity.
2. If the athlete exhibits breathing problems or altered responsiveness, send for emergency medical assistance.
3. Monitor breathing, and provide CPR if needed.
4. Place an unresponsive athlete in the recovery position (if uninjured).
5. For an athlete with suspected depressant overdose who is in respiratory arrest, begin rescue breathing immediately. For further instructions, refer to CPR and AED training as outlined by your certification.

It is also reasonable for responders to administer intramuscular or intranasal naloxone whenever anyone presents with the signs of opioid overdose or when opioid overdose is suspected (see figure 10.1 at the end of the chapter). Naloxone saves lives because it can quickly restore normal breathing in situations where a person's breathing has slowed or stopped as a result of overdose on prescription opioid medications, heroin, or drugs that are adulterated and contaminated with an opioid-like fentanyl (e.g., cocaine, methamphetamine) (CDC 2024).

**Playing Status**

The athlete cannot return to activity until examined and released by a health care provider.

## PREVENTION

- Drug abuse education
- Monitoring of athletes who show signs of depressant abuse

# STIMULANT OVERDOSE OR REACTION

Stimulant overdose or reaction is a dangerous and possibly life-threatening response to using a stimulant (reaction) or taking an excessive amount of a stimulant (overdose).

## Signs and Symptoms

- Lack of fatigue
- Irritability
- Hyperstimulation
- Restlessness
- Anxiety
- Dilated pupils
- Increased body temperature
- Rapid pulse
- Hallucinations
- Paranoia (high doses of cocaine)
- Confusion
- Mood changes
- Cardiac arrest (extreme cases)

## FIRST AID

1. Rest the athlete from all activity.
2. If symptoms don't improve, or if the athlete has breathing difficulties, send for emergency medical assistance.
3. Monitor breathing, and provide CPR if needed.
4. Place an unresponsive athlete in the recovery position (if uninjured).
5. Treat for shock if signs of shock are present, and send for emergency medical assistance.
6. If the athlete recovers quickly, have the parent or guardian take the athlete to an appropriate health care provider.

## Playing Status

The athlete cannot return to activity until examined and released by a health care provider.

## PREVENTION

- Drug abuse education
- Monitoring of athletes who show signs of stimulant abuse

# MDMA (ECSTASY) OVERDOSE OR REACTION

MDMA (ecstasy) overdose or reaction is a dangerous and possibly life-threatening response caused by using ecstasy (reaction) or taking an excessive amount of ecstasy (overdose).

## Signs and Symptoms

- Depression and anxiety
- Nausea
- Feeling faint
- Blurred vision
- Muscle tension
- Involuntary teeth clenching
- Insomnia
- Paranoia
- Chills
- Sweating
- Increased heart rate
- Confusion

## FIRST AID

1. Rest the athlete from all activity.
2. If symptoms don't improve, or if the athlete has breathing difficulties, send for emergency medical assistance.
3. Monitor breathing, and provide CPR if needed.
4. Place an unresponsive athlete in the recovery position (if uninjured).
5. Treat for shock if necessary, and send for emergency medical assistance if shock occurs.
6. If the athlete recovers quickly, speak to the parent or guardian and send the athlete to the appropriate health care provider.

## Playing Status

The athlete cannot return to activity until examined and released by a health care provider.

## PREVENTION

- Drug abuse education
- Monitoring of athletes showing signs of ecstasy abuse

## Supplement Reactions

Touted to enhance performance by boosting strength, decreasing fatigue, and improving endurance, supplements are becoming increasingly popular among athletes. However, because nutritional supplements are not regulated by the U.S. Food and Drug Administration(FDA), they may contain substances that are not listed on the label. This lack of precise labeling can be especially problematic for athletes who have severe allergies to certain substances, such as bee pollen (a common supplement). Although a variety of options are available to athletes, this section focuses on two common supplements: creatine and anabolic steroids.

### Creatine

Creatine is a substance made from amino acids (the building blocks of protein). It is primarily found in the muscles, where it is used to help release the energy needed for short bouts of physical activity. Although creatine is synthesized in the body and also found in foods (primarily lean meat and fish), it has become very popular as a manufactured supplement.

Creatine supplements are widely used by athletes in an effort to improve their performance in brief, high-intensity exercise or sports. Taken at certain dosages, creatine has been found to enhance intense, brief exercise performance in weightlifting, sprint cycling, and jumping.

Creatine use is widespread, but it is difficult to quantify because the available data are limited to self-report surveys, which are limited by response error. The CDC's National Health Interview Survey (CDC 2011) found creatine use among children and adolescents to be 34.1 percent, with the purpose of enhancing sport performance. The long-term effects of creatine use on adolescents is unknown, so it is possible that this statistic indicates a problem. In addition, supplements are not subjected to the same rigorous restrictions placed on over-the-counter and prescription medications (they are not regulated for content or purity), and some athletes have adverse effects from taking creatine. Therefore, you are advised to play it safe; protect your athletes by prohibiting the use of performance-enhancing supplements such as creatine.

# CREATINE REACTION

Creatine reaction is gastrointestinal distress, muscle cramps, weight gain, or dehydration caused by creatine use.

## Signs and Symptoms

- Nausea
- Stomach discomfort (gas)
- Loss of appetite
- Weight gain (due to water retention in the muscles)
- Muscle cramps
- Dehydration
- Diarrhea

## FIRST AID

1. Rest the athlete from activity until signs and symptoms subside.
2. Monitor the athlete for signs and symptoms of a more serious condition such as an abdominal injury (chapter 9) or heat illness (chapter 11), and provide appropriate first aid as needed.

## Playing Status

If the athlete exhibits signs of dehydration (see chapter 11), do not allow them to return to activity until they are adequately rehydrated.

## PREVENTION

- Sport supplement education to athletes and parents or guardians
- Monitoring of athletes who exhibit creatine side effects

## Anabolic Steroids

Anabolic steroids are manufactured substances derived from the male reproductive hormone testosterone. While these substances can be used for medical purposes, their use is legal only with a prescription. Steroids can increase muscle size, lean muscle mass, and muscle strength, so athletes use them illegally to enhance their athletic performance and appearance. According to the Taylor Hooten Foundation (n.d.), in the United States, 7 percent of high school students admit to using steroids, and 21 percent of high school students know a friend who uses steroids. According to the foun-

dation, anabolic steroid use is prevalent among all students; 62.5 percent of users said they do it to improve their looks, and 57 percent admitted they would take a powder or pill if it guaranteed them reaching their athletic goal regardless of the possibility of it shortening their life.

Despite their ability to enhance performance, anabolic steroids cause serious health effects. They can lead to high blood pressure, increased cholesterol, cardiovascular disease, liver damage, and infertility (in males). If used by adolescents, steroids may prematurely stop growth and result in shorter stature.

# ANABOLIC STEROID ABUSE

While anabolic steroids can be used for medical purposes, their use is legal only with a prescription. Anabolic steroid abuse is the illegal use, use for purposes other than those for which they are meant, or use in excessive amounts of anabolic steroids. Drug abuse may lead to social, physical, emotional, and job-related problems.

### Signs and Symptoms

- Baldness, increased breast size, and decreased testicular size in males
- Swollen feet or ankles (signs of cardiovascular disease)
- Increased facial hair, deepened voice, reduced breast size, and menstrual cycle changes in females
- Mood swings
- Aching joints
- Nervousness and trembling
- Yellowish skin (sign of jaundice)
- Bad breath
- Increased acne

## FIRST AID

1. Monitor the athlete for symptoms or signs of more serious illnesses or injuries, and refer to the appropriate health care provider if necessary.
2. Speak to the athlete and their parent or guardian about the suspected steroid use.
3. Require that the athlete see the appropriate health care provider.

### Playing Status

The athlete cannot return to activity until examined and released by a health care provider.

## PREVENTION

- Steroid abuse education for athletes and parents or guardians
- Monitoring of and communication with athletes who show symptoms or signs of steroid use

## Other Acute Illnesses

Other sudden illnesses you may encounter as a coach include insect sting allergies, fainting, gastroenteritis, and airborne diseases. Anaphylactic shock (covered in chapter 7) may occur in athletes who are allergic to certain insect stings. Fainting in athletes is most often caused by illness or dehydration. Influenza, COVID-19, and some cases of gastroenteritis can happen at any time, and they can quickly spread to other athletes. Each of these acute illnesses requires quick and accurate assessment and first aid intervention.

# FAINTING

Fainting is temporary unresponsiveness that is not caused by a head injury. Caused by extreme fatigue, dehydration, low blood pressure, or illness, fainting can be classified as a mild form of shock.

### Signs and Symptoms

- Nausea
- Weakness
- Headache
- Fatigue
- Dizziness
- Pale, cool, clammy skin
- Shallow, rapid breathing
- Loss of responsiveness

### FIRST AID

If the athlete is responsive, do the following:

1. If the athlete is feeling faint, dizzy, or uneasy, instruct the athlete to lie on their back with their feet elevated or in a comfortable position.
2. Monitor the athlete, treat them for shock if necessary, and send for emergency medical assistance if shock occurs.
3. If the athlete does not recover within a few minutes, send for emergency medical assistance.

If the athlete is unresponsive, do the following:

1. Monitor breathing, and provide CPR if needed.
2. If the athlete does not recover within a few minutes, send for emergency medical assistance.
3. Place the athlete in the recovery position (if uninjured).
4. Monitor the athlete, treat them for shock if necessary, and send for emergency medical assistance if shock occurs.

### Playing Status

Rest the athlete for the remainder of the day, and inform the athlete's parent or guardian. If the athlete is ill, they must be examined by the appropriate health care provider. The athlete cannot return to activity until released by a health care provider.

### PREVENTION

- Eat regular meals, and avoid skipping meals
- Drink enough water every day
- If you need to stand in one place for a long time, be sure to move your legs and don't lock your knees
- If you're prone to anxiety, find a coping strategy that works for you
- If you have sudden anxiety and feel like you might faint, take deep breaths

# GASTROENTERITIS

Gastroenteritis is sudden infection or toxin exposure affecting the stomach and intestines. People often call it the stomach flu or food poisoning. It is caused by direct contact with bacteria, viruses, and certain parasites or germs, which can be spread through inhalation, personal contact, contact with contaminated surfaces, consumption of contaminated food or fluids, and handling of contaminated pets or animals.

## Signs and Symptoms

- Nausea or vomiting
- Headache
- Muscle aches
- Weakness
- Chills
- Diarrhea
- Abdominal pain and stomach cramps
- Low-grade fever (99.1-100.4 °F)
- Dehydration (dry and parched lips, dry skin, extreme thirst, no urination in 6 hours)

## FIRST AID

1. Rest the athlete from all activity.
2. Suggest that the athlete avoid solid foods.
3. If the athlete is vomiting, encourage them to consume only ice chips until vomiting stops and then to drink clear fluids.
4. Immediately send the athlete to the appropriate health care provider if any of the following are present:
   - Severe abdominal pain, particularly in the right lower abdomen
   - Forceful vomiting
   - Fever greater than 101 °F
   - Bloody stool or vomit
   - Signs and symptoms lasting more than 48 hours
   - Signs of dehydration
   - Possibility of food poisoning

## Playing Status

The athlete cannot return to activity until signs and symptoms have been gone for 48 hours, or until examined and released by a health care provider.

## PREVENTION

- No direct contact of an infected athlete with other athletes
- No indirect contact with an infected athlete via shared water bottles, towels, or eating utensils
- Reminders to wash hands

# AIRBORNE DISEASES (COVID-19 AND INFLUENZA)

Airborne diseases are diseases that can transmit through coughs or sneezes, spraying liquid, or dust. According to the Centers for Disease Control and Prevention (CDC 2011), airborne diseases can spread through a direct or an indirect form of transmission, depending on the germ involved. Many airborne diseases exist, and the symptoms, treatment, and outlook vary according to the disease. This section concentrates only on COVID-19 and influenza.

## Signs and Symptoms

- Muscle or joint achiness
- Headache
- Fatigue
- Fever
- Cough
- Nasal congestion
- Sore throat
- Runny nose
- Watery eyes
- New loss of taste or smell
- Shortness of breath
- Nausea or vomiting
- Diarrhea

## FIRST AID

1. Rest the athlete from all activity.
2. Encourage the athlete to drink liquids.
3. Refer to the appropriate health care provider.
4. Monitor other athletes.
5. Sanitize any and all equipment as needed.

## Playing Status

The athlete cannot return to activity until examined and released by a health care provider.

## PREVENTION

- Social distancing and avoiding direct contact of infected athlete with others
- Avoiding indirect contact with infected athlete
- Washing or sanitizing of hands and surfaces
- Wearing of face covering according to regulations

# Chapter 10 Recap

❏ What quick first aid care can you provide to help treat hypoglycemia or hyperglycemia?

❏ What are the signs and symptoms of a minor (petit mal) seizure?

❏ What are the signs and symptoms of a major (grand mal) seizure?

❏ What are some substances that depress the central nervous system?

❏ What are the signs and symptoms of an overdose or adverse reaction to depressants?

❏ What are the signs and symptoms of an overdose or adverse reaction to stimulants?

❏ Can you describe the first aid techniques for an overdose or adverse reaction to depressants and stimulants?

❏ Describe the first aid care for fainting.

❏ What can you do to help prevent the spread of infectious disease among your athletes?

# DIRECTIONS

## NARCAN®
Naloxone HCl Nasal Spray 4 mg

**Emergency Treatment of Opioid Overdose**

**Important:**
- For use in the nose only
- Do not test nasal spray device before use
- 1 nasal spray device contains 1 dose of medicine
- Each device sprays 1 time only

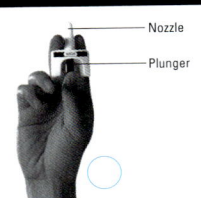
Nozzle
Plunger

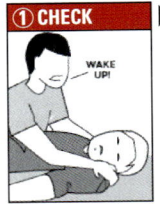
① CHECK

**Step 1: CHECK if you suspect an overdose:**

- **CHECK** for a <u>suspected overdose:</u> the person will not wake up or is very sleepy or not breathing well
  - yell "Wake up!"
  - shake the person gently
  - if the person is not awake, go to Step 2

**Unfold for *Directions***

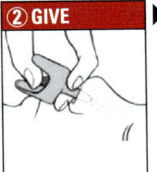
② GIVE

**Step 2: Give 1st dose in the nose**

- **HOLD** the nasal spray device with your thumb on the bottom of the plunger
- **INSERT** the nozzle into either NOSTRIL
- **PRESS** the plunger firmly to give the 1st dose
- 1 nasal spray device contains 1 dose

**Unfold for *Directions***

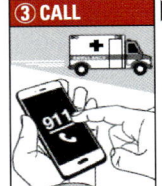
③ CALL

**Step 3: Call 911**

- **CALL 911** immediately after giving the 1st dose

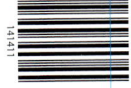

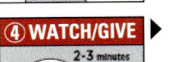
④ WATCH/GIVE
2-3 minutes

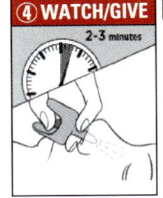

**Step 4: WATCH & GIVE**

- **WAIT** 2-3 minutes after the 1st dose to give the medicine time to work
- if the person <u>wakes up</u>: Go to Step 5
- if the person does <u>not wake up</u>:
  - **CONTINUE TO GIVE** doses every 2-3 minutes until the person wakes up
  - it is safe to keep giving doses

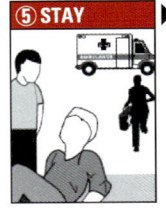
⑤ STAY

**Step 5: STAY**

- **STAY** until ambulance arrives: even if the person wakes up
- **GIVE** another dose if the person becomes very sleepy again
- You may need to give all the doses in the pack

**EMERGENT®**

<u>For opioid emergencies, call 911.</u> For questions on NARCAN, call 1-844-4NARCAN (1-844-462-7226) or go to www.narcan.com.
©2023 Emergent Devices Inc. EMERGENT® and NARCAN® are registered trademarks of Emergent BioSolutions Inc, or its subsidiaries.

A1162

**Figure 10.1** Narcan (naloxone) quick start guide.

NARCAN® Nasal Spray is a registered trademark of Emergent Operations Ireland Limited. Human Kinetics, Inc., is not affiliated with, sponsored by or endorsed by Emergent Operations Ireland Limited or Emergent BioSolutions Inc.

# WEATHER-RELATED INJURIES AND ILLNESSES

## IN THIS CHAPTER, YOU WILL LEARN THE FOLLOWING:

- How to prevent injuries and illnesses related to heat, cold, and lightning
- How to identify the symptoms and signs of heat cramps
- How to identify and differentiate between the symptoms and signs of heat exhaustion and heatstroke
- How to identify the symptoms and signs of first-, second-, and third-degree frostbite, and mild to severe hypothermia
- What first aid care to provide for heat cramps, heat exhaustion, heatstroke, frostbite, hypothermia, and lightning injuries

### INJURIES AND CONDITIONS IN THIS CHAPTER

Searing lightning, sweltering heat, and numbing cold are an accepted part of outdoor seasons in sports. Even so, coaches should not overlook the serious illnesses and injuries that can result from these conditions. Lightning, heatstroke, and hypothermia can be life-threatening, and frostbite can lead to disfiguration. Fortunately, almost all of these conditions can be prevented. As a coach, you play a key role in not only preventing but also quickly identifying and providing appropriate first aid care for temperature-related illnesses and lightning injuries.

## Temperature-Related Illnesses

Before learning the sport first aid specifics for temperature-related illnesses, you need to first understand how body temperature is regulated. The body's temperature changes through several processes, including metabolism, convection, conduction, radiation, and evaporation (see figure 11.1). These methods of temperature regulation are described as follows:

*Metabolism*—As the body's cells work and use energy (metabolism), heat is produced. When a person is active, the body temperature rises due to an increase in metabolic rate.

*Convection*—In convection, heat is lost or gained by air (wind) circulating around the body. If the air temperature is warmer than the body, the body will gain heat; if the air temperature is cooler, the body will lose heat.

*Conduction*—When the body touches warmer or colder objects, it gains or loses heat; this process is called conduction. For example, sitting in a warm whirlpool will cause body temperature to rise; sitting on a cold, metal bench will lower body temperature.

*Radiation*—Radiation occurs when heat is gained through contact with electromagnetic waves, such as from the sun. The degree of cloudiness and the angle of the sun can influence the sun's radiative effects. Heat can be lost through radiation from the body to the environment whenever the environmental temperature is less than body temperature.

*Evaporation*—Sweating is the body's built-in mechanism for cooling itself. However, it's only effective if the sweat actually evaporates from the skin. Humidity (the amount of moisture already in the air) directly influences how much sweat will evaporate. The more humid the environment, the less sweat will evaporate, and the more difficult it is for the body to lose heat. Equipment and type of clothing can also affect sweat evaporation. For example, a helmet will prevent heat from the head from being dissipated through radiation, evaporation, and convection.

With this understanding of body temperature regulation, the following sections explore what can happen when body temperature goes awry.

## Exertional Heat-Related Illnesses

Consider the following examples of heat-related illnesses:

After experiencing heat exhaustion and leaving practice early the day before, perhaps he felt he couldn't afford to take it easy during drills and conditioning, even though it was another

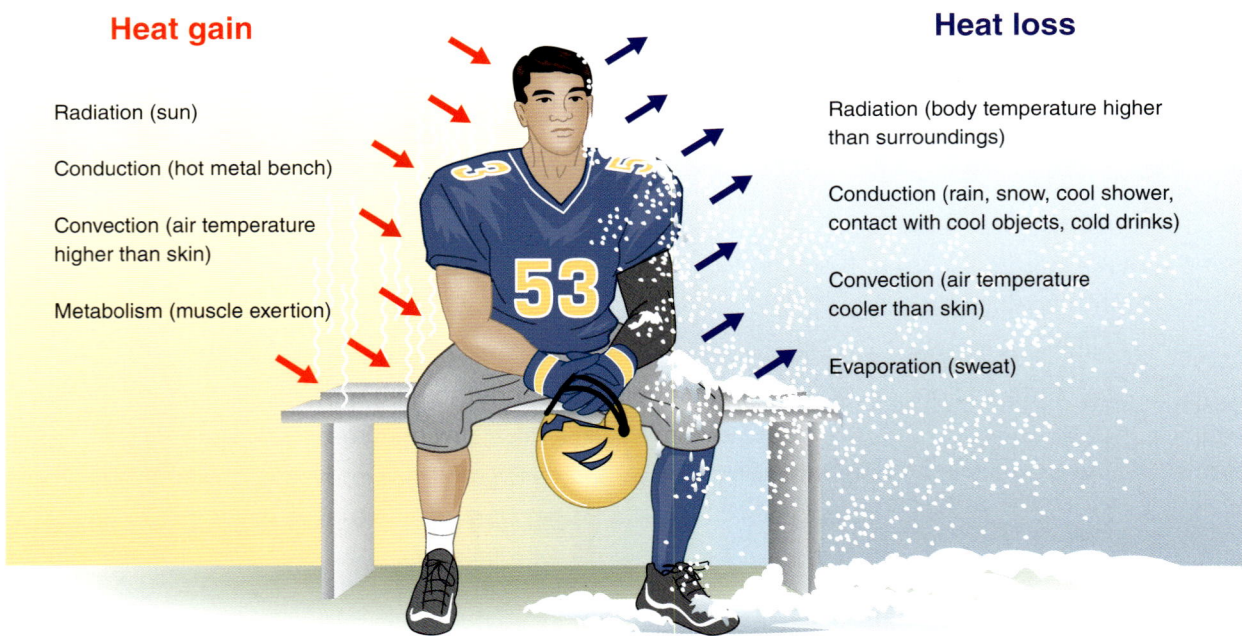

**Heat gain**

Radiation (sun)

Conduction (hot metal bench)

Convection (air temperature higher than skin)

Metabolism (muscle exertion)

**Heat loss**

Radiation (body temperature higher than surroundings)

Conduction (rain, snow, cool shower, contact with cool objects, cold drinks)

Convection (air temperature cooler than skin)

Evaporation (sweat)

**Figure 11.1** Methods of body temperature change.

day of stifling heat. So, he pushed himself through practice. It was hard; he vomited several times. Finally, it was time to head inside to the long-awaited air-conditioned environment. There, he developed symptoms of heatstroke, including weakness and rapid breathing. Although he was immediately evaluated and treated by athletic trainers and then transported to a hospital, Korey Stringer, offensive tackle for the Minnesota Vikings, was unresponsive at the time of arrival. His body temperature had soared to over 108 degrees Fahrenheit, resulting in multiorgan system failure and, finally, death.

In 1997, within the span of one month, three college wrestlers died trying to make weight. The February 20, 1998, issue of the *Morbidity and Mortality Weekly Report,* published by the Centers for Disease Control and Prevention (CDC), concluded that all three victims wore vapor-impermeable suits and exercised vigorously in hot environments. "These conditions promoted dehydration and heat-related illness," stated the report, which noted that the body temperature of one of the wrestlers was 108 degrees Fahrenheit at the time of death.

Athletes can limit heat-related injuries and illnesses by taking proper precautions before participating in outdoor activity. Some of these precautions are outlined next.

### Prevention of Exertional Heat-Related Illnesses

The Korey Stringer Institute recommends five pillars of exertional heatstroke prevention (NFHS and Korey Stringer Institute 2015). They include hydration, body cooling, work-to-rest ratios, acclimatization, and education. Key factors related to these pillars include the following:

### Monitor Weather Conditions, and Adjust Practices Accordingly

Wet-bulb globe temperature (WBGT) is considered the gold standard of environmental monitoring. Multiple organizations, including the U.S. Department of Defense and the American College of Sports Medicine, recommend this method for environmental monitoring (Cooper et al. 2017). WBGT relies on humidity, radiant heat, ambient air temperature, and wind speed to display a more accurate temperature. Most U.S. high schools have developed plans for practice modifications according to the WBGT tem-

perature. Typically, an athletic trainer (on staff or assigned to the school) monitors the WBGT temperature in real time and alerts the coach of practice or game modifications if needed.

Figure 11.2 shows the specific air temperature and humidity percentages that can be hazardous. This information can be used to help determine playing modifications in the absence of a WBGT device. Keep in mind that exertional heat-related deaths have occurred in football players at temperatures as low as 82 degrees Fahrenheit with a relative humidity index at only 40 percent. If heat and humidity are equal to or higher than these conditions, make sure athletes are acclimated to the weather and are wearing light practice clothing. Schedule practices for early morning and evening to avoid higher heat in the middle of the day. In addition, remember that information presented in figure 11.2 is less accurate than an onsite WBGT device, and it does not account for all factors that the device would use; however, it can still serve as a guideline for activity planning and modifications. Table 11.1 is an example of the NJSIAA (New Jersey State Interscholastic Athletic Association) heat participation policy. You can use this sample to create your own heat participation policy and help prevent exertional heat-related illness; it is important to first research your state's policies and procedures.

In addition, having appropriate work-to-rest ratios (the amount of time spent involved in exercise versus the amount of time spent in recovery) should be modified as environmental conditions become extreme. Environmental extremes should be measured using WBGT, for an accurate measure of the heat stress that the athlete will be experiencing during exercise in the heat. Modifications of work-to-rest ratios in extreme environmental conditions include increasing the number of rest breaks, the duration of rest breaks, and having unlimited access to hydration.

### Acclimate Athletes to Exercising in High Heat and Humidity

If you are located in a warm-weather climate or have practices during the summer, athletes need time (about 7-10 days) to adjust to high heat and humidity. During this time, hold short practices at low to moderate activity levels, and provide fluid and rest breaks every 15 to 20 minutes. The

| Relative humidity (%) | Temperature (°F) 80 | 82 | 84 | 86 | 88 | 90 | 92 | 94 | 96 | 98 | 100 | 102 | 104 | 106 | 108 | 110 |
|---|---|---|---|---|---|---|---|---|---|---|---|---|---|---|---|---|
| 40 | 80 | 81 | 83 | 85 | 88 | 91 | 94 | 97 | 101 | 105 | 109 | 114 | 119 | 124 | 130 | 136 |
| 45 | 80 | 82 | 84 | 87 | 89 | 93 | 96 | 100 | 104 | 109 | 114 | 119 | 124 | 130 | 137 | |
| 50 | 81 | 83 | 85 | 88 | 91 | 95 | 99 | 103 | 108 | 113 | 118 | 124 | 131 | 137 | | |
| 55 | 81 | 84 | 86 | 89 | 93 | 97 | 101 | 106 | 112 | 117 | 124 | 130 | 137 | | | |
| 60 | 82 | 84 | 88 | 91 | 95 | 100 | 105 | 110 | 116 | 123 | 129 | 137 | | | | |
| 65 | 82 | 85 | 89 | 93 | 98 | 103 | 108 | 114 | 121 | 128 | 136 | | | | | |
| 70 | 83 | 86 | 90 | 95 | 100 | 105 | 112 | 119 | 126 | 134 | | | | | | |
| 75 | 84 | 88 | 92 | 97 | 103 | 109 | 116 | 124 | 132 | | | | | | | |
| 80 | 84 | 89 | 94 | 100 | 106 | 113 | 121 | 129 | | | | | | | | |
| 85 | 85 | 90 | 96 | 102 | 110 | 117 | 126 | 135 | | | | | | | | |
| 90 | 86 | 91 | 98 | 105 | 113 | 122 | 131 | | | | | | | | | |
| 95 | 86 | 93 | 100 | 108 | 117 | 127 | | | | | | | | | | |
| 100 | 87 | 95 | 103 | 112 | 121 | 132 | | | | | | | | | | |

Caution   Extreme caution   Danger   Extreme danger

**Figure 11.2** Heat index chart.

Source: National Weather Service. Available: https://www.weather.gov/ama/heatindex.

**Table 11.1** Sample Heat Participation Policy*

| WBGT reading | Flag | Risk for heat illness | Activity and rest break guidelines |
|---|---|---|---|
| Under 80 °F | Green | Very low | Normal activities—Provide at least three separate rest breaks each hour (minimum duration: 3 min each). |
| 80.0-85.0 °F | Yellow | Low | Use discretion for intense or prolonged exercise; watch at-risk players carefully; provide at least three separate rest breaks each hour (minimum duration: 4 min each). |
| 85.1-88.0 °F | Orange | Moderate | Maximum practice time is 2 hours. For football, lacrosse, and field hockey: All helmets and shoulder pads must be removed for practice and conditioning activities. If the WBGT rises to this level during practice, football players may continue to work out wearing football pants without changing into shorts. For all sports: Provide at least four separate rest breaks each hour (minimum duration: 4 min each). |
| 88.1-90.0 °F | Red | High | Maximum duration of practice is 1 hour. For football, lacrosse, and field hockey: No protective equipment may be worn during practice, and no conditioning activities are allowed. For all sports: No conditioning is allowed, and you must have 20 minutes of rest breaks distributed throughout the hour of practice. |
| >90.0 °F | Black | Very high | No outdoor workouts are allowed. Delay practice until a cooler WBGT level is reached. |

*Please note that these WBGTs may vary depending on the location.

Adapted by permission from Guidelines, Policies and Procedures, 2022-2023, NJSIAA, accessed January 31, 2024, https://www.njsiaa.org/sites/default/files/documents/2022-08/NJSIAA%20Policies%20and%20Procedures%20%2722-%2723%20-%20With%20accepted%20changes.pdf.

National Athletic Trainers' Association's Position Statement: Exertional Heat Illnesses (Casa et. al. 2015) offers more specific guidelines for acclimating high school athletes to hot environmental conditions; the recommendations are as follows:

- *Days 1 and 2*: Single 3-hour practice, or one 2-hour practice and one 1-hour field session with helmets only
- *Days 3 and 4*: Single 3-hour practice, or one 2-hour practice and one 1-hour field session with helmets and shoulder pads
- *Day 5*: Single 3-hour practice, or one 2-hour practice and one 1-hour field session with full pads
- *After day 5*: One day between days with multiple practices; less than 5 hours total practice time; and less than 2 hours walk through

The NATA specifies that any athlete who misses a practice for any reason must still complete acclimation guidelines as listed previously. Therefore, the athlete must pick up where they left off before missing a practice.

### Switch to Light Clothing and Less Equipment

Athletes stay cooler if they wear shorts, white T-shirts, and less equipment (particularly helmets and pads). Equipment blocks the ability of sweat to evaporate. It's especially important for athletes to wear light clothing and minimal equipment while they are acclimating to the heat.

### Prepare for Hot Practices

If practice must happen during times when heat may be an issue, plan accordingly for the conditions. Having access to cooling methods is essential for treating heat-related conditions; these methods include the following:

*Cold-water immersion*—This method is the most effective way to cool an athlete in an emergency. It uses a tub, such as a small inflatable pool filled with water or any other vessel big enough to submerge an athlete up to their neck. Ideally, the tub should be filled with water before practice, and ice should be available to be added if needed. Water in the tub should be approximately 33.8 to 78.8 degrees Fahrenheit.

*Tarp-assisted cooling oscillation*—This method, called the taco method, should be used when cold-water immersion is not available. In lieu of a rigid cold tub, many organizations recommend the taco method. The athlete lies on a tarp while volunteers hold the sides up. The tarp is then filled with ice water. The volunteers then use their knees to oscillate the water in the tarp to aid with cooling.

*Cold shower*—This method is another way to cool an athlete in the event that cold-water immersion is not available. This method requires the athlete to remove unnecessary clothing, be positioned under a shower or hose, and get drenched in cold water.

*Ice towels*—This method uses towels completely soaked in ice water; when an athlete needs cooling, the towel is placed over their shoulders. Although ice towels are easier to acquire and transport than a cold-water immersion tub, they are less effective at cooling.

Other cooling methods may include instant ice bags; ice packs placed on the inner thighs, armpits, and head; or ice vests. While these methods may help in an emergency, cold-water immersion should still be considered the primary choice for emergency cooling. In addition, you should ensure the drinking water provided to the athletes has ice in it; if individual bottles are used, keep them in a cooler.

### Identify and Monitor Athletes Prone to Heat Illness

Athletes who are particularly prone to exertional heat illness include those who have previously experienced a heat illness and those with the sickle-cell trait. These athletes should be continuously monitored during activity. Dehydrated, overweight, heavily muscled, or deconditioned athletes, as well as athletes taking certain medications (antihistamines, decongestants, some asthma medications, certain supplements, and attention-deficit/hyperactivity disorder medications) are at risk. Closely monitor these athletes, and make sure they drink plenty of fluids. Rest dehydrated athletes until they have become rehydrated (see the following section on adequate hydration).

### Strictly Enforce Adequate Hydration

Athletes can lose a great deal of water through sweat. If this fluid is not replaced, the body will have less water to cool itself and will become dehydrated. Dehydration not only increases athletes' risk for heat illness, but it also decreases their performance. In fact, athletic performance may worsen after only 2 percent of the body weight is lost through sweat. For example, dehydrated athletes may experience decreased muscle strength, increased fatigue, decreased mental function (e.g., concentration), and decreased endurance. Signs and symptoms of dehydration include the following:

- Thirst
- Flushed skin
- Fatigue
- Muscle cramps
- Apathy
- Dry lips and mouth
- Dark urine (should be clear or light yellow)
- Feeling weak

Most athletes don't feel thirsty until they have lost 3 percent or more of their body weight in sweat (water). By that time, their performance will have started to decrease, and their risk of exertional heat illness will have increased. Therefore, instead of relying on athletes to drink enough fluids on their own, you should remind them to drink fluids at regular intervals. In addition, athletes may not drink enough fluid to replenish the water lost through sweat during activity in high heat and humidity. The most effective way to determine the amount of fluid lost through sweat is for athletes to weigh themselves with minimal clothing on before and after practices and competitions that take place

in high heat and humidity. For every pound lost, an athlete should drink 16 to 24 ounces of water (DHS 2021). For additional aid in proper hydration, see your organization's licensed health care provider (athletic trainer, team physician). If hydration is a persistent issue, consult with the athlete's parent or guardian, or the appropriate health care provider.

### Replenish Electrolytes Lost Through Sweat

During activities lasting longer than 50 minutes, substantial amounts of electrolytes such as sodium (salt) and potassium are lost in sweat. These electrolytes are used in muscle contraction, fluid balance, and other body functions, so they must be replaced. In addition, sodium plays a role in activating the body's thirst mechanism, so it can stimulate athletes to keep hydrated. The best way for athletes to replace these nutrients is by drinking a sports beverage (containing sodium) and eating their usual diet. It might be tempting to advise athletes to take salt tablets or other supplements. However, they can replenish sodium and the other necessary electrolytes (like potassium and calcium) through proper nutrition and hydration choices, so using salt tablets is not recommended. Only a small amount of potassium is lost in sweat. Oranges and bananas are good sources of potassium. Having them available during practices and competitions can help athletes replenish the minimal potassium lost through sweat.

### Prohibit Artificial Means of Quick Weight Reduction

Athletes looking for the quick and easy way to lose weight may try to cut corners and use

---

# Sports Drinks Versus Water

If athletes are engaged in any vigorous or high-intensity activity, practicing or competing for more than an hour, competing or practicing more than once per day, or are dehydrated, then sports drinks (with 6% to 7% carbohydrate solution and containing sodium) are preferred because they

- stimulate thirst,
- promote fluid retention,
- replenish carbohydrates utilized for energy,
- help to reduce muscle cramping, and
- appeal to athletes (because of the flavor), which causes them to drink more.

---

unsafe and unhealthy methods to do so. Weight loss should be accomplished by eating healthy, and safely reducing your caloric intake while increasing your caloric expenditure. The 2023-24 NFHS Wrestling Rule Book (Rule 1, Section 5, Articles 1-3) outlines the process for discouraging excessive weight loss and establishing a safe minimum weight, which involves the wrestler, parents or guardians, the appropriate health care provider, and coach (Hopkins 2023).

### Identifying and Treating Exertional Heat Illnesses

During physical activity, the body can produce 10 to 20 times the amount of heat that it produces at rest; this heat production occurs through metabolism. Approximately 75 percent of this heat must be eliminated. If the air temperature is less than the body temperature, radiation, conduction, and convection can help dissipate 65 to 75 percent of the heat. However, if the air temperature is near the body temperature, these modes of heat loss are less effective, and the body must rely more on perspiration. High humidity reduces the amount of sweat evaporation, leaving exercising athletes at risk of exertional heat illness.

This section covers three types of exertional heat illness: heat cramps, heat exhaustion, and heatstroke. Each has different signs and symptoms, and each has different first aid interventions. Heatstroke is life-threatening, whereas heat exhaustion and heat cramps typically are not. Therefore, it is important that you learn to evaluate the signs and symptoms and learn to apply the first aid techniques that are appropriate for each illness. For a summary of first aid care for these conditions, see the Heat Cramp, Heat Exhaustion, and Heatstroke flowcharts in the appendix.

# HEAT CRAMPS

Heat cramps are sudden muscle spasms that usually occur in the quadriceps, hamstrings, or calves. Causes include dehydration, electrolyte (sodium and potassium) loss, decreased blood flow to the muscles, or fatigue.

## Signs and Symptoms

- Pain
- Fatigue
- Severe muscle spasms, often in the quadriceps, hamstrings, or calves
- Heavy sweating

## FIRST AID

1. Rest the athlete in a cool place.
2. Assist the athlete with stretching the affected muscle.
3. Give the athlete a sports beverage (containing sodium) to drink. If a sports drink is not available, provide the athlete with regular water.
4. If the spasms do not stop with stretching or after a few minutes of rest, look for other possible causes.
5. Monitor the athlete for worsening signs and symptoms, or any signs of dehydration, and send the athlete to the appropriate health care provider if worsening occurs. If spasms continue, or if other injuries are found, inform the athlete's parent or guardian and send the athlete to the appropriate health care provider.
6. Seek medical attention for an athlete who has heart problems, is on a low-sodium diet, or continues to experience cramps for more than an hour.

## Playing Status

The athlete can return to activity once the spasms stop and the athlete can run, jump, and cut without limping or experiencing pain. If the athlete is referred to a health care provider, they cannot return to activity until examined and released by the health care provider.

## PREVENTION

- Adequate hydration for athletes
- Rest for athletes with signs of dehydration

# HEAT EXHAUSTION

Heat exhaustion is a shocklike condition caused by dehydration, which occurs when the body's water and electrolyte supplies are depleted through sweating.

## Signs and Symptoms

- Headache
- Nausea
- Dizziness
- Chills

- Fatigue
- Thirst
- Muscle cramps
- Pale, cool, and clammy skin

- Rapid, weak pulse
- Loss of coordination
- Dilated pupils
- Profuse sweating

## FIRST AID

1. Remove the athlete from the hot environment, and rest them from activity and exertion.
2. Remove excess clothing.
3. Send for emergency medical assistance.
4. Have a medical professional take a rectal temperature to differentiate exertional heat exhaustion from the more serious heatstroke. With heat exhaustion, core body temperature (measured rectally) would usually be less than 104 degrees Fahrenheit. Rectal temperature should only be obtained by a trained medical professional. In the event that an athlete has a suspected raised core temperature, full-body cooling should take place immediately and you should send for emergency medical assistance regardless of the actual core temperature.
5. Immediately initiate active cooling by using whole-body cooling (from the neck down). Water should be approximately 33.8 to 78.8 degrees Fahrenheit. If cold-water immersion is unavailable, other cooling methods should be initiated such as commercial ice packs, a cold shower, ice sheets or towels, cooling vests and jackets, or fanning.
6. Give the athlete a sports beverage (containing sodium) to drink. If a sports drink is not available, provide the athlete with water.
7. Monitor breathing, and provide CPR if needed.
8. Monitor and treat for shock as needed.

## Playing Status

An athlete must not return to activity on the same day that they experienced heat exhaustion. If the athlete is sent to a health care provider or does not quickly recover, they cannot return to activity until examined and released by the health care provider. The athlete cannot return to activity until the weight lost through sweat is regained.

## PREVENTION

- Adequate hydration
- Rest for athletes with signs of dehydration
- Scheduling of activity during cooler times

# HEATSTROKE

Heatstroke is a life-threatening condition in which the body temperature rises dangerously high. It is caused by a malfunction in the brain's temperature control center, which results from severe dehydration, fever, or inadequate balance of the body's temperature regulation.

## Signs and Symptoms

- Feeling extremely hot
- Nausea or vomiting
- Irritability
- Fatigue
- Hot and flushed or red skin
- Lack of sweat

- Very high body temperature
- Rapid pulse
- Rapid breathing
- Constricted pupils
- Diarrhea
- Confusion

- Possible seizures
- Possible unresponsiveness
- Possible respiratory or cardiac arrest

## FIRST AID

1. Send for emergency medical personnel.
2. Quickly move the athlete to a cool, shaded area, and rest the athlete from activity and exertion.
3. Place the athlete in a semireclining position. If the athlete is unresponsive, raise their head or roll them on their side as necessary to allow fluids and vomit to drain from the mouth.
4. Remove excess clothing.
5. Have a trained medical professional take a rectal temperature to differentiate exertional heat exhaustion from the more serious heatstroke. With heat exhaustion, core body temperature (measured rectally) would normally be less than 104 degrees Fahrenheit. In the event that an athlete has a suspected raised core temperature, full-body cooling should take place immediately and you should send for emergency medical assistance regardless of the actual core temperature.
6. Immediately initiate active cooling by using full-body cooling (from the neck down). Water should be approximately 33.8 to 78.8 degrees Fahrenheit. If cold-water immersion is unavailable, initiate other cooling methods, such as commercial ice packs, a cold shower, ice sheets or towels, cooling vests and jackets, or fanning.
7. If the athlete is responsive and able to ingest fluids, give them a sports beverage (containing sodium). If a sports drink is not available, provide the athlete with regular water.
8. Monitor breathing, and provide CPR if needed.
9. Monitor and treat for shock as needed.

## Playing Status

The athlete cannot return to activity until examined and released by a health care provider; at that point, they should return to activity gradually.

## PREVENTION

- Adequate hydration
- Rest for athletes with signs of dehydration

## Cold-Related Illnesses

As with heat-related illnesses, cold-related illnesses are caused by an imbalance in the factors that affect body temperature. Exposure to cold weather and cold equipment causes body temperature to drop below normal. To counteract this drop, the body tries to gain or conserve heat by shivering (increases metabolism) and reducing blood flow to the skin and extremities (to conserve heat and blood flow to the brain, heart, and lungs). This response can result in frostbite or hypothermia.

### *Prevention of Cold-Related Illnesses*

The body best withstands cold temperatures when it is prepared to handle them. Following are guidelines to reduce the risk of cold-related illnesses.

### Ensure Athletes Wear Appropriate Protective Clothing

Athletes should dress in layers to allow sweat to evaporate and to protect against the cold. Wool, Gore-Tex, and spandex are excellent materials to wear. Also, be sure the head and neck are covered to prevent excessive heat loss. Mittens are preferable to gloves because they allow the fingers to warm each other.

### Keep Athletes Active to Maintain Body Heat

Athletes who must stand along the sidelines should keep moving to help produce body heat. Jumping up and down and jogging in place are good sideline exercises.

### Monitor Windchill, and Adjust Cold Exposure Accordingly

The combination of wind, cold temperatures, and wet conditions increases athletes' risk of hypothermia (see figure 11.3 for the U.S. National Weather Service's windchill temperature index). Figure 11.4 is an example of a cold participation policy; it is important to first research your state's individual policies and procedures for cold weather participation.

### Monitor Athletes At Risk for Cold-Related Illness

Thin, highly conditioned athletes may be prone to cold-related illness because they have less fat to help insulate their bodies. Dehydrated athletes are also at risk.

| | | | | | | | | | | Temperature (°F) | | | | | | | | |
|---|---|---|---|---|---|---|---|---|---|---|---|---|---|---|---|---|---|---|
| **Calm** | **40** | **35** | **30** | **25** | **20** | **15** | **10** | **5** | **0** | **-5** | **-10** | **-15** | **-20** | **-25** | **-30** | **-35** | **-40** | **-45** |
| **5** | 36 | 31 | 25 | 19 | 13 | 7 | 1 | -5 | -11 | -16 | -22 | -28 | -34 | -40 | -46 | -52 | -57 | -63 |
| **10** | 34 | 27 | 21 | 15 | 9 | 3 | -4 | -10 | -16 | -22 | -28 | -35 | -41 | -47 | -53 | -59 | -66 | -72 |
| **15** | 32 | 25 | 19 | 13 | 6 | 0 | -7 | -13 | -19 | -26 | -32 | -39 | -45 | -51 | -58 | -64 | -71 | -77 |
| **20** | 30 | 24 | 17 | 11 | 4 | -2 | -9 | -15 | -22 | -29 | -35 | -42 | -48 | -55 | -61 | -68 | -74 | -81 |
| **25** | 29 | 23 | 16 | 9 | 3 | -4 | -11 | -17 | -24 | -31 | -37 | -44 | -51 | -58 | -64 | -71 | -78 | -84 |
| **30** | 28 | 22 | 15 | 8 | 1 | -5 | -12 | -19 | -26 | -33 | -39 | -46 | -53 | -60 | -67 | -73 | -80 | -87 |
| **35** | 28 | 21 | 14 | 7 | 0 | -7 | -14 | -21 | -27 | -34 | -41 | -48 | -55 | -62 | -69 | -76 | -82 | -89 |
| **40** | 27 | 20 | 13 | 6 | -1 | -8 | -15 | -22 | -29 | -36 | -43 | -50 | -57 | -64 | -71 | -78 | -84 | -91 |
| **45** | 26 | 19 | 12 | 5 | -2 | -9 | -16 | -23 | -30 | -37 | -44 | -51 | -58 | -65 | -72 | -79 | -86 | -93 |
| **50** | 26 | 19 | 12 | 4 | -3 | -10 | -17 | -24 | -31 | -38 | -45 | -52 | -60 | -67 | -74 | -81 | -88 | -95 |
| **55** | 25 | 18 | 11 | 4 | -3 | -11 | -18 | -25 | -32 | -39 | -46 | -54 | -61 | -68 | -75 | -82 | -89 | -97 |
| **60** | 25 | 17 | 10 | 3 | -4 | -11 | -19 | -26 | -33 | -40 | -48 | -55 | -62 | -69 | -76 | -84 | -91 | -98 |

The left axis is labeled **Wind (mph)**.

Frostbite times: ☐ 30 minutes ☐ 10 minutes ■ 5 minutes

Wind Chill (°F) = $35.74 + 0.6215T - 35.75(V^{0.16}) + 0.4275T(V^{0.16})$
Where T = Air Temperature (°F); V = Wind Speed (mph)

**Figure 11.3** National Weather Service windchill temperature index.

Source: National Weather Service. Available: https://www.weather.gov/safety/cold-wind-chill-chart.

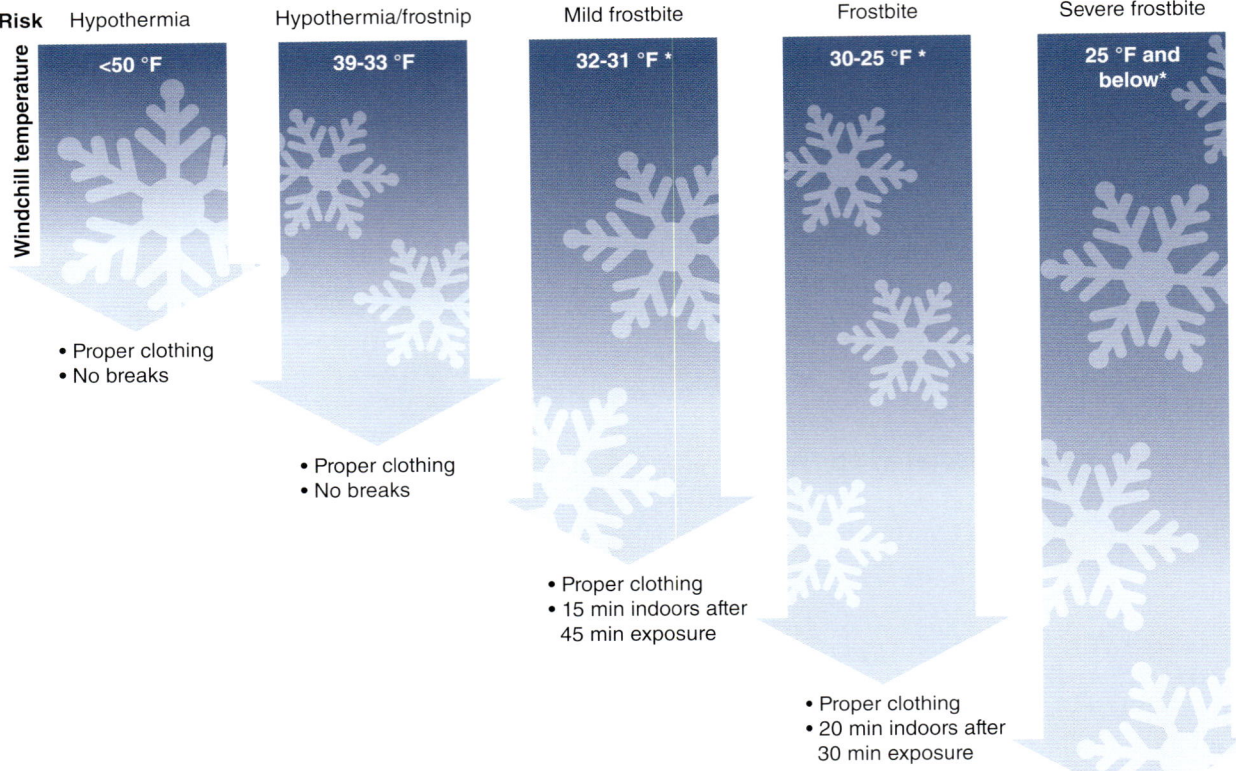

| Risk | Hypothermia | Hypothermia/frostnip | Mild frostbite | Frostbite | Severe frostbite |
|---|---|---|---|---|---|

*When windchill is below 31 °F, modify activity and rewarming procedures as necessary.

**Figure 11.4**   Sample cold participation policy.

Adapted from Castellani et al. (2006).

## Identifying and Treating Cold-Related Illnesses

Frostbite and hypothermia occur in varying degrees of severity, advancing from mild to severe. Each stage has specific signs and symptoms that will dictate the first aid that you administer. For first aid protocols for these illnesses, see the Frostbite and Hypothermia flowcharts in the appendix.

**SAFETY MEASURE**

**For Frostbite**

Do not rub or massage frostbitten areas, apply ice to frostbitten areas, or allow frostbitten tissue to refreeze. Doing any of these things can worsen an athlete's condition.

# FROSTBITE

Frostbite is a condition in which tissues freeze and blood vessels constrict. It is caused by exposure of body parts to cold. There are three stages of frostbite: frostnip (first degree), superficial frostbite (second degree), and deep frostbite (third degree).

When experiencing frostnip, the skin will turn red and feel cold to the touch. Superficial frostbite involves localized freezing of the skin and the superficial tissues below it. The nose, ears, toes, and fingers are especially prone to superficial frostbite and may include red or flushed skin that turns white, gray, or pale. Additional signs and symptoms of superficial frostbite include firm, white, and waxy skin; and blisters. The skin may appear tinted purple when the area is rewarmed. Deep frostbite begins superficially, then it advances to deep tissues such as muscles and tendons. Deep frostbite may present with blisters and bluish skin, and the frostbitten area may seem very cold and stiff.

First aid for potential first- or second-degree frostbite includes moving the athlete to a warm area, not allowing the athlete to walk on frostbitten feet, and removing wet and cold clothing. Call the athlete's parent or guardian immediately. Monitor and treat the athlete for shock if necessary, and call for emergency medical assistance if shock occurs. Rewarming should take place only if medical assistance will be delayed or if no risk of refreezing exists. If rewarming is initiated and the area refreezes, it could cause more damage. For potential third-degree frostbite, send for emergency medical assistance immediately, then proceed with guidelines for first- and second-degree frostbite. Monitor breathing, and provide CPR if needed.

An athlete suspected of sustaining a frostbite injury should be released by the appropriate health care provider before returning to activity. To prevent frostbite in athletes, monitor weather conditions during practice and halt practice or change to an indoor location if the weather is cold; ensure athletes wear appropriate clothing during practice; and encourage athletes to stay active at practice.

# HYPOTHERMIA

Hypothermia is a condition in which the body temperature drops below 95 degrees Fahrenheit. It is caused by prolonged exposure to a wet, windy, and cold environment; extreme fatigue, such as that experienced after competition in a marathon or triathlon; or dehydration. Mild hypothermia (core temperature of 95 to 90 degrees Fahrenheit) can show the following signs and symptoms: loss of coordination, loss of sensation, drowsiness, shivering, pale and hard skin, numbness, irritability, mild confusion, depression, withdrawn behavior, slow and irregular pulse, slowed breathing, sluggish movements, inability to walk, and difficulty speaking. Moderate hypothermia (core temperature of 89 to 86 degrees Fahrenheit) can show the following signs and symptoms: hallucinations, dilated pupils, decreasing pulse rate, or decreasing respiratory rate. Severe hypothermia (core temperature of 85 degrees Fahrenheit and below) could show unresponsiveness, respiratory arrest, or erratic or no pulse.

First aid for hypothermia includes checking for responsiveness and normal breathing, sending for emergency medical assistance regardless of severity, and providing CPR if the athlete is not responsive. Move the athlete to a warm area, gently remove cold and wet clothing, and wrap the athlete in blankets. Monitor breathing, and treat for shock as needed.

An athlete with suspected hypothermia cannot return to activity until examined and released by a health care provider. Prevention of hypothermia includes monitoring weather conditions at practices or games, ensuring athletes wear proper clothing during practices or games, and moving practice to a different location if conditions require.

## Lightning-Related Injuries

According to the U.S. National Weather Service, individuals in recreation activities and sports comprise two-thirds of all lightning injuries in the United States (NWS n.d.-b). Common sites for these injuries include athletic fields, golf courses, and swimming pools. Metal bats, fences, benches and bleachers, trees, and water are good conductors of lightning. Athletes, staff, and spectators are vulnerable to lightning while around these objects. Because lightning tends to strike taller objects, standing in an open playing field increases the risk of a lightning injury. Seeking shelter under a tree is also risky because lightning can travel through the tree to nearby objects. To minimize the risk of lightning injuries, develop a lightning safety policy.

# LIGHTNING INJURY

A direct or indirect hit by lightning can cause a wide variety of injuries, such as burns, fractures, or cardiac arrest. Signs and symptoms of lightning injury could include headache, dizziness, disorientation, burns at the point of entry and exit, or unresponsiveness. First aid should include quickly moving the athlete to a safe area, away from lightning, while also being mindful of any other injuries. Send for emergency medical assistance, monitor breathing, and provide CPR if needed. You should monitor and treat for shock as needed, and remove smoldering clothing, shoes, and accessories such as a belt to prevent burns. If breathing is present and no fractures are suspected, place an unresponsive or incoherent athlete in the recovery position (see chapter 4) to allow fluids and vomit to drain from the mouth.

An athlete cannot return to activity until examined and released by a health care provider. To help prevent lightning injuries, develop a lightning injury prevention plan, and stop activities when thunder occurs (even without lightning). If you hear thunder or see lightning, move everyone to a safe location. Wait 30 minutes after the last lightning strike or clap of thunder before continuing activity.

## Chapter 11 Recap

❑ What are the five pillars of heat injury prevention?

❑ What are the three common types of heat illness and what are their signs and symptoms?

❑ What steps can be taken to prevent all heat-related illnesses?

❑ What steps can be taken to prevent cold-related illnesses?

❑ Define hypothermia and list the first steps for managing hypothermia.

❑ How can you prevent the possibility of a lightning strike?

# CHAPTER 12

# UPPER BODY MUSCULOSKELETAL INJURIES

## IN THIS CHAPTER, YOU WILL LEARN THE FOLLOWING:

- How to recognize various upper body musculoskeletal injuries
- What first aid care to provide for each of these injuries
- How to prevent various upper body musculoskeletal injuries
- What conditions are required before an injured athlete can return to play

## INJURIES IN THIS CHAPTER

Sports that involve throwing, swinging, lifting, catching, pushing, or pulling place a lot of demand on the upper body, shoulders, arms, wrists, and hands. Consider this scenario: You are a high school boys' baseball coach. A youth baseball pitcher has been going to pitching lessons with a private coach all year while playing club baseball. He wants to play on your team also, but he is complaining of pain on the inside of his elbow; he states that his pitching coach is concerned about his lack of velocity lately. What would you do in this situation?

Before discussing the details of injuries in this chapter, here is an overview of the common areas of injury in the upper body:

- Acute shoulder injuries are those that occur suddenly, and they typically occur in football and wrestling. Chronic shoulder injuries are those that develop gradually, and they typically occur in volleyball, swimming, baseball, and softball. In the 2021-22 school year, shoulder injuries accounted for 14 percent of injuries among high school wrestlers, and they accounted for 11.8 percent of all injuries sustained by high school baseball players (Collins, Robison, and Burus 2022). For a summary of first aid care for these injuries, see the flowcharts titled Shoulder Fracture or Sprain, and Shoulder Strain in the appendix.

- The upper arm bone (humerus) and the muscles that span its length are subject to direct blows, twisting (torsion), and tension injuries in sports. Specifically, acute injuries to the upper arm include fractures, and biceps and triceps strains. In addition, repetitive pushing, pulling, and lifting activities can irritate muscle tendons over time, leading to chronic upper arm injuries such as biceps or triceps tendinitis.

- In contact sports, the ribs are subjected to being jabbed by elbows; crunched by helmets; pelted by pucks, baseballs, or softballs; and crushed by the weight of other players. As a coach, you need to be able to tell the difference between a potentially life-threatening rib fracture and a simple contusion.

- The elbow is injured most often in tennis, baseball, softball, and wrestling. Tennis, baseball, and softball players are particularly susceptible to chronic injuries such as tennis elbow, whereas wrestlers and gymnasts are more prone to acute injuries such as dislocation. In the 2021-22 school year, 9.6 percent of all injuries in high school wrestlers occurred at the elbow, and baseball players had an elbow injury rate of 19.9 percent (Collins, Robison, and Burus 2022). For the first aid care protocol for these injuries, see the Acute Elbow Injury flowchart in the appendix.

- Almost all of the sport injuries involving the forearm, wrist, and hand are acute. In the 2021-22 school year, forearm, wrist, and hand injuries accounted for the following: boys' basketball (7.4%), girls' basketball (6.6%), baseball (9.6%), and football (8.9%) (Collins, Robison, and Burus 2022). For a summary of these injuries, see the Acute Forearm, Wrist, or Hand Injury flowchart in the appendix.

First aid decisions for musculoskeletal injuries often depend on the severity of the injury, which is classified as mild (Grade I), moderate (Grade II), or severe (Grade III). (To review the definitions and illustrations of Grade I, II, and III strains and sprains, see chapter 3.) In addition, many of the first aid protocols in this chapter include icing and immobilizing (splinting) the injured part. To review guidelines for ice application and splinting, see chapter 5.

# CLAVICLE FRACTURE

A clavicle fracture is a crack or break in the collarbone (clavicle). It is caused by a direct blow to the front or side of the shoulder.

**Signs and Symptoms**

- Pain in front of the shoulder along the clavicle
- Pain when raising the arm
- Grating sensation
- Deformity
- Swelling
- Point tenderness

## FIRST AID

1. Immobilize the arm with a sling, and secure the arm to the body with an elastic wrap (see figure 12.1).
2. If bones are grossly displaced or protruding through the skin, or if the athlete is experiencing shock, send for emergency medical assistance.
3. After immobilizing, apply ice to the injury for 15 minutes, then send the athlete to the appropriate health care provider (if shock does not occur).

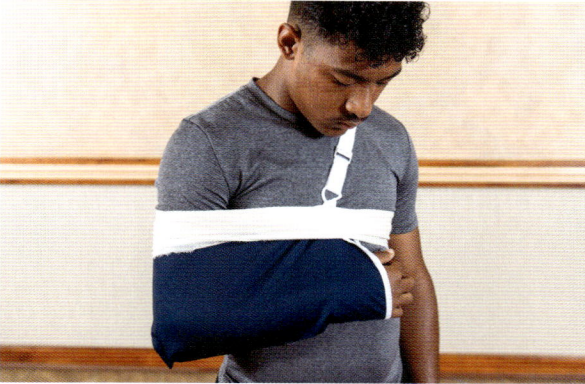

**Figure 12.1**    Sling and wrap immobilization for a clavicle fracture.

**Playing Status**

The athlete cannot return to activity until examined and released by a health care provider; the shoulder is free of pain; and they have full strength, flexibility, and range of motion in the shoulder.

## PREVENTION

- Requirement for wearing properly fitted shoulder pads (if applicable to the sport)

# ACROMIOCLAVICULAR (AC) JOINT SPRAIN

Acromioclavicular (AC) joint sprain (also called shoulder separation or AC joint separation) is a stretch or tear of the ligaments that connect the clavicle to the shoulder blade (AC joint) (see figure 12.2). Causes include a direct blow to the top or side of the shoulder, or a fall on an outstretched arm.

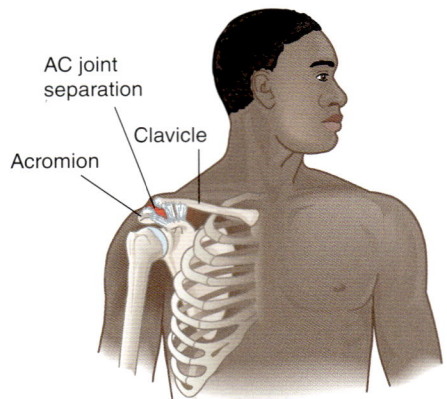

AC joint separation

Clavicle

Acromion

**Figure 12.2** AC joint sprain.

## Signs and Symptoms

### Grade I

- Mild pain or tenderness along the outer edge of the clavicle
- Mild pain with raising the arm overhead
- Mild pain with reaching the arm across the body
- Slight elevation of the outer edge of the clavicle

### Grades II and III

- Moderate to severe pain or tenderness along the outer edge of the clavicle
- Moderate to severe pain with raising the arm overhead
- Moderate to severe pain with reaching the arm across the body
- Moderate to severe elevation of the outer edge of the clavicle

## FIRST AID

### Grade I

1. Rest the athlete from painful activities.
2. Apply ice for 15 minutes.
3. Refer the athlete to the appropriate health care provider if symptoms and signs worsen (or occur more often, especially with daily activities) or do not subside within a few days.

### Grades II and III

1. Immobilize the arm with a sling, and secure the arm to the body with an elastic wrap (see figure 12.1).
2. Monitor the athlete, treat them for shock if needed, and send for emergency medical assistance if shock occurs.
3. Apply ice for 15 minutes, and send the athlete to the appropriate health care provider (if shock does not occur).

### Playing Status

- For a Grade I AC joint sprain, the athlete can return to activity if signs and symptoms subside; the shoulder is free of pain; and the athlete has full strength, flexibility, and range of motion in the shoulder. If the athlete is sent to a health care provider, they cannot return to activity until examined and released by the health care provider. When returning to activity, the athlete may benefit from wearing a protective pad over the injury.

- For a Grade II or Grade III AC joint sprain, the athlete cannot return to activity until examined and released by a health care provider; the shoulder is free of pain; and they have full strength, flexibility, and range of motion in the shoulder. When returning to activity, the athlete may benefit from wearing a protective pad over the injury.

## PREVENTION

- Requirement for wearing properly fitted shoulder pads (if applicable to the sport)

# STERNOCLAVICULAR (SC) SPRAIN

Sternoclavicular (SC) sprain (also called shoulder separation) is a stretch or tear of the ligaments that connect the clavicle to the breastbone (sternum). It is caused by a direct blow that pushes the clavicle forward or backward or by falling on an outstretched arm (see figure 12.3). Signs and symptoms of a Grade I SC sprain include mild pain at the attachment of the clavicle to the sternum when moving the arm across the chest, when reaching the arm backward while raised to shoulder level, and when shrugging the shoulders; or slight deformity at the attachment of the clavicle to the sternum. Signs and symptoms of Grade II and Grade III SC sprains include dizziness (if the clavicle is pushed backward at the SC joint, it can potentially damage major blood vessels to the brain); moderate to severe pain at the attachment of the clavicle to the sternum when moving the arm across the chest, when reaching the arm backward while raised to shoulder level, and when shrugging the shoulders; moderate to severe deformity at the attachment of the clavicle to the sternum; or unresponsiveness, or respiratory or cardiac arrest (if the clavicle is displaced backward toward the neck).

First aid for forward-displaced Grade I SC sprain includes resting the athlete from painful activity, applying ice for 15 minutes, and referring the athlete to the appropriate health care provider if symptoms and signs worsen (or occur more often, especially with daily activities) or do not subside within a few days. For backward displacement of the clavicle, rest the athlete from all activity, apply ice to the injury for 15 minutes, and refer the athlete to the appropriate health care provider.

First aid for forward-displaced Grade II and Grade III SC sprains includes immobilizing the arm with a sling and securing the arm to the body with an elastic wrap, monitoring the athlete and treating them for shock if needed, sending for emergency medical assistance (if shock occurs), applying ice for 15 minutes, and referring the athlete to the appropriate health care provider (if shock does not occur). For a backward-displaced Grade II or Grade III SC sprain, you should send for emergency medical assistance, monitor breathing and provide CPR if needed, monitor the athlete and treat them for shock if needed, and keep the athlete from moving the arm.

The athlete cannot return to activity until examined and released by a health care provider, and must demonstrate full range of motion and strength of the shoulder. The athlete should also consider wearing a protective pad over the injury site. To help prevent SC sprains, encourage athletes to wear properly fitted shoulder pads in sports that require them. Shoulder pads should be regularly maintained in accordance with National Operating Committee on Standards for Athletic Equipment (NOCSAE) or the manufacturer's instructions.

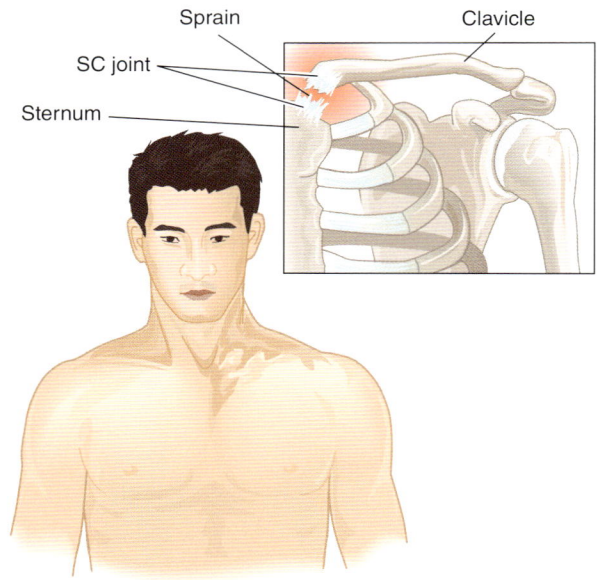

**Figure 12.3**   SC sprain.

# SHOULDER DISLOCATION OR SUBLUXATION

In a shoulder dislocation, the upper arm bone (humerus) pops out of the shoulder socket; in a shoulder subluxation, the humerus pops out of the shoulder socket and then spontaneously shifts back into the socket. Causes of these injuries include a backward blow to the upper arm while it is raised to the side (see figure 12.4), a forceful contraction of the shoulder muscles, or a fall on an outstretched arm. Signs and symptoms of a subluxation or dislocation could include intense pain where the humerus connects to the clavicle, a sense of looseness or giving away, tingling in the arm or hand, or the athlete reporting that they felt or heard a pop. A dislocation could present with inability to move the arm, flat (not rounded) appearance of the shoulder, the arm being held slightly out from the body, lack of sensation in the arm or hand (caused by the displaced bone pinching a nerve), or a bluish arm or hand (caused by the displaced bone pinching the blood supply).

To provide first aid for a subluxated shoulder, immobilize the arm with a sling, and secure the arm to the body with an elastic wrap. Monitor the athlete, treat them for shock if necessary, and send for emergency medical assistance if shock occurs. If shock does not occur, apply ice to the injury for 15 minutes, and refer the athlete to the appropriate health care provider. To provide first aid for a dislocated shoulder, send for emergency medical assistance. If emergency medical assistance is delayed more than 20 minutes, stabilize the arm in the position found. Do not try to put the humerus back into the socket. Apply ice for 15 minutes, and monitor and treat for shock if needed until help arrives.

The athlete cannot return to activity until examined and released by a health care provider, and must demonstrate full range of motion and strength of the shoulder. To help prevent shoulder subluxations and dislocations, athletes should participate in shoulder-strengthening programs.

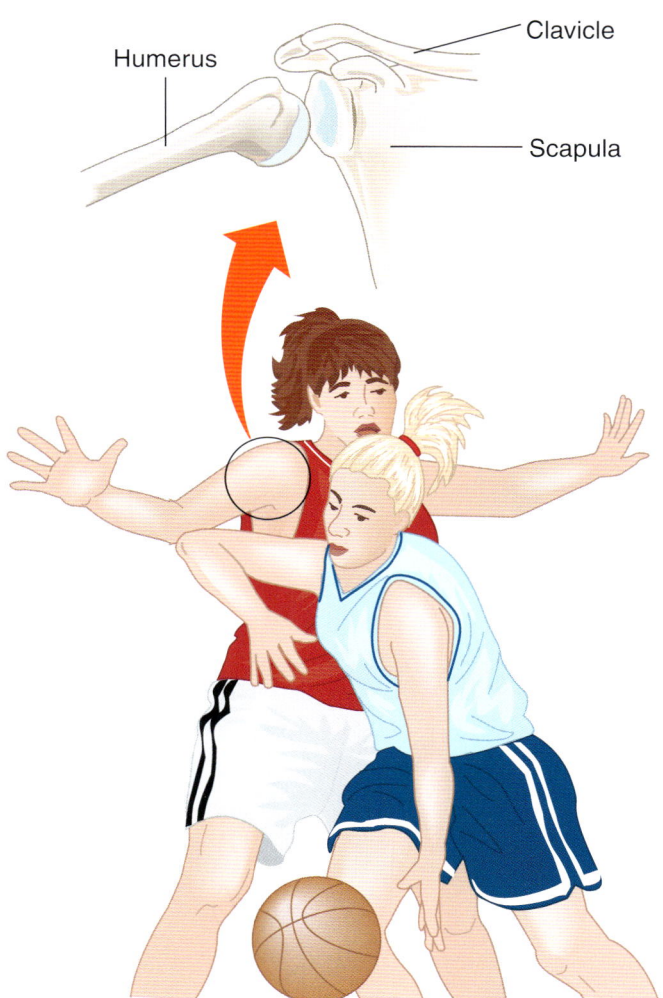

**Figure 12.4** A shoulder can be dislocated if the athlete sustains a backward blow to the upper arm while it is raised to the side.

# ROTATOR CUFF STRAIN

A rotator cuff strain is a stretch or tear of the muscles used in throwing, swimming, and hitting motions and essential to holding the humerus in the socket (see figure 12.5). Causes include throwing sidearm, swinging a racket or throwing with just the arm and not the body, weak and tight shoulder muscles, or overuse.

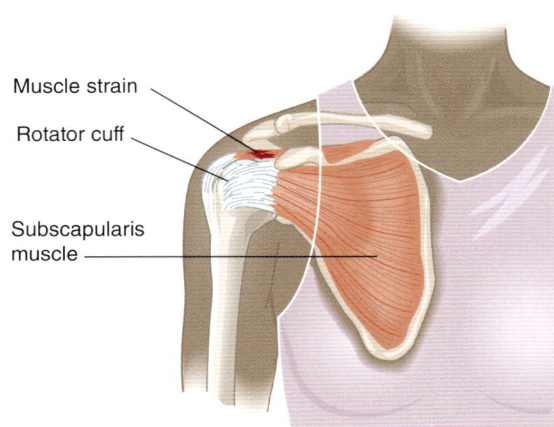

Muscle strain

Rotator cuff

Subscapularis muscle

**Figure 12.5**    Rotator cuff strain.

### Signs and Symptoms

### All Grades

- Pain with swimming, throwing, spiking, serving, and forehand and backhand motions
- Pain with lifting the arm overhead

### Grade I

- Mild tenderness over the front of the shoulder, just below the outer edge of the clavicle, along the scapula, or the outside of the shoulder
- Muscle tightness

### Grades II and III

- Indentation or lump where the muscle or tendon is torn
- Inability to throw, spike, serve, or hit a forehand or backhand with a normal motion
- Moderate to severe tenderness over the front of the shoulder, just below the outer edge of the clavicle, along the scapula, or the outside of the shoulder
- Arm weakness
- Swelling
- Muscle spasm

## FIRST AID

### Grade I

1. Rest the athlete from painful activities.
2. Apply ice for 15 minutes.
3. Refer the athlete to the appropriate health care provider if symptoms and signs worsen (or occur more often, especially with daily activities) or do not subside within a few days.

### Grades II and III

1. Immobilize the arm with a sling, and secure the arm to the body with an elastic wrap (see figure 12.1).
2. Monitor and treat for shock if needed, and send for emergency medical assistance if shock occurs.
3. Apply ice for 15 minutes, and send the athlete to the appropriate health care provider (if shock does not occur).

### Playing Status

- For a Grade I rotator cuff strain, the athlete can return to activity if signs and symptoms subside; the shoulder is free of pain; and the athlete has full strength, flexibility, and range of motion in the shoulder. If the athlete is sent to a health care provider, they cannot return to activity until examined and released by the health care provider.
- For a Grade II or Grade III rotator cuff strain, the athlete cannot return to activity until examined and released by a health care provider; the shoulder is free of pain; and they have full strength, flexibility, and range of motion in the shoulder.

## PREVENTION

- Preseason strengthening and stretching exercises for the shoulder
- Throwing progressions for distance and speed

# PECTORAL MUSCLE STRAIN

Pectoral muscle strain is a stretch or tear of the muscles used in moving the arm across the chest (see figure 12.6). Causes include throwing sidearm, swinging a racket or throwing with the arm only, weak and inflexible chest and shoulder muscles, or lifting weights that are too heavy or using incorrect technique (e.g., lowering the elbows too far) in the bench press.

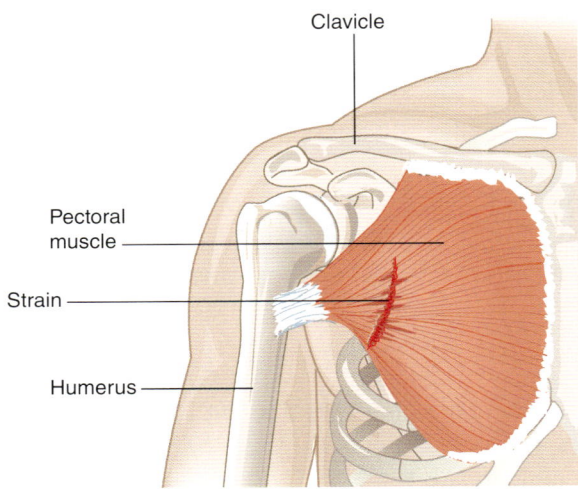

**Figure 12.6**    Pectoral muscle strain.

## Signs and Symptoms

### All Grades

- Pain with swimming, spiking, serving, sidearm throwing, forehand motions, push-ups, and bench and incline presses
- Pain with reaching the arm across the chest
- Pain when the arm is stretched straight out to the side
- Pain over the front of the shoulder or chest, below the clavicle
- Slight muscle tightness

### Grade I

- Mild point tenderness

### Grades II and III

- Indentation or lump where the muscle or tendon is torn
- Inability to throw, spike, serve, or hit a forehand with normal motion
- Arm weakness
- Moderate to severe point tenderness
- Swelling
- Muscle spasm

## FIRST AID

### Grade I

1. Rest the athlete from painful activities.
2. Apply ice for 15 minutes.
3. Refer the athlete to the appropriate health care provider if symptoms and signs worsen (or occur more often, especially with daily activities) or do not subside within a few days.

### Grades II and III

1. Immobilize the arm with a sling, and secure the arm to the body with an elastic wrap (see figure 12.1).
2. Monitor and treat for shock if needed, and send for emergency medical assistance if shock occurs.
3. Apply ice for 15 minutes, and send the athlete to the appropriate health care provider (if shock does not occur).

### Playing Status

- For a Grade I pectoral muscle strain, the athlete can return to activity if signs and symptoms subside; the shoulder is free of pain; and the athlete has full strength, flexibility, and range of motion in the shoulder. If the athlete is sent to a health care provider, they cannot return to activity until examined and released by the health care provider.
- For a Grade II or Grade III pectoral muscle strain, the athlete cannot return to activity until examined and released by a health care provider; the shoulder is free of pain; and they have full strength, flexibility, and range of motion in the shoulder.

## PREVENTION

- Preseason strengthening and stretching exercises for the shoulder and pectoral muscles
- Gradual throwing progressions for distance and speed

# DELTOID MUSCLE STRAIN

A deltoid muscle strain is a stretch or tear of the muscles around the front, back, or side of the shoulder (see figure 12.7). Causes include weak and inflexible shoulder muscles and throwing sidearm.

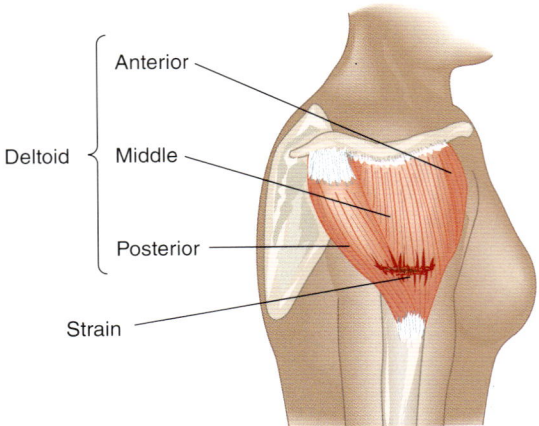

**Figure 12.7**    Deltoid muscle strain.

## Signs and Symptoms

### All Grades

- Pain with throwing, spiking, serving, and swimming
- Pain when raising the arm forward, to the side, or backward
- Slight muscle tightness

### Grade I

- Mild point tenderness over the front, side, or back of the shoulder below the clavicle or the spine of the scapula

### Grades II and III

- Indentation or lump where the muscle or tendon is torn
- Inability to throw, spike, or serve with a normal motion
- Moderate to severe point tenderness over the front, side, or back of the shoulder below the clavicle or the spine of the scapula
- Arm weakness
- Swelling
- Muscle spasm

## FIRST AID

### Grade I

1. Rest the athlete from painful activities.
2. Apply ice for 15 minutes.
3. Refer the athlete to the appropriate health care provider if symptoms and signs worsen (or occur more often, especially with daily activities) or do not subside within a few days.

### Grades II and III

1. Immobilize the arm with a sling, and secure the arm to the body with an elastic wrap (see figure 12.1).
2. Monitor and treat for shock if needed, and send for emergency medical assistance if shock occurs.
3. Apply ice to the injury for 15 minutes, and send the athlete to the appropriate health care provider (if shock does not occur).

### Playing Status

- For a Grade I deltoid muscle strain, the athlete can return to activity if signs and symptoms subside; the shoulder is free of pain; and the athlete has full strength, flexibility, and range of motion in the shoulder. If the athlete is sent to a health care provider, they cannot return to activity until examined and released by the health care provider.
- For a Grade II or Grade III deltoid muscle strain, the athlete cannot return to activity until examined and released by a health care provider; the shoulder is free of pain; and they have full strength, flexibility, and range of motion in the shoulder.

## PREVENTION

- Preseason strengthening and stretching exercises for the shoulder

# UPPER TRAPEZIUS MUSCLE STRAIN

Upper trapezius muscle strain is a stretch or tear of the trapezius muscle. The trapezius (also called trap) muscle extends from the base of the skull to the outer tips of the shoulders and down to just above the low back. Different portions of the muscle shrug the shoulders, extend the head backward, and squeeze the shoulder blades together (see figure 12.8). Causes for strain in this muscle include weak upper back or neck muscles, tight chest muscles, lifting weights that are too heavy, or performing weighted shoulder shrugs incorrectly.

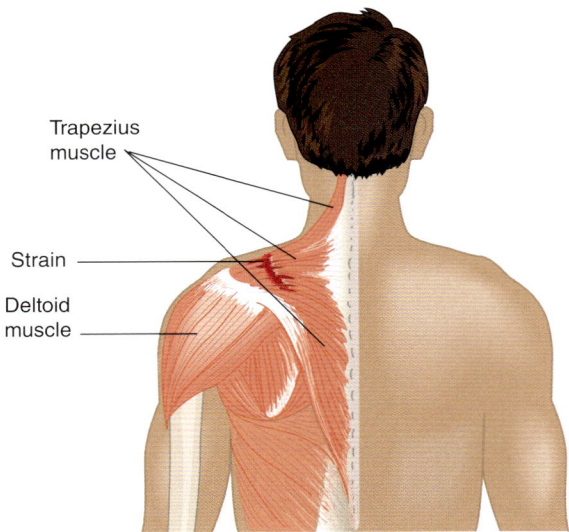

**Figure 12.8**   Upper trapezius muscle strain.

## Signs and Symptoms

### Grade I

- Mild pain with shrugging the shoulders, extending the head backward, and squeezing the shoulder blades together
- Mild pain with stretching the arm across the chest
- Slight muscle tightness at the back of the neck, just above the shoulder blade, or down the upper and mid back
- Mild point tenderness at the neck, just above the shoulder blades, or down the upper and mid back

### Grades II and III

- Moderate to severe pain with shrugging the shoulders, extending the head backward, and squeezing the shoulder blades together
- Moderate to severe pain with stretching the arm across the chest
- Indentation or lump where the muscle or tendon is torn
- Inability to throw, spike, serve, or hit a forehand with a normal motion
- Moderate to severe point tenderness at the neck, just above the shoulder blades, or down the upper and mid back
- Weakness in extending the upper arm backward or pushing the head backward
- Swelling
- Muscle spasm

## FIRST AID

### Grade I

1. Rest the athlete from painful activities.
2. Apply ice for 15 minutes.
3. Refer the athlete to the appropriate health care provider if symptoms and signs worsen (or occur more often, especially with daily activities) or do not subside within a few days.

### Grades II and III

1. Immobilize the arm with a sling, and secure the arm to the body with an elastic wrap (see figure 12.1).
2. Monitor and treat for shock if needed, and send for emergency medical assistance if shock occurs.
3. Apply ice to the injury for 15 minutes, and send the athlete to the appropriate health care provider (if shock does not occur).

### Playing Status

- For a Grade I upper trapezius muscle strain, the athlete can return to activity if signs and symptoms subside; the neck, shoulder, and upper back are free of pain; and the athlete has full strength, flexibility, and range of motion in the neck, shoulder, and upper back. If the athlete is sent to a health care provider, they cannot return to activity until examined and released by the health care provider.
- For a Grade II or Grade III upper trapezius muscle strain, the athlete cannot return to activity until examined and released by a health care provider; the neck, shoulder, and upper back are free of pain; and the athlete has full strength, flexibility, and range of motion in the neck, shoulder, and upper back.

## PREVENTION

- Preseason strengthening exercises for neck and upper back muscles
- Preseason stretching exercises for pectoral and latissimus dorsi muscles

# RIB FRACTURE OR CONTUSION

A rib fracture or contusion is a break or bruise of a rib. It is caused by a direct blow to the rib cage (see figure 12.9).

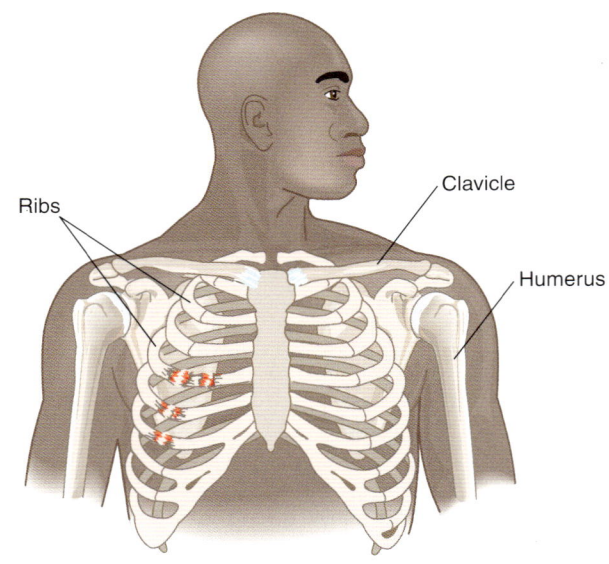

**Figure 12.9**  Rib fracture.

## Signs and Symptoms

### Contusion

- Mild pain with breathing, coughing, sneezing, or laughing
- Swelling
- Bruising
- Mild point tenderness over the site of the injury

### Fracture

- Moderate to severe pain with breathing, coughing, sneezing, or laughing
- Deformity
- Pain when the rib cage is gently compressed on either side of the injury
- Moderate to severe point tenderness over the site of the injury
- Swelling
- Breathing difficulties (if fractured rib punctures lung)

## FIRST AID

### Contusion

1. Rest the athlete from all activities.
2. Apply ice for 15 minutes, and send the athlete to the appropriate health care provider.

### Fracture

1. Rest the athlete from all activities.
2. If the athlete has breathing difficulties, has an open chest wound, has a backward-displaced (toward internal organs) rib, or is experiencing shock, call for emergency medical assistance.
3. If none of the previous signs and symptoms are present, then apply ice for 15 minutes, and send the athlete to the appropriate health care provider.

### Playing Status

The athlete cannot return to activity until examined and released by a health care provider. If the athlete returns to contact sports, the injured area should be padded.

### PREVENTION

- Requirement to wear rib pads (if applicable to the sport)

# RHOMBOID MUSCLE STRAIN

Rhomboid muscle strain is a stretch or tear of the rhomboid, a muscle between the shoulder blade (scapula) and spine that pulls the scapula toward the spine (see figure 12.10). This injury is caused by weak upper back muscles and tight chest muscles. Signs and symptoms of a Grade I rhomboid strain can include mild pain when shrugging the shoulders and squeezing the scapulae together, mild pain when stretching the arm across the chest, or mild muscle tightness and point tenderness between the scapula and spine. Signs and symptoms of a Grade II or Grade III rhomboid muscle strain may include moderate to severe pain when shrugging the shoulders and squeezing the scapulae together, moderate to severe pain when stretching the arm across the chest, moderate to severe pain or point tenderness between the scapula and spine, an indentation or lump where the muscle or tendon is torn, inability to swim or hit a backhand with a normal motion, weakness in squeezing the scapulae together and reaching the upper arm backward (while raised out to the side at shoulder level), swelling, or muscle spasm.

First aid for a Grade I rhomboid muscle strain includes resting the athlete from painful activities, applying ice for 15 minutes, and referring the athlete to the appropriate health care provider if symptoms and signs worsen (or occur more often, especially with daily activities) or do not subside within a few days. First aid for a Grade II or Grade III rhomboid strain includes immobilizing the arm with a sling and securing the arm to the body with an elastic wrap, monitoring and treating the athlete for shock if needed and sending for emergency medical assistance if shock occurs, or applying ice to the injury for 15 minutes and sending the athlete to the appropriate health care provider (if shock does not occur).

For a Grade I rhomboid muscle strain, the athlete can return to activity if signs and symptoms subside; the shoulder is free of pain; and the athlete has full strength, flexibility, and range of motion in the shoulder. If the athlete is sent to a health care provider, they cannot return to activity until examined and released by the health care provider. For a Grade II or Grade III strain, the athlete cannot return to activity until examined and released by a health care provider; the muscle is free of pain; and the athlete has full strength, flexibility, and range of motion in the shoulder. To help prevent rhomboid strains, encourage athletes to participate in strengthening exercises for the upper back and shoulders.

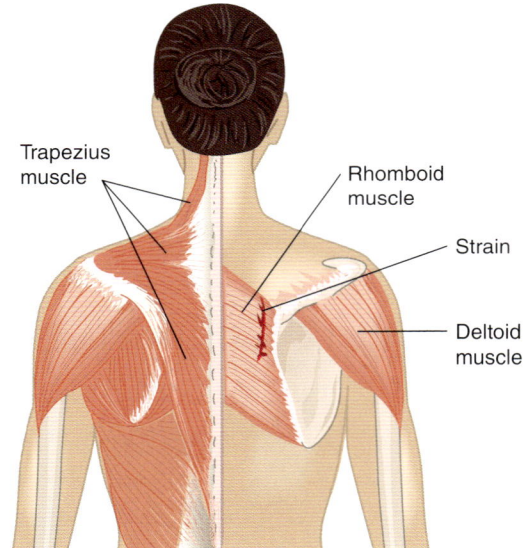

**Figure 12.10**  Rhomboid muscle strain.

# HUMERUS FRACTURE

A humerus fracture is a crack or break in the upper arm bone (humerus). It is caused by a direct blow, torsion, or compression (see figure 12.11). A humerus fracture could show the following signs and symptoms: severe pain and point tenderness; deformity; swelling; inability to move the arm; bluish skin on the forearm, wrist, hand, or fingers; or loss of sensation and tingling in the forearm, wrist, hand, or fingers.

First aid for a humerus fracture should include sending for emergency medical assistance, immobilizing the injury in the position found, monitoring breathing, and providing CPR if necessary. Monitor and treat for shock if needed, and apply ice for 15 minutes if shock does not occur.

The athlete cannot return to activity until examined and released by a health care provider. To help prevent humerus fractures, teach athletes to tuck their arm when they fall.

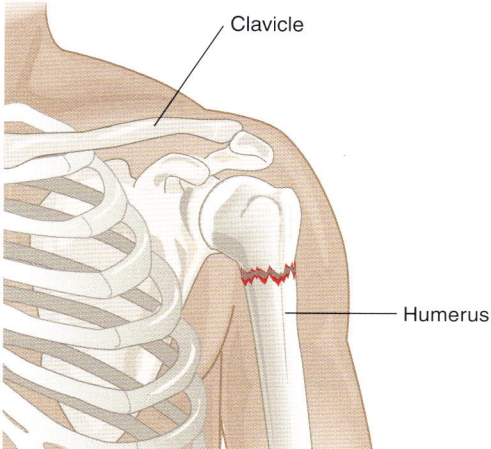

**Figure 12.11**    Humerus fracture.

# BICEPS MUSCLE STRAIN

A biceps muscle strain is a stretch or tear of the biceps, a muscle that bends the elbow. It is caused by a sudden forceful contraction or stretch of the muscle (see figure 12.12).

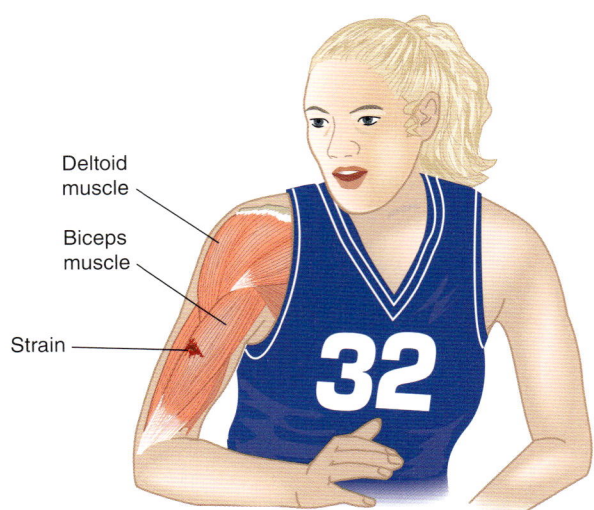

Deltoid muscle

Biceps muscle

Strain

**Figure 12.12**   Biceps muscle strain.

## Signs and Symptoms

### Grade I

- Mild pain or slight muscle tightness along the front of the upper arm
- Mild point tenderness
- Mild pain when bending the elbow
- Mild pain when the elbow is straight and the arm extends back past the body
- Mild pain when raising the upper arm forward

### Grades II and III

- Moderate to severe pain along the front of the upper arm
- Moderate to severe point tenderness
- Moderate to severe pain when bending the elbow
- Moderate to severe pain when the elbow is straight and the arm extends back past the body

- Moderate to severe pain when raising the upper arm forward
- Indentation or lump where the muscle or tendon is torn
- Inability to lift objects while bending the elbow (arm curl)
- Inability to bend or fully straighten the elbow
- Inability to raise the upper arm forward
- Swelling
- Discoloration (occurs several days after a partial or complete tear of the muscle)
- Muscle spasm

## FIRST AID

### Grade I

1. Rest the athlete from painful activities.
2. Apply ice for 15 minutes.
3. Refer the athlete to the appropriate health care provider if symptoms and signs worsen (or occur more often, especially with daily activities) or do not subside within a few days.

### Grades II and III

1. Immobilize the arm with a sling if tolerated.
2. Monitor and treat for shock if needed, and send for emergency medical assistance if shock occurs.
3. Apply ice for 15 minutes, and send the athlete to the appropriate health care provider (if shock does not occur).

### Playing Status

- For a Grade I biceps muscle strain, the athlete can return to activity if signs and symptoms subside; the biceps is free of pain; and the athlete has full range of motion in the shoulder and elbow, and full strength and flexibility in the biceps. If the athlete is sent to a health care provider, they cannot return to activity until examined and released by the health care provider.
- For a Grade II or Grade III biceps muscle strain, the athlete cannot return to activity until examined and released by a health care provider; the biceps is free of pain; and they have full range of motion in the shoulder and elbow, and full strength and flexibility in the biceps.

## PREVENTION

- Preseason strengthening and stretching exercises for the upper arm

# TRICEPS MUSCLE STRAIN

A triceps muscle strain is a stretch or tear of the triceps, a muscle that straightens the elbow and extends the upper arm backward (see figure 12.13). Causes include repeated forceful contraction or stretch of the triceps, and weak or inflexible triceps.

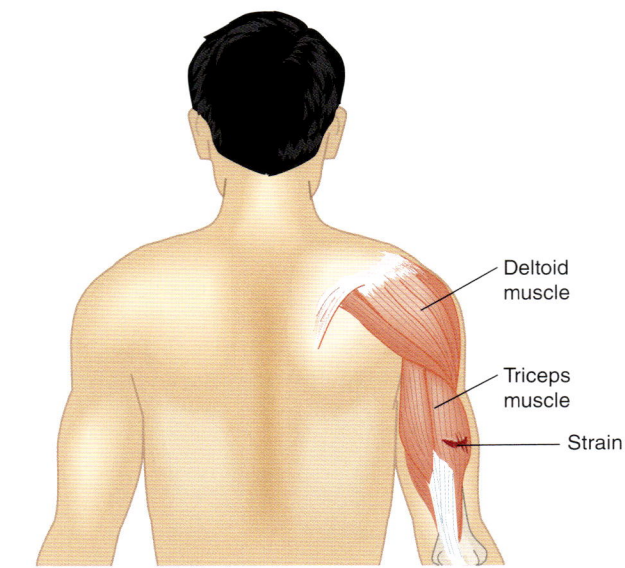

Deltoid muscle

Triceps muscle

Strain

**Figure 12.13**    Triceps muscle strain.

## Signs and Symptoms

### Grade I

- Mild pain or slight muscle tightness along the back of the upper arm
- Mild point tenderness
- Mild pain when extending the upper arm backward past the body
- Mild pain when straightening the elbow against resistance (triceps extension)
- Mild pain when the elbow is bent and the upper arm is stretched forward and up toward the head

### Grades II and III

- Moderate to severe pain along the back of the upper arm
- Moderate to severe point tenderness
- Moderate to severe pain when extending the upper arm backward past the body
- Moderate to severe pain when straightening the elbow against resistance (triceps extension)

- Moderate to severe pain when the elbow is bent and the upper arm is stretched forward and up toward the head
- Indentation or lump where the muscle or tendon is torn
- Inability to fully straighten or bend the elbow
- Swelling
- Discoloration (occurs several days after a partial or complete tear of the muscle)
- Muscle spasm

## FIRST AID

### Grade I

1. Rest the athlete from painful activities.
2. Apply ice for 15 minutes.
3. Refer the athlete to the appropriate health care provider if symptoms and signs worsen (or occur more often, especially with daily activities) or do not subside within a few days.

### Grades II and III

1. Immobilize the arm with a sling, if tolerated.
2. Monitor the athlete, treat them for shock if needed, and send for emergency medical assistance if shock occurs.
3. Apply ice for 15 minutes, and send the athlete to the appropriate health care provider (if shock does not occur).

### Playing Status

- For a Grade I triceps muscle strain, the athlete can return to activity if signs and symptoms subside; the triceps is free of pain; and the athlete has full range of motion in the shoulder and elbow, and full strength and flexibility in the triceps. If the athlete is sent to a health care provider, they cannot return to activity until examined and released by the health care provider.
- For a Grade II or Grade III triceps muscle strain, the athlete cannot return to activity until examined and released by a health care provider; the triceps is free of pain; and they have full range of motion in the shoulder and elbow, and full strength and flexibility in the triceps.

## PREVENTION

- Preseason strengthening and stretching exercises for the upper arm

# BICEPS TENDINITIS

Biceps tendinitis is inflammation in the biceps tendon. It is caused by repeated forceful contraction or stretch of the biceps, or a weak or inflexible biceps (see figure 12.14).

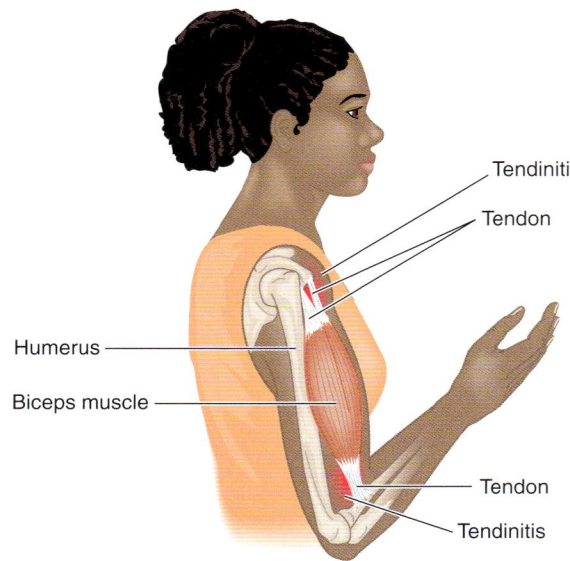

**Figure 12.14**   Biceps tendinitis.

## Signs and Symptoms

### Mild

- Mild pain or slight tenderness along the front of the upper arm near the shoulder or elbow
- Mild pain when raising the upper arm forward
- Mild pain when the elbow is straight and the arm is extended back past the body

### Moderate to Severe

- Moderate to severe pain or point tenderness along front of the upper arm near the shoulder or elbow
- Moderate to severe pain when raising the upper arm forward
- Moderate to severe pain when the elbow is straight and the arm is extended back past the body
- Decreased ability or inability to lift objects while bending the elbow and raising the upper arm
- Swelling

## FIRST AID

### Mild

1. Rest the athlete from painful activities.
2. Apply ice for 15 minutes.
3. Refer the athlete to the appropriate health care provider if symptoms and signs worsen (or occur more often, especially with daily activities) or do not subside within a few days.

### Moderate to Severe

1. Rest the arm from all activities.
2. Apply ice to the injury for 15 minutes, and send the athlete to the appropriate health care provider.

### Playing Status

- For mild biceps tendinitis, the athlete can return to activity if signs and symptoms subside; the tendon is free of pain; and the athlete has full range of motion in the shoulder and elbow, and full strength and flexibility in the biceps. If the athlete is sent to a health care provider, the athlete cannot return to activity until examined and released by the health care provider.
- For moderate to severe biceps tendinitis, the athlete cannot return to activity until examined and released by a health care provider; the tendon is free of pain; and the athlete has full range of motion in the shoulder and elbow, and full strength and flexibility in the biceps.

## PREVENTION

- Preseason strengthening and stretching exercises for the upper arm

# TRICEPS TENDINITIS

Triceps tendinitis is inflammation in the triceps tendon. It is caused by repeated forceful contraction or stretch of the triceps, or a weak or inflexible triceps (see figure 12.15).

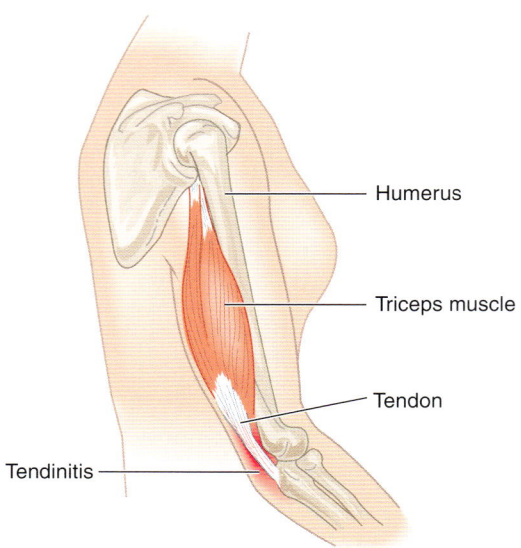

Humerus

Triceps muscle

Tendon

Tendinitis

**Figure 12.15** Triceps tendinitis.

## Signs and Symptoms

### Mild

- Mild pain along the back of the upper arm near the shoulder or elbow
- Slight point tenderness along the back of the elbow
- Mild pain when straightening the elbow
- Mild pain when the elbow is bent and the upper arm is stretched forward and up toward the head
- Mild pain when extending the upper arm backward

### Moderate to Severe

- Moderate to severe pain along the back of the upper arm near the shoulder or elbow
- Moderate to severe point tenderness along the back of the elbow
- Moderate to severe pain when straightening the elbow
- Moderate to severe pain when the elbow is bent and the upper arm is stretched forward and up toward the head
- Moderate to severe pain when extending the upper arm backward

- Decreased ability or inability to straighten the elbow against resistance (triceps extension)
- Decreased ability or inability to extend the upper arm backward
- Swelling

## FIRST AID

### Mild

1. Rest the athlete from painful activities.
2. Apply ice for 15 minutes.
3. Refer the athlete to the appropriate health care provider if symptoms and signs worsen (or occur more often, especially with daily activities) or do not subside within a few days.

### Moderate to Severe

1. Rest the arm from all activities.
2. Apply ice to the injury for 15 minutes, and send the athlete to the appropriate health care provider.

### Playing Status

- For mild triceps tendinitis, the athlete can return to activity if signs and symptoms subside; the elbow and triceps are free of pain; and the athlete has full range of motion in the elbow, and full strength and flexibility in the triceps. If the athlete is sent to a health care provider, the athlete cannot return to activity until examined and released by the health care provider.
- For moderate to severe triceps tendinitis, the athlete cannot return to activity until examined and released by a health care provider; the elbow and triceps are free of pain; and the athlete has full range of motion in the elbow, and full strength and flexibility in the triceps.

## PREVENTION

- Preseason strengthening and stretching exercises for the upper arm

# ELBOW FRACTURE

An elbow fracture is a break of any or all of the three elbow bones: the bottom of the humerus (figure 12.16), the radius, and the ulna. (The humerus is the upper arm bone; the radius and ulna make up the forearm.) This fracture can be caused by a direct blow to the area or by falling on an outstretched arm. Signs and symptoms of an elbow fracture include numbness around the area or down the forearm and hand (if the fracture injures nerves); severe pain; grating sensation at the site of injury; deformity; swelling; severe point tenderness at the site of injury; inability to bend or straighten the elbow; and bluish skin on the forearm, wrist, hand, or fingers (if the fracture injures blood vessels).

First aid for an elbow fracture should include sending for emergency medical assistance, splinting the arm in the position found, and securing the arm to the body with an elastic wrap. Monitor and treat for shock as needed or apply ice for 15 minutes after immobilization if shock does not occur (while avoiding the ulnar nerve, which runs to the hand), and send the athlete to the appropriate health care provider.

The athlete cannot return to activity until examined and released by a health care provider; the elbow is free of pain; and they have full strength, flexibility, and range of motion in the elbow.

To help prevent elbow fractures, teach proper tackling technique in the preseason and instruct athletes to avoid landing on their outstretched arm.

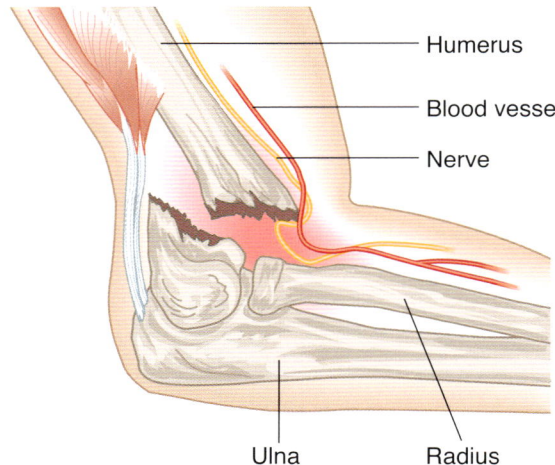

**Figure 12.16**    Fracture of the lower humerus.

# ELBOW DISLOCATION OR SUBLUXATION

In an elbow dislocation, the bones of the elbow joint move out of place. In an elbow subluxation, the bones of the elbow joint move out of place and then spontaneously shift back into position. Causes of these injuries include a direct blow, falling on an outstretched arm, a severe elbow sprain, or an elbow being forcefully extended backward. Signs and symptoms of an elbow subluxation may include tingling down the forearm and hand (if the subluxated bone pinches nerves), lack of sensation in the hand (if the subluxated bone pinches nerves), feeling or hearing a pop, a sense of looseness or giving away, extreme tenderness around the elbow, and swelling. Signs and symptoms of an elbow dislocation could include deformity; the elbow in a slightly bent position; intense pain, swelling, or another deformity around the elbow area; tingling down the forearm and hand (if the dislocated bone pinches nerves); lack of sensation in the hand (if the dislocated bone pinches nerves); feeling or hearing a pop; a sense of looseness or giving away; inability to bend or straighten the elbow; and extreme tenderness around the elbow.

First aid for an elbow subluxation should include resting the athlete from all activity, immobilizing the arm with a sling, and securing the arm to the body with an elastic wrap. Monitor the athlete, treat them for shock if needed, and send for emergency medical assistance if shock occurs. Apply ice for 15 minutes after immobilization (while avoiding the ulnar nerve, which runs to the hand), and send the athlete to the appropriate health care provider. First aid for an elbow dislocation should include resting the athlete from all activity, immobilizing the arm with a sling, and securing the arm to the body with an elastic wrap. Monitor and treat the athlete for shock as needed, and send for emergency medical assistance if shock occurs. Apply ice for 15 minutes after immobilization if shock does not occur (avoiding the ulnar nerve, which runs to the hand), and send the athlete to the appropriate health care provider.

The athlete cannot return to activity until examined and released by a health care provider; the elbow is free of pain; and they have full range of motion in the elbow, and full strength and flexibility in the elbow, wrist, and hand. When returning to activity, the athlete may need to use protective taping or bracing. To help prevent elbow subluxation and dislocation, encourage athletes to perform preseason exercises that strengthen and stretch the biceps, triceps, and forearm muscles.

# ULNAR NERVE CONTUSION

An ulnar nerve contusion is a bruise of the ulnar nerve, which is on the back of the elbow joint and runs from the shoulder to the hand. The injury is caused by a direct blow to the inside of the back of the elbow (see figure 12.17). This injury is commonly described as hitting your funny bone.

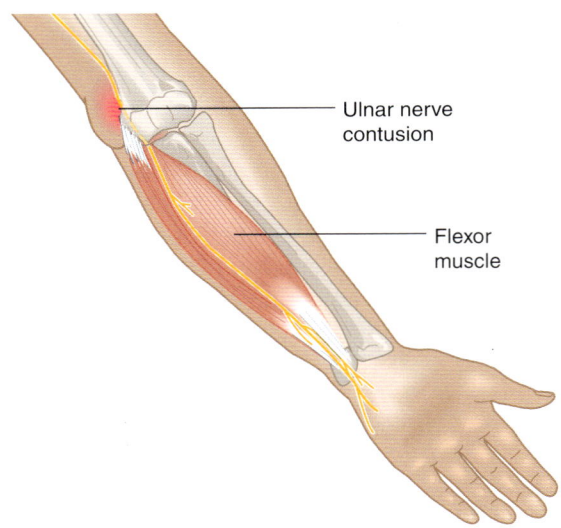

**Figure 12.17**    Ulnar nerve contusion.

## Signs and Symptoms

### Mild

- Tingling down the forearm and hand that lasts a few minutes
- Mild pain shooting from the elbow down to the forearm
- Mild point tenderness

### Moderate to Severe

- Tingling down the forearm and hand that lasts more than 5 minutes
- Loss of sensation in the ring and little fingers
- Moderate to severe pain shooting from the elbow down to the forearm
- Moderate to severe point tenderness
- Hand weakness or loss of grip strength
- Swelling
- Discoloration

# FIRST AID

## Mild

1. Rest the athlete from activity until numbness and tingling are gone, and until the athlete has full elbow range of motion and full hand strength.

## Moderate to Severe

1. Rest the athlete from all activity.
2. Immobilize the arm with a sling, if tolerated.
3. Monitor the athlete, treat them for shock if needed, and send for emergency medical assistance if shock occurs.
4. Send the athlete to the appropriate health care provider (if shock does not occur).

## Playing Status

- For mild ulnar nerve contusion, the athlete can return to activity if numbness and tingling disappear within a few minutes and grip strength is equal to the other side.
- For moderate to severe ulnar nerve contusion, the athlete cannot return to activity until examined and released by a health care provider, the elbow is free of pain, and they have full elbow range of motion and hand strength.

# PREVENTION

- Protective elbow pads for high-impact sports

# ELBOW SPRAIN

An elbow sprain is a stretch or tear of the ligaments holding the bones of the elbow together. It is caused by a direct blow or torsion injury that forces the elbow sideways or backward (see figure 12.18).

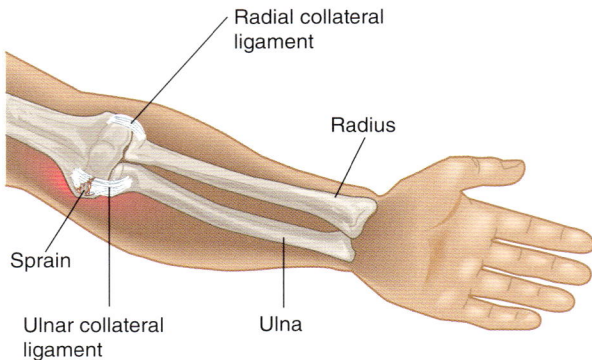

**Figure 12.18**   Elbow sprain.

## Signs and Symptoms

### Grade I

- Mild pain or point tenderness along the sides, back, or front of the elbow
- Mild pain when bending and straightening the elbow

### Grades II and III

- Moderate to severe pain or point tenderness along the sides, back, or front of the elbow
- Moderate to severe pain when bending and straightening the elbow
- Loose or unstable feeling in the elbow
- Inability to fully bend or straighten the elbow
- Swelling

## FIRST AID

### Grade I

1. Rest the athlete from painful activities.
2. Apply ice for 15 minutes.
3. Refer the athlete to the appropriate health care provider if symptoms and signs worsen (or occur more often, especially with daily activities) or do not subside within a few days.

### Grades II and III

1. Rest the arm from all activities.
2. Immobilize the arm with a sling, if tolerated.
3. Monitor the athlete, treat them for shock if needed, and send for emergency medical assistance if shock occurs.
4. Apply ice for 15 minutes (avoid the ulnar nerve, which runs to the hand), and send the athlete to the appropriate health care provider (if shock does not occur).

### Playing Status

- For a Grade I elbow sprain, the athlete can return to activity if pain subsides and if they have full range of motion in the elbow, and full strength and flexibility in the elbow and wrist. If an athlete was sent to a health care provider, they cannot return to activity until examined and released by the health care provider.
- For a Grade II or Grade III elbow sprain, the athlete cannot return to activity until examined and released by a health care provider; the elbow is free of pain; and they have full range of motion in the elbow, and full strength and flexibility in the elbow and wrist.

## PREVENTION

- Preseason training for arm and forearm strength and flexibility

# TENNIS ELBOW

Tennis elbow is chronic strain or inflammation where the wrist muscles attach to the outside of the elbow joint (see figure 12.19). Causes of this injury include weak or inflexible wrist muscles, using incorrect stroke technique (particularly backhand) in racket sports (such as using the wrist instead of the shoulder and body for all the force of a swing), or using a racket that is strung too tightly.

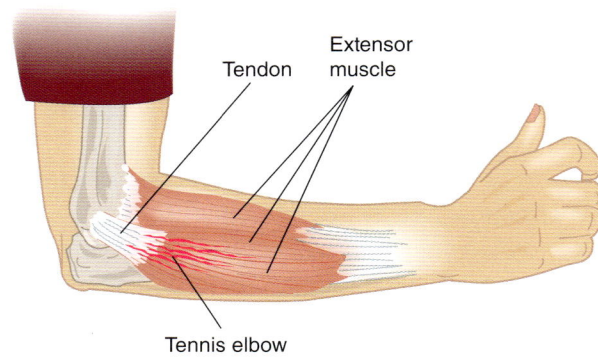

**Figure 12.19**   Tennis elbow.

## Signs and Symptoms

### Mild

- Mild pain during backhand strokes in racket sports
- Slight point tenderness over the outside of the elbow
- Mild pain when gripping or making a fist
- Mild pain when lifting objects with the palm facing down

### Moderate to Severe

- Moderate to severe pain during backhand strokes in racket sports
- Moderate to severe point tenderness over the outside of the elbow
- Moderate to severe pain when gripping or making a fist
- Moderate to severe pain when lifting objects with the palm facing down
- Inability to lift objects when the palm is facing down
- Swelling over the outside of the elbow

## FIRST AID

### Mild

1. Rest the arm from painful activities.
2. Apply ice for 15 minutes.
3. Refer the athlete to the appropriate health care provider if symptoms and signs worsen (or occur more often, especially with daily activities) or do not subside.

### Moderate to Severe

1. Rest the arm from all activities.
2. Apply ice for 15 minutes, and send the athlete to the appropriate health care provider.

### Playing Status

- For mild tennis elbow, the athlete can return to activity if signs and symptoms subside; the elbow is free of pain; and the athlete has full strength, flexibility, and range of motion in the elbow and wrist. If the athlete is sent to a health care provider, they cannot return to activity until examined and released by the health care provider.
- For moderate to severe tennis elbow, the athlete cannot return to activity until examined and released by a health care provider; the elbow is free of pain; and they have full strength, flexibility, and range of motion in the elbow and wrist.

## PREVENTION

- Preseason training for upper arm and forearm strength and flexibility
- Use of the shoulder and body for power during a backhand stroke

# GOLFER'S ELBOW

Golfer's elbow is chronic strain or inflammation where the wrist muscles attach to the inside of the elbow joint (see figure 12.20). Causes of this injury include overuse of weak or inflexible wrist muscles, throwing sidearm, or using only the forearm and wrist for power in a forehand racket stroke.

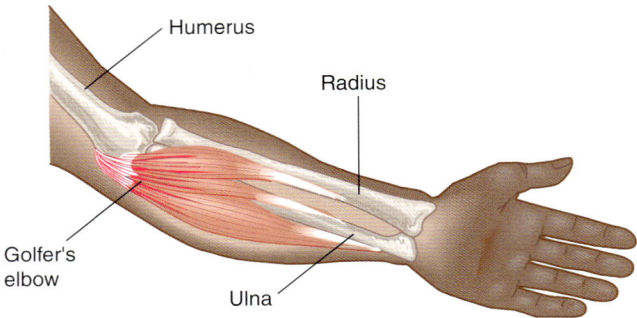

Humerus

Radius

Golfer's elbow

Ulna

**Figure 12.20**   Golfer's elbow.

## Signs and Symptoms

### Mild

- Mild pain during forehand strokes in racket sports
- Slight point tenderness over the inside of the elbow
- Mild pain when gripping or making a fist
- Mild pain when lifting objects with the palm facing up

### Moderate to Severe

- Moderate to severe pain during forehand strokes in racket sports
- Moderate to severe point tenderness over the inside of the elbow
- Moderate to severe pain when gripping or making a fist
- Moderate to severe pain when lifting objects with the palm facing up
- Inability to lift objects when the palm is facing up
- Swelling over the inside of the elbow

## FIRST AID

### Mild

1. Rest the arm from painful activities.
2. Apply ice for 15 minutes (while avoiding the ulnar nerve, which runs to the hand).
3. Refer the athlete to the appropriate health care provider if symptoms and signs worsen (or occur more often, especially with daily activities) or do not subside.

### Moderate to Severe

1. Rest the arm from all activities.
2. Apply ice for 15 minutes (while avoiding the ulnar nerve, which runs to the hand), and send the athlete to the appropriate health care provider.

### Playing Status

- For mild golfer's elbow, the athlete can return to activity if signs and symptoms subside; the elbow is free of pain; and the athlete has full strength, flexibility, and range of motion in the elbow and wrist. If the athlete is sent to a health care provider, they cannot return to activity until examined and released by the health care provider.
- For moderate to severe golfer's elbow, the athlete cannot return to activity until examined and released by a health care provider; the elbow is free of pain; and they have full strength, flexibility, and range of motion in the elbow and wrist.

## PREVENTION

- Preseason training for upper arm and forearm strength and flexibility
- Use of shoulder and body for power during a forehand stroke

# ELBOW EPIPHYSEAL (GROWTH PLATE) STRESS FRACTURE

An elbow epiphyseal stress fracture is a break in the growth plate of the humerus at the elbow. This injury is caused by repetitive and forceful throwing, which weakens the growth plate until it breaks. Signs and symptoms of an elbow epiphyseal fracture may include pain over the inside edge of the elbow that gradually worsens with activity, point tenderness over the inside of the elbow, swelling over the inside of the elbow, or achiness in the elbow when at rest.

First aid for an elbow epiphyseal stress fracture includes resting the athlete from all activities and immobilizing the arm with a sling (if tolerated). Monitor the athlete, treat them for shock if needed, and send for emergency medical assistance if shock occurs. Apply ice for 15 minutes after immobilization (while avoiding the ulnar nerve, which runs to the hand), and send the athlete to the appropriate health care provider if shock does not occur.

The athlete cannot return to activity until examined and released by a health care provider. To help prevent elbow epiphyseal stress fractures, encourage athletes to do preseason training for strength and flexibility in the upper arm and forearm. Also follow league guidelines for limiting forceful throwing by growing athletes.

# ELBOW BURSITIS

Elbow bursitis is irritation of the elbow bursa. This irritation is caused by a single blow to the elbow, repetitive blows to the elbow, or an infection.

## Signs and Symptoms

- Pain along the back of the elbow
- Gradual or sudden localized swelling on the back of the elbow
- Noticeable bump on the back of the elbow
- Warmth over the elbow area (indicates possible infection)

## FIRST AID

1. Rest the elbow from all activities.
2. Apply ice for 15 minutes, and send the athlete to the appropriate health care provider. Monitor the lower arm for numbness or tingling, and remove ice if numbness or tingling are present.

## Playing Status

The athlete cannot return to activity until examined and released by a health care provider; the elbow is free of pain; and they have full strength, flexibility, and range of motion in the elbow. When returning to activity, the athlete should wear a protective elbow pad.

## PREVENTION

- Protective elbow pads for high-impact sports

# FOREARM FRACTURE

A forearm fracture is a break in the radius, the ulna, or both bones. This injury is caused by a direct blow or by falling on an outstretched hand (see figure 12.21).

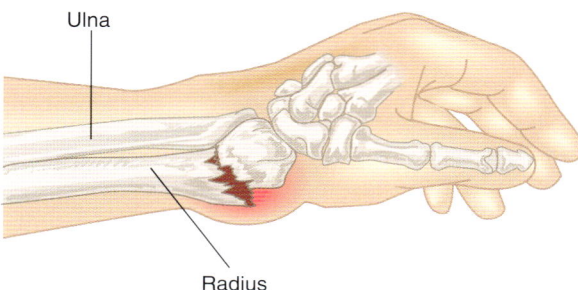

**Figure 12.21**   In a forearm fracture, the radius, ulna, or both forearm bones may be broken.

## Signs and Symptoms

- Pain and severe point tenderness
- Swelling
- Deformity
- Inability to rotate or twist the forearm to turn the palm up or down
- Inability to bend or straighten the wrist or elbow (depending on the site of the injury along the forearm)
- Bluish skin on the hand or fingers (if the fracture injures blood vessels)
- Loss of sensation and tingling in the hand and fingers (if the fracture injures nerves)

## FIRST AID

Send for emergency medical assistance if bones are grossly displaced or sticking through the skin, if you see signs of nerve damage or disrupted circulation, or if the athlete is experiencing shock.
   If none of those signs or symptoms are present, do the following:

1. Splint the arm in the position found.
2. Apply ice for 15 minutes (while avoiding the ulnar nerve, which runs to the hand), and send the athlete to the appropriate health care provider.

## Playing Status

The athlete cannot return to activity until examined and released by a health care provider; the forearm is free of pain; they have full strength, flexibility, and range of motion in the elbow and wrist; and they have equal grip strength.

## PREVENTION

- Protective forearm pads for football and ice hockey

# WRIST SPRAIN

A wrist sprain is a stretch or tear of the ligaments that hold the wrist bones together. It is caused by torsion or by falling on an outstretched hand (see figure 12.22).

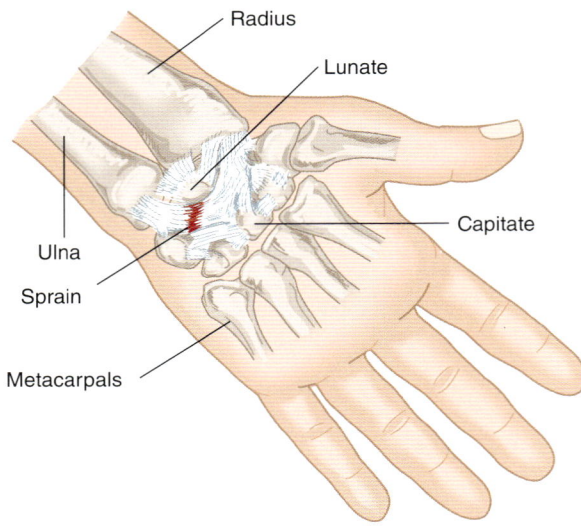

**Figure 12.22** Wrist sprain.

## Signs and Symptoms

### Grade I

- Mild pain or point tenderness along sides, back, or front of the wrist
- Mild pain when bending the wrist to the extremes
- Mild pain when rotating the palm up or down

### Grades II and III

- Moderate to severe pain or point tenderness along the sides, back, or front of the wrist
- Moderate to severe pain when bending the wrist to extremes
- Moderate to severe pain when rotating the palm up or down
- Deformity (if the sprain results in the wrist bone shifting out of position)
- Feeling loose or unstable in the wrist
- Decreased grip strength
- Swelling

## FIRST AID

### Grade I

1. Rest the athlete from painful activities.
2. Apply ice for 15 minutes.
3. Refer the athlete to the appropriate health care provider if symptoms and signs worsen (or occur more often, especially with daily activities) or do not subside within a few days.

### Grades II and III

1. Rest the arm from all activities.
2. Splint the wrist and hand, and secure them to the body with a sling.
3. Monitor the athlete, treat them for shock as needed, and send for emergency medical assistance if shock occurs.
4. Apply ice for 15 minutes, and send the athlete to the appropriate health care provider (if shock does not occur).

### Playing Status

- For a Grade I wrist sprain, the athlete can return to activity if the pain subsides; they have full strength, flexibility, and range of motion in the wrist; and they have equal grip strength in the hands. If the athlete is sent to a health care provider, they cannot return to activity until examined and released by the health care provider.

- For a Grade II or Grade III wrist sprain, the athlete cannot return to activity until examined and released by a health care provider; the wrist is free of pain; and the athlete has full strength, flexibility, and range of motion in the wrist; and they have equal grip strength in the hands.

### PREVENTION

- Preseason training for arm and forearm strength and flexibility

# WRIST FRACTURE

A wrist fracture is a break in one or more of the small wrist bones. This injury is caused by a direct blow or by falling on an outstretched hand (see figure 12.23).

## Signs and Symptoms

- Pain when rotating or bending the wrist
- Pain when tilting the wrist from side to side
- Swelling
- Deformity
- Point tenderness
- Inability to rotate or twist the forearm and wrist
- Inability to bend the wrist
- Bluish skin on the hand and fingers (if the fracture injures blood vessels)
- Loss of sensation and tingling in the hand and fingers (if the fracture injures nerves)

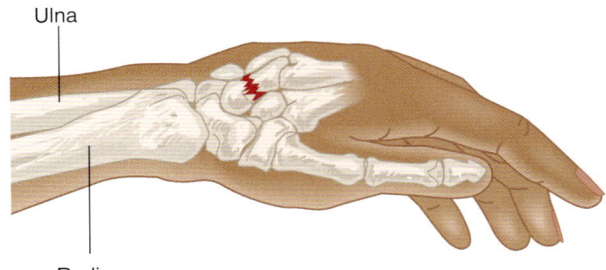

**Figure 12.23**    Fractured wrist bone.

## FIRST AID

Send for emergency medical assistance if the bones are grossly displaced or sticking through the skin, if you see signs of nerve damage or disrupted circulation, or if the athlete is experiencing shock.

If none of those signs or symptoms are present, do the following:

1. Splint the forearm and hand in the position found.
2. Apply a sling, if tolerated.
3. Apply ice for 15 minutes, and send the athlete to the appropriate health care provider.

## Playing Status

The athlete cannot return to activity until examined and released by a health care provider; the wrist is free of pain; they have full range of motion in the wrist, and full strength and flexibility in the hand and forearm.

## PREVENTION

- Preseason program for strengthening the wrist
- Training for proper technique
- Healthy diet to mitigate severity of potential fractures

# HAND FRACTURE

A hand fracture is a break in one or more of the bones of the hand. This injury is caused by a direct blow or by falling on an outstretched hand (see figure 12.24).

## Signs and Symptoms

- Pain localized around the injured area
- Grating sensation
- Pain or weakness when gripping or making a fist
- Point tenderness
- Swelling
- Deformity
- Loss of function

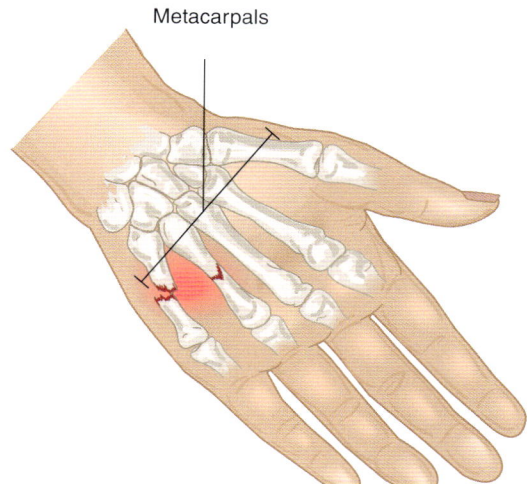
Metacarpals

**Figure 12.24**   In a hand fracture, one or more of the bones of the hand are broken.

## FIRST AID

Send for emergency medical assistance if bones are grossly displaced or sticking through the skin, if you see signs of nerve damage or disrupted circulation, or if the athlete is experiencing shock.

If none of those signs or symptoms are present, do the following:

1. Immobilize the hand and fingers.
2. Secure the hand to the body by applying an arm sling.
3. Apply ice for 15 minutes, and send the athlete to the appropriate health care provider.

## Playing Status

The athlete cannot return to activity until examined and released by a health care provider; the hand is free of pain; and they have full range of motion in the wrist, and full strength and flexibility in the wrist and hand.

## PREVENTION

- Protective hand pads in football, lacrosse, and ice hockey

# FINGER DISLOCATION

In a finger dislocation, finger bones move out of position. This injury is caused by a direct blow to the end of the finger, or by a forceful crushing or pinching of the finger between two objects (see figure 12.25).

**Signs and Symptoms**

- Intense pain
- Tingling in the finger (if dislocated bone pinches nerves)
- Lack of sensation in the finger (if dislocated bone pinches nerves)
- Extreme tenderness around the finger joint
- Feeling or hearing a pop
- Sense of looseness or giving away
- Finger stuck in a bent position
- Inability to bend or straighten the finger
- Swelling
- Deformity

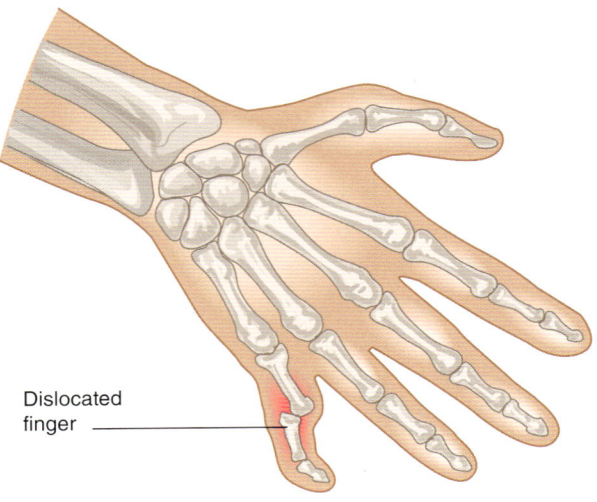

Dislocated finger

**Figure 12.25**    Finger dislocation.

## FIRST AID

Send for emergency medical assistance if the athlete is experiencing shock, or if you see signs of nerve damage or disrupted circulation.

If none of those signs or symptoms are present, do the following:

1. Immobilize the hand and finger (in the position found).
2. Apply ice for 15 minutes, and send the athlete to the appropriate health care provider.

**Playing Status**

The athlete cannot return to activity until examined and released by a health care provider; the finger is free of pain; and they have full strength, flexibility, and range of motion in the wrist, hand, and finger. When returning to activity, the athlete may need protective taping for the finger. Tape the finger to an adjacent uninjured finger toward the midline of the hand (called buddy taping; see figure 12.26).

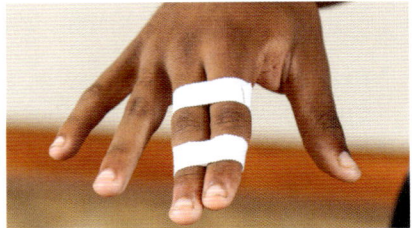

**Figure 12.26**    Protective taping (buddy taping) for a finger.

## PREVENTION

- Preseason exercises to strengthen and stretch the wrist and hand muscles
- Taping of previously injured fingers before practices and games

# FINGER OR THUMB FRACTURE

A finger or thumb fracture is a break of one or more of the finger or thumb bones. This injury is caused by a direct blow to the end of the finger or thumb or by a forceful crushing or pinching of the finger or thumb between two objects (see figure 12.27).

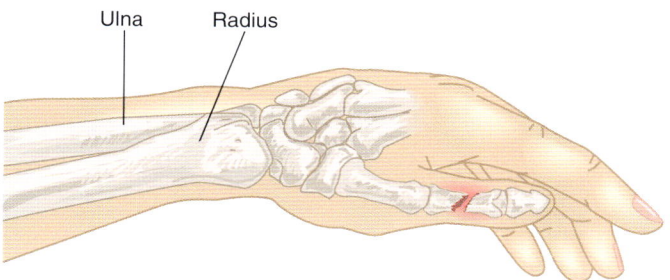

**Figure 12.27**    Thumb fracture.

## Signs and Symptoms

- Pain when bending or straightening the finger or thumb
- Pain when the end of the finger or thumb is tapped
- Swelling
- Deformity
- Inability to bend or straighten the finger or thumb

## FIRST AID

Send for emergency medical assistance if bones are sticking through the skin, if you see signs of nerve damage or disrupted circulation, or if the athlete is experiencing shock.

    If none of those signs or symptoms are present, do the following:

1. Immobilize the hand and fingers.
2. Secure the hand to the body by applying an arm sling.
3. Apply ice for 15 minutes, and send the athlete to the appropriate health care provider.

## Playing Status

The athlete cannot return to activity until examined and released by a health care provider; the finger or thumb is free of pain; and they have full strength, flexibility, and range of motion in the wrist, hand, and finger or thumb. When returning to activity, the athlete may need protective taping (see figure 12.26).

## PREVENTION

- Taping of previously injured fingers or thumbs before practices and games

# FINGER OR THUMB SPRAIN

A finger or thumb sprain occurs when finger or thumb joint ligaments are stretched or torn. This injury is caused by a direct blow to the end of the finger or thumb, or by torsion of the finger or thumb joint (see figure 12.28).

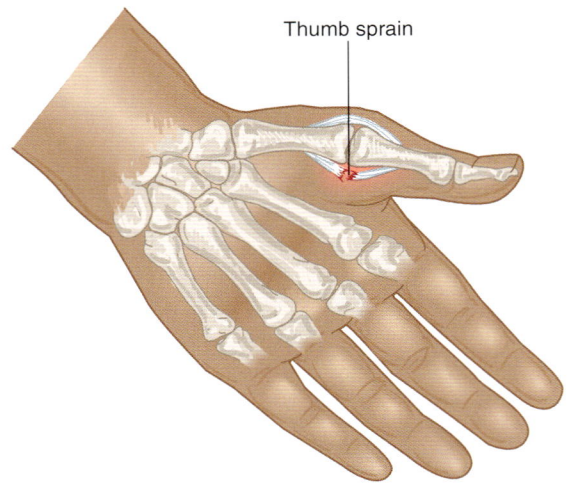

Thumb sprain

**Figure 12.28**    In a thumb sprain, the ligaments are torn (shown here) or stretched.

## Signs and Symptoms

### Grade I

- Mild pain when bending or straightening the injured joint
- Mild pain or point tenderness along the sides, back, or front of the injured joint

### Grades II and III

- Moderate to severe pain when bending or straightening the injured joint
- Moderate to severe pain or point tenderness along the sides, back, or front of the injured joint
- Feeling of looseness or instability at the injured joint
- Grating sensation
- Feeling or hearing a pop
- Inability to bend or straighten the injured joint
- Decreased grip strength
- Swelling

## FIRST AID

### Grade I

1. Rest the athlete from painful activities.
2. Apply ice for 15 minutes.
3. Refer the athlete to the appropriate health care provider if symptoms and signs worsen (or occur more often, especially with daily activities) or do not subside within a few days.

### Grades II and III

1. Rest the hand from all activities.
2. Splint the finger or thumb.
3. Monitor the athlete, treat them for shock if needed, and send for emergency medical assistance if shock occurs.
4. Apply ice for 15 minutes, instruct the athlete to elevate the injury, and send the athlete to the appropriate health care provider (if shock does not occur).

### Playing Status

- For a Grade I finger or thumb sprain, the athlete can return to activity if pain subsides, and if the athlete has full strength and range of motion in the joint. If the athlete is sent to a health care provider, the athlete cannot return to activity until examined and released by the health care provider. When the athlete returns to activity, protective taping may be applied to the finger (does not apply to thumb sprain).

- For a Grade II or Grade III finger or thumb sprain, the athlete cannot return to activity until examined and released by a health care provider, the joint is free of pain, and the athlete has full strength and range of motion in the joint. When returning to activity, the athlete may need protective taping (see figure 12.26).

## PREVENTION

- Preseason strengthening exercises for the forearm and hand
- Taping of previously injured fingers and thumbs before practices and games

## Chapter 12 Recap

❏ Why is it potentially life-threatening if the clavicle is pushed back in an SC joint sprain?

❏ What sports and types of actions may cause pain for an athlete who has a rotator cuff strain?

❏ If applying ice for a potential lower humerus fracture, what portion of the elbow should be avoided? Why?

❏ Where is the ulnar nerve located?

❏ Where is the pain typically felt with tennis elbow?

❏ What are the signs of elbow bursitis?

❏ How would you immobilize a finger or thumb fracture?

# LOWER BODY MUSCULOSKELETAL INJURIES

## IN THIS CHAPTER, YOU WILL LEARN THE FOLLOWING:

- How to recognize various lower body musculoskeletal injuries
- What first aid care to provide for each of these injuries
- How to prevent various lower body musculoskeletal injuries
- What conditions are required before an injured athlete can return to play

## INJURIES AND CONDITIONS IN THIS CHAPTER

From the waist down, the lower body has to withstand some amazingly large forces. For example, when running, the hip absorbs a force that is seven times greater than the body's weight. In basketball, landing from a layup or jump shot produces vertical forces from five to seven times the body's weight (Cavanaugh and Robison 1989). These forces can take a toll on the back and abdominal muscles as well as the hips, thighs, knees, lower legs, ankles, feet, and toes.

Your ability to quickly evaluate injuries to these areas and provide first aid care will help minimize the amount of time these injuries sideline your athletes. Consider this scenario: You are a high school girls' basketball coach. During practice, an athlete landed from a jump on another athlete's foot, causing excessive inversion of the ankle. At the time of the injury, she felt severe pain on the outside of the ankle. Now, the athlete has pain with movement of the ankle, and she has difficulty walking. Do you know what the athlete's injury is and what the first aid procedures are for this injury?

Before discussing the details of each specific injury, here is an overview of the common areas of injury in the lower body from the abdomen down to the feet:

- Abdominal and back muscles help support the body during all movements. Therefore, injuries to these areas can become debilitating and chronic if they are not caught quickly and provided appropriate care. The Abdominal Injury and Low Back Strain flowcharts in the appendix summarize first aid care for these injuries.
- Hip injuries can be extremely painful and debilitating; and thigh injuries, especially muscle strains and contusions, are common to most sports. Early in the season, many athletes experience strains to the quadriceps, hamstrings, and groin muscles of the thigh because they are out of shape and may have weak, inflexible muscles. In a survey of high school sport injuries during the 2021-22 school year, there was a high incidence of hip, thigh, and upper leg inju-

ries out of all injuries in both female and male soccer athletes (13.5% and 21.8%, respectively) (Collins, Robison, and Burus 2022). To learn the first aid protocols for various hip and thigh injuries, see the Acute Hip Injury and the Acute Thigh Injury flowcharts in the appendix.

- The knee is probably the second most injured area in all of sports. In high school soccer, girls experience a proportionally higher rate of knee injuries than boys; in the 2021-22 school year, female soccer players experienced a higher rate (20.7% of total injuries) compared to male soccer players (15.9% of total injuries) (Collins, Robison, and Burus 2022). To learn the first aid protocols for common knee injuries in sports, see the Acute Knee Injury and Chronic Knee Injury flowcharts in the appendix.
- Ankle injuries are probably the most common injuries in sports. In the 2021-22 school year, high school basketball ankle injuries accounted for a total of 36.8 percent of boys' injuries and 24.4 percent of girls' injuries. In high school girls' volleyball, the ankle was the site of 33.9 percent of all injuries (Collins, Robison, and Burus 2022).
- Because of the prevalence of calf, shin, ankle, and foot injuries in sports, you should become well-versed in first aid techniques for the injuries in these areas. To learn first aid protocols for injuries in these areas, see the Acute Leg, Foot, or Ankle Injury and the Chronic Leg, Foot, or Ankle Injury flowcharts in the appendix.

First aid decisions for musculoskeletal injuries often depend on the severity of the injury; they can be mild (Grade I), moderate (Grade II), or severe (Grade III). (To review the definitions and illustrations of Grade I, II, and III strains and sprains, see chapter 3.) In addition, many of the first aid protocols in this chapter include icing and immobilizing (splinting) the injured part. To review guidelines for ice application and splinting, see chapter 5.

# SIDE STITCH

A side stitch is a cramping or spasm felt in either the right or left side. Although the cause is unknown, it is most often experienced by runners or athletes who lack cardiorespiratory (aerobic) endurance.

## Signs and Symptoms

- Sharp pain in the side during activity
- Pain that usually disappears after the athlete rests

## FIRST AID

1. Instruct the athlete to bend forward and push their fingertips into the painful side.
2. Have the athlete take a deep breath and blow it out through tight lips.
3. Instruct the athlete to stretch the muscles by placing the same-side arm overhead and bending at the waist over to the opposite side.

## Playing Status

The athlete can return to activity once the pain subsides, and breathing and heart rate are normal. If the pain does not subside, the athlete cannot return to activity until examined and released by a health care provider.

## PREVENTION

- Adequate aerobic warm-up before activity
- No eating within 2 hours before strenuous activity

# ABDOMINAL STRAIN

Abdominal strain is a stretch or tear of abdominal muscle fibers. This injury is caused by a sudden stretch or contraction of the abdominal muscles, or weak or inflexible abdominal muscles (see figure 13.1).

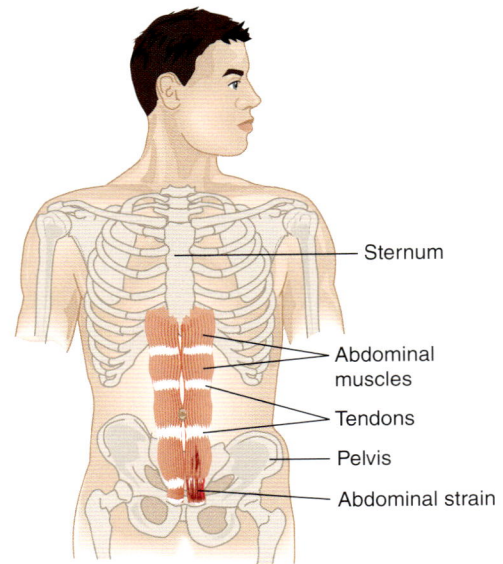

**Figure 13.1**    Abdominal strain.

## Signs and Symptoms

### Grade I

- Mild pain when abdominal muscles contract
- Mild tenderness
- Mild pain with rising to a sitting position from lying down
- Mild pain with abdominal crunches

### Grades II and III

- Moderate to severe pain when abdominal muscles contract
- Moderate to severe pain with rising to a sitting position from lying down
- Moderate to severe pain with abdominal crunches
- Moderate to severe tenderness
- Lump or indentation where the muscle is torn
- Abdominal weakness
- Bruising (appears a day or two after initial injury)

## FIRST AID

### Grade I

1. Rest the athlete from painful activities.
2. Apply ice for 15 minutes.
3. Refer the athlete to the appropriate health care provider if symptoms and signs worsen (or occur more often, especially with daily activities) or do not subside within a few days.

### Grades II and III

1. Rest the athlete from all activities.
2. Monitor the athlete, treat them for shock if needed, and send for emergency medical assistance if shock occurs.
3. Send for emergency medical assistance if the athlete has symptoms and signs of a constricted muscle hernia (bulge in the abdominal wall accompanied by nausea or vomiting) or the injury was caused by a direct blow and the athlete has symptoms and signs of internal injury (shock, vomiting, bloody urine, or referred pain).
4. Apply ice to the injury for 15 minutes, and send the athlete to the appropriate health care provider (if emergency medical assistance is not involved).

### Playing Status

- For a Grade I abdominal strain, the athlete can return to activity if signs and symptoms subside, the abdomen is free of pain, and they have full abdominal muscle flexibility and strength. If the athlete is sent to a health care provider, they cannot return to activity until examined and released by the health care provider.
- For a Grade II or Grade III abdominal strain, the athlete cannot return to activity until examined and released by a health care provider; the abdomen is free of pain; and they have full abdominal and hip muscle flexibility and strength, and full trunk and hip range of motion.

## PREVENTION

- Preseason exercises to strengthen and stretch abdominal, lower back, and hip muscles

# LOW BACK STRAIN

Low back strain is a stretch or tear of back muscle fibers. It is caused by a sudden stretch or contraction of the low back muscles, weak abdominal muscles, or tight low back and hip muscles (see figure 13.2).

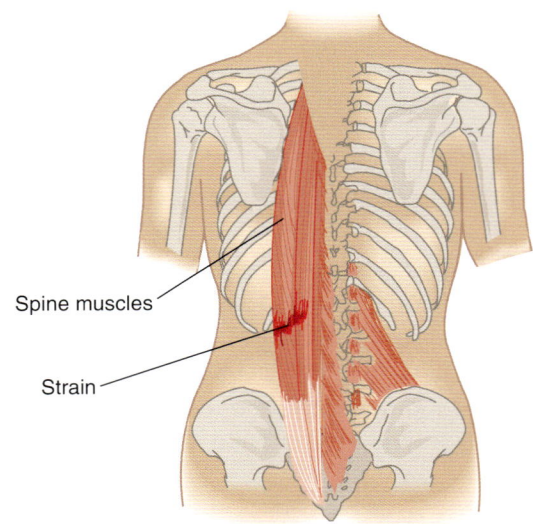

Spine muscles

Strain

**Figure 13.2**   Low back strain.

## Signs and Symptoms

### Grade I

- Mild tenderness over the site of injury (toward either side of the spine)
- Mild pain when low back muscles contract
- Mild pain with rising from lying down to sitting
- Mild pain when bending forward, arching the back, or twisting at the waist

### Grades II and III

- Moderate to severe tenderness over the site of injury (toward either side of the spine)
- Moderate to severe pain when the low back muscles contract
- Moderate to severe pain when rising from lying down to sitting
- Moderate to severe pain when bending forward, arching the back, or twisting at the waist
- Lump or indentation where the muscle is torn
- Back weakness
- Bruising (appears a day or two after initial injury)

## FIRST AID

### Grade I

1. Rest the athlete from painful activities.
2. Apply ice for 15 minutes.
3. Refer the athlete to the appropriate health care provider if symptoms and signs worsen (or occur more often, especially with daily activities) or do not subside within a few days.

### Grades II and III

1. Rest the athlete from all activities.
2. Monitor the athlete, treat them for shock as needed, and send for emergency medical assistance if shock occurs.
3. Send for emergency medical assistance if the injury was caused by a direct blow and resulted in spine deformity or tenderness directly over the spine, or if the athlete has signs and symptoms of nerve damage (sharp and shooting pain, numbness or tingling down one leg, leg weakness, lower extremity paralysis, or incontinence).
4. Apply ice to the injury for 15 minutes, and send the athlete to the appropriate health care provider (if emergency medical assistance is not sent for).

### Playing Status

- For a Grade I low back strain, the athlete can return to activity if signs and symptoms subside; the back is free of pain; and they have full range of motion in the trunk and hip, and full flexibility and strength in the back muscles. If the athlete is sent to a health care provider, they cannot return to activity until examined and released by the health care provider.
- For a Grade II or Grade III low back strain, the athlete cannot return to activity until examined and released by a health care provider; the back is free of pain; and they have full range of motion in the trunk and hip, and full flexibility and strength in the back, hip, and abdominal muscles.

## PREVENTION

- Preseason exercises to strengthen and stretch the lower back, abdominal, and hip muscles

# HIP CONTUSION (HIP POINTER)

A hip contusion (also called a pointer) is a bruise high to the front of the hip bone. This injury is caused by a direct blow (see figure 13.3).

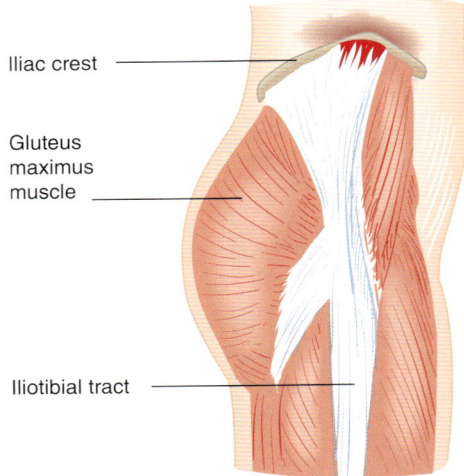

Iliac crest

Gluteus maximus muscle

Iliotibial tract

**Figure 13.3**    Hip contusion.

## Signs and Symptoms

### Mild

- Slight point tenderness over the front of the hip bone
- Mild pain when raising the thigh forward
- Mild pain when arching the back

### Moderate to Severe

- Moderate to severe point tenderness over the front of the hip bone
- Moderate to severe pain when walking
- Moderate to severe pain when raising the thigh forward
- Inability to raise the thigh forward
- Moderate to severe pain when arching the back
- Swelling
- Bruising (appears a day or two after initial injury)
- Limping or inability to walk

## FIRST AID

### Mild

1. Rest the athlete from painful activities.
2. Apply ice to the injury for 15 minutes.
3. Refer the athlete to the appropriate health care provider if symptoms and signs worsen (or occur more often, especially with daily activities) or do not subside within a few days.

### Moderate to Severe

1. Rest the athlete from all activities.
2. Prevent the athlete from walking on the injured leg.
3. Monitor the athlete, treat them for shock if needed, and send for emergency medical assistance if shock occurs.
4. Apply ice to the injury for 15 minutes, and send the athlete to the appropriate health care provider (if shock does not occur).

### Playing Status

- For a mild hip contusion, the athlete can return to activity if signs and symptoms subside; the hip is free of pain; and they have full range of motion in the hip, and full strength and flexibility in the hip and thigh muscles. If the athlete is sent to a health care provider, they cannot return to activity until examined and released by the health care provider. When returning to activity, the athlete should wear a protective pad over the hip.
- For a moderate to severe hip contusion, the athlete cannot return to activity until examined and released by a health care provider; the hip is free of pain; and they have full range of motion in the hip, and full flexibility and strength in the hip and thigh muscles. When returning to activity, the athlete should wear a protective pad over the hip.

## PREVENTION

- Protective hip pads for football, volleyball, ice hockey, baseball, and softball

# HIP FLEXOR STRAIN

A hip flexor strain is a stretch or tear of the muscles located high on the front of the thigh or pelvis. This injury is caused by forceful contraction or stretch of the muscles, or weak or inflexible hip and thigh muscles (see figure 13.4).

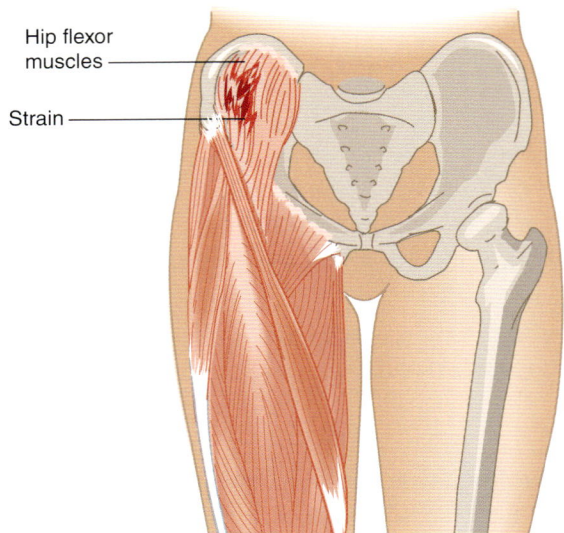

Hip flexor muscles

Strain

**Figure 13.4** Hip flexor strain.

## Signs and Symptoms

### Grade I

- Mild pain high on the front of the thigh
- Mild tenderness over the front of the hip
- Mild pain when trying to raise the thigh forward
- Mild pain when running

### Grades II and III

- Moderate to severe pain high on the front of the thigh
- Moderate to severe tenderness over the front of the hip
- Moderate to severe pain when trying to raise the thigh forward
- Moderate to severe pain when running
- Hearing or feeling a pop
- Lump or indentation where the muscle is torn
- Weakness in the hip and thigh
- Bruising (appears a day or two after initial injury)

- Inability to raise the thigh forward
- Swelling
- Limping

## FIRST AID

### Grade I

1. Rest the athlete from painful activities.
2. Apply ice to the injury for 15 minutes.
3. Refer the athlete to the appropriate health care provider if symptoms and signs worsen (or occur more often, especially with daily activities) or do not subside within a few days.

### Grades II and III

1. Rest the athlete from all activities.
2. Monitor the athlete, treat them for shock if needed, and send for emergency medical assistance if shock occurs.
3. Send for emergency medical assistance if the muscle is completely torn (rolled up).
4. Prevent the athlete from walking on the injured leg.
5. Apply ice to the injury for 15 minutes, and send the athlete to the appropriate health care provider (if emergency medical assistance is not sent for).

### Playing Status

- For a Grade I hip flexor strain, the athlete can return to activity if signs and symptoms subside; the hip is free of pain; and they have full strength, flexibility, and range of motion in the hip. If the athlete is sent to a health care provider, they cannot return to activity until examined and released by the health care provider. When returning to activity, the athlete may benefit from wearing an elastic wrap to support the hip and thigh and from stretching the upper hip and quadriceps muscles daily.
- For a Grade II or Grade III hip flexor strain, the athlete cannot return to activity until examined and released by a health care provider; the hip is free of pain; and they have full strength, flexibility, and range of motion in the hip. When returning to activity, the athlete may benefit from wearing an elastic wrap to support the hip and thigh and from stretching the upper hip and quadriceps muscles daily.

## PREVENTION

- Preseason strengthening and stretching exercises for the core, hip, and thigh
- Adequate aerobic warm-up before activity

# HIP DISLOCATION OR SUBLUXATION

In a hip dislocation, the head of the thigh bone (femur) pops out of the socket on the pelvis (figure 13.5). In a hip subluxation, the head of the femur pops out of the socket on the pelvis and spontaneously shifts back into the socket. Typically, these injuries occur when an athlete lands on a bent knee while the thigh is rotated inward and positioned close to the midline of the body. An example is a running football player who is tackled and falls forward on a bent knee. Signs and symptoms of hip subluxations and dislocations could include severe pain in the hip and thigh; tingling in the leg and foot (if the displaced bone pinches nerves); a sense of looseness or instability; feeling or hearing a pop; pain in the knee, lower leg, or back; inability to move the thigh; the leg appearing shorter; and inability to walk.

First aid for a hip subluxation or dislocation should include preventing the athlete from moving the entire leg, applying ice for 15 minutes, and calling for emergency medical assistance. Monitor the athlete, and treat them for shock if needed.

The athlete cannot return to activity until examined and released by a health care provider; the hip is free of pain; and they have full range of motion in the hip, and full strength and flexibility in the hip and thigh. To help prevent hip subluxations and dislocations, encourage athletes to do preseason exercises to strengthen the core and hips.

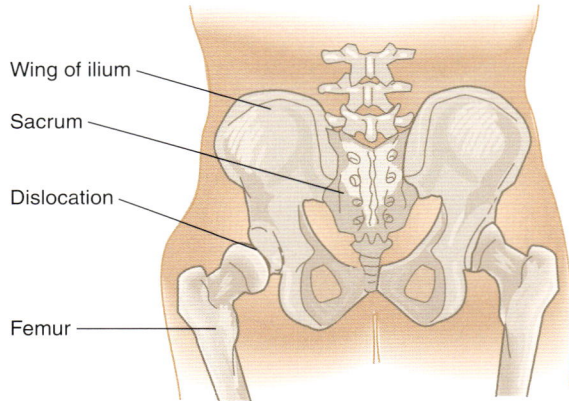

Wing of ilium

Sacrum

Dislocation

Femur

**Figure 13.5**    In most hip dislocations, the head of the thighbone slips backward out of its socket in the pelvis.

# FEMUR FRACTURE

A femur fracture is a break of the thigh bone. It is caused by compression or torsion (twisting). A femur fracture is a medical emergency; if you suspect one has occurred, send for emergency medical assistance immediately. Signs and symptoms of a femur fracture may include hearing or feeling a pop or snap; a grating sensation; pain at the site of the injury when gently squeezing the thigh above and then below the injury; severe pain with any movement; deformity; inability to move the thigh; lack of sensation in the leg, foot, or toes (if the displaced bone pinches nerves); bluish leg, foot, or toes (if the displaced bone disrupts blood supply); and muscle spasm.

First aid for a femur fracture should include preventing the athlete from moving the hip and entire leg, and sending for emergency medical assistance. You should monitor the athlete, and treat them for shock if needed.

The athlete cannot return to activity until examined and released by a health care provider and they have full range of motion in the hip and knee, and full strength and flexibility in the quadriceps and hamstrings. When returning to contact sports, the athlete should wear a protective pad over the thigh. To help prevent a thigh fracture, athletes should wear protective thigh pads for football and ice hockey.

# INNER THIGH STRAIN

Inner thigh strain is a stretch or tear of the adductor (inner thigh) muscles. It is caused by forceful contraction or stretch of the inner thigh muscles, weak or inflexible inner thigh muscles, or twisting of the upper body while the foot is planted (see figure 13.6).

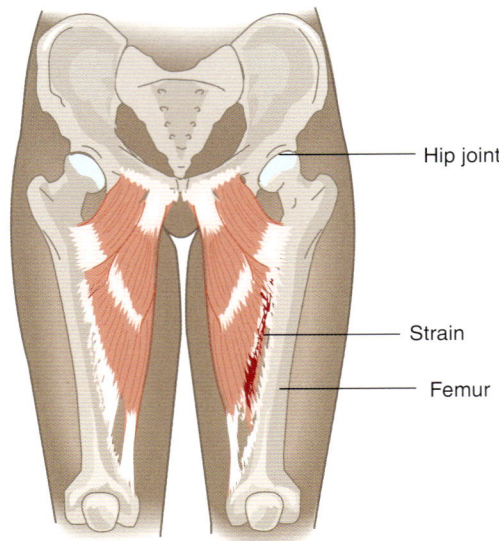

Hip joint

Strain

Femur

**Figure 13.6**    Inner thigh strain.

## Signs and Symptoms

### Grade I

- Mild pain along the inside of the thigh
- Mild tenderness along the inner thigh
- Mild pain when trying to move the thigh inward toward the other leg (such as when kicking the leg across the body)
- Mild pain when running
- Mild pain during cutting and pivoting maneuvers
- Mild pain when moving sideways

### Grades II and III

- Moderate to severe pain along the inside of the thigh
- Moderate to severe tenderness along the inner thigh
- Moderate to severe pain when trying to move the thigh inward toward the other leg (such as when kicking the leg across the body)
- Moderate to severe pain when running
- Moderate to severe pain during cutting and pivoting maneuvers
- Moderate to severe pain when moving sideways

- Hearing or feeling a pop
- Lump or indentation where the muscle is torn
- Inner thigh weakness
- Bruising down the inner thigh or knee (appears a day or two after initial injury)
- Inability to move the thigh inward toward the other thigh (such as when kicking the leg across the body)
- Inability to stretch the legs apart
- Swelling
- Limping

## FIRST AID

### Grade I

1. Rest the athlete from painful activities.
2. Apply ice to the injury for 15 minutes.
3. Refer the athlete to the appropriate health care provider if symptoms and signs worsen (or occur more often, especially with daily activities) or do not subside within a few days.

### Grades II and III

1. Rest the athlete from all activities.
2. Monitor the athlete, treat them for shock if needed, and send for emergency medical assistance if shock occurs.
3. Send for emergency medical assistance if the muscle is completely torn (rolled up).
4. Prevent the athlete from walking on the injured leg.
5. Apply ice to the injury for 15 minutes, and send the athlete to the appropriate health care provider (if emergency medical assistance is not sent for).

### Playing Status

- For a Grade I inner thigh strain, the athlete can return to activity if signs and symptoms subside; the thigh is free of pain; and they have full range of motion in the hip, and full strength and flexibility in the hip and thigh. If the athlete is sent to a health care provider, they cannot return to activity until examined and released by the health care provider. When returning to activity, the athlete may benefit from wearing an elastic wrap or neoprene (rubberized) thigh sleeve to support the inner thigh and from stretching the inner thigh muscles daily.
- For a Grade II or Grade III inner thigh strain, the athlete cannot return to activity until examined and released by a health care provider; the thigh is free of pain; and they have full range of motion in the hip, and full flexibility and strength in the hip and thigh. When returning to activity, the athlete may benefit from wearing an elastic wrap or neoprene (rubberized) thigh sleeve to support the thigh and from stretching the inner thigh muscles daily.

## PREVENTION

- Preseason strengthening and stretching exercises for the core, hip, and thigh
- Adequate aerobic warm-up before activity

# THIGH CONTUSION

A thigh contusion is a bruise to the soft tissues or bones of the thigh. This injury is caused by a direct blow (see figure 13.7).

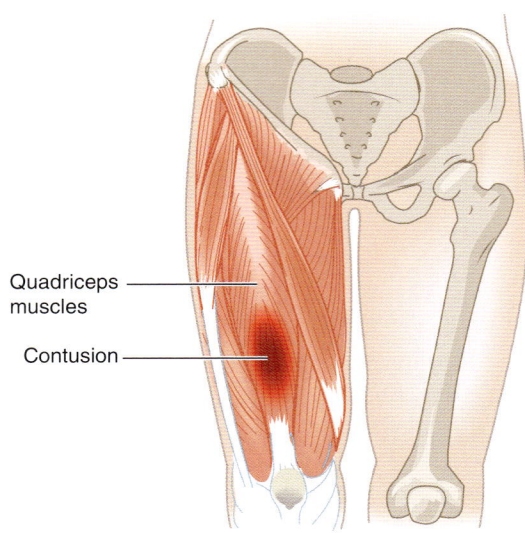

Quadriceps
muscles

Contusion

**Figure 13.7**    Thigh contusion.

## Signs and Symptoms

### Mild

- Slight point tenderness over the injury site
- Mild pain when raising the thigh forward or moving it backward (depending on the injury site)
- Mild pain when walking or running
- Mild pain when bending or straightening the knee

### Moderate to Severe

- Moderate to severe point tenderness over the injury site
- Moderate to severe pain when raising the thigh forward or moving it backward (depending on the injury site)
- Inability to raise the thigh forward or move it backward (depending on the site of the injury)
- Inability to bend or straighten the knee
- Moderate to severe pain when walking or running

- Moderate to severe pain when bending or straightening the knee
- Swelling
- Bruising (appears a day or two after initial injury)
- Muscle spasm
- Decreased thigh strength
- Limping

## FIRST AID

### Mild

1. Rest the athlete from painful activities.
2. Apply ice to the injury for 15 minutes, then apply a compression wrap.
3. Refer the athlete to the appropriate health care provider if symptoms and signs worsen (or occur more often, especially with daily activities) or do not subside within a few days.

### Moderate to Severe

1. Rest the athlete from all activities.
2. Prevent the athlete from walking on the injured leg.
3. Monitor the athlete, treat them for shock if needed, and send for emergency medical assistance if shock occurs.
4. Apply ice to the injury for 15 minutes, and send the athlete to the appropriate health care provider (if shock does not occur).

### Playing Status

- For a mild thigh contusion, the athlete can return to activity if signs and symptoms subside; the thigh is free of pain; and they have full range of motion in the hip and knee, and full flexibility and strength in the thigh muscle. If the athlete is sent to a health care provider, they cannot return to activity until examined and released by the health care provider. When returning to contact sports, the athlete should wear a protective pad over the area; repeated blows could cause calcification of the muscle tissue.
- For a moderate to severe thigh contusion, the athlete cannot return to activity until examined and released by a health care provider; the thigh is free of pain; and they have full range of motion in the hip and knee, and full flexibility and strength in the thigh muscle. When returning to activity, the athlete should wear a protective pad over the area; repeated blows could cause calcification of the muscle tissue.

## PREVENTION

- Protective thigh pads for football and ice hockey

# QUADRICEPS STRAIN

A quadriceps strain is a stretch or tear of the quadriceps muscles. This injury is caused by a forceful contraction or stretch of the quad muscles, or by weak or inflexible muscles (see figure 13.8).

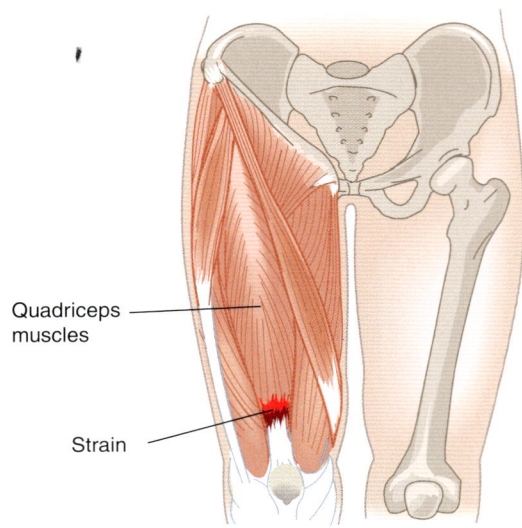

Quadriceps
muscles

Strain

**Figure 13.8**  Quadriceps strain.

## Signs and Symptoms

### Grade I

- Mild pain on the front of the thigh
- Mild tenderness over the front of the thigh
- Mild pain when trying to raise the thigh forward or straighten the knee
- Mild pain when running
- Mild pain when extending the thigh backward while the knee is bent

### Grades II and III

- Moderate to severe pain on the front of the thigh
- Moderate to severe tenderness over the front of the thigh
- Moderate to severe pain when trying to raise the thigh forward or straighten the knee
- Moderate to severe pain when running
- Moderate to severe pain when extending the thigh backward while the knee is bent
- Hearing or feeling a pop
- Pain while going up and down stairs

- Lump or indentation where the muscle is torn
- Bruising down the thigh, knee, or lower leg (appears a day or two after initial injury)
- Decreased ability or inability to flex the thigh forward or straighten the knee
- Swelling
- Limping

## FIRST AID

### Grade I

1. Rest the athlete from painful activities.
2. Apply ice to the injury for 15 minutes.
3. Refer the athlete to the appropriate health care provider if symptoms and signs worsen (or occur more often, especially with daily activities) or do not subside within a few days.

### Grades II and III

1. Rest the athlete from all activities.
2. Monitor the athlete, treat them for shock as needed, and send for emergency medical assistance if shock occurs.
3. Send for emergency medical assistance if the muscle is completely torn (rolled up).
4. Prevent the athlete from walking on the injured leg.
5. Apply ice to the injury for 15 minutes, and send the athlete to the appropriate health care provider (if emergency medical assistance is not sent for).

### Playing Status

- For a Grade I quadriceps strain, the athlete can return to activity if signs and symptoms subside; the thigh is free of pain; and they have full range of motion in the hip and knee, and full strength and flexibility in the quadriceps. If the athlete is sent to a health care provider, they cannot return to activity until examined and released by the health care provider. When returning to activity, the athlete may benefit from wearing an elastic wrap or neoprene (rubberized) thigh sleeve to support the thigh and from stretching the quadriceps daily.
- For a Grade II or Grade III quadriceps strain, the athlete cannot return to activity until examined and released by a health care provider; the thigh is free of pain; and they have full range of motion in the hip and knee, and full strength and flexibility in the quadriceps. When returning to activity, the athlete may benefit from wearing an elastic wrap or neoprene (rubberized) thigh sleeve to support the thigh and from stretching the quadriceps daily.

## PREVENTION

- Preseason exercises to strengthen and stretch the core, knee, hip, and thigh muscles
- Adequate aerobic warm-up before activity

# HAMSTRING STRAIN

A hamstring strain is a stretch or tear of the hamstring muscles. It is caused by forceful contraction or stretch of the hamstring muscles, or weak or inflexible hamstrings (see figure 13.9).

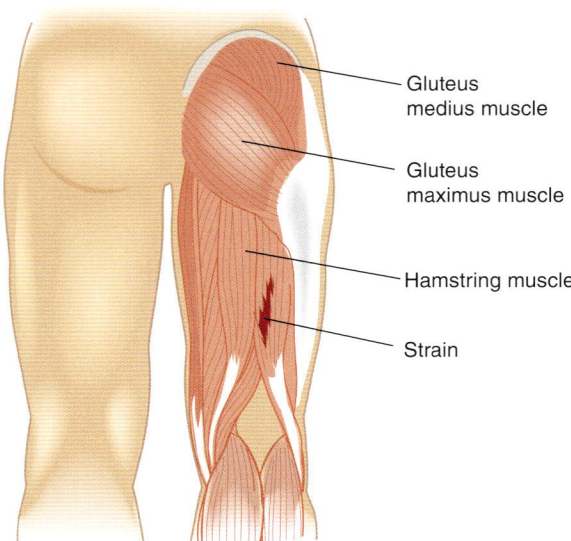

Gluteus medius muscle

Gluteus maximus muscle

Hamstring muscle

Strain

**Figure 13.9** Hamstring strain.

## Signs and Symptoms

### Grade I

- Mild pain on the back of the thigh
- Mild tenderness over the back of the thigh
- Mild pain when trying to extend the thigh backward or bend the knee
- Mild pain when running
- Mild pain when flexing the thigh forward while straightening the knee

### Grades II and III

- Moderate to severe pain on the back of the thigh
- Moderate to severe tenderness over the back of the thigh
- Moderate to severe pain when trying to extend the thigh backward or bend the knee
- Moderate to severe pain when walking
- Moderate to severe pain when flexing the thigh forward while straightening the knee
- Hearing or feeling a pop
- Lump or indentation where the muscle is torn
- Bruising down the back of the thigh, knee, or lower leg (appears a day or two after initial injury)

- Decreased ability or inability to extend the thigh backward or bend the knee
- Swelling
- Limping

## FIRST AID

### Grade I

1. Rest the athlete from painful activities.
2. Apply ice to the injury for 15 minutes.
3. Refer the athlete to the appropriate health care provider if symptoms and signs worsen (or occur more often, especially with daily activities) or do not subside within a few days.

### Grades II and III

1. Rest the athlete from all activities.
2. Monitor the athlete, treat for shock if needed, and send for emergency medical assistance if shock occurs.
3. Send for emergency medical assistance if the muscle is completely torn (rolled up).
4. Prevent the athlete from walking on the injured leg.
5. Apply ice to the injury for 15 minutes, and send the athlete to the appropriate health care provider (if emergency medical assistance is not sent for).

### Playing Status

- For a Grade I hamstring strain, the athlete can return to activity if signs and symptoms subside; the affected hamstring muscle is free of pain; and they have full range of motion in the hip and knee, and full strength and flexibility in the hamstrings. If the athlete is sent to a health care provider, they cannot return to activity until examined and released by the health care provider. When returning to activity, the athlete may benefit from wearing an elastic wrap or neoprene (rubberized) thigh sleeve to support the thigh and from stretching the hamstring muscles daily.
- For a Grade II or Grade III hamstring strain, the athlete cannot return to activity until examined and released by a health care provider; the affected hamstring muscle is free of pain; and they have full range of motion in the hip and knee, and full strength and flexibility in the hamstrings. When returning to activity, the athlete may benefit from wearing an elastic wrap or neoprene (rubberized) thigh sleeve to support the thigh and from stretching the hamstring muscles daily.

## PREVENTION

- Preseason exercises to strengthen and stretch the core, thigh, hip, and knee
- Adequate aerobic warm-up before activity

# KNEE SPRAIN

A knee sprain is a stretch or tear of the ligaments that hold the knee bones in place. It is caused by compression to either the front, side, or back of the knee; torsion at the knee joint; hyperextension or hyperflexion of the knee; or weak thigh muscles (see figure 13.10, a-d).

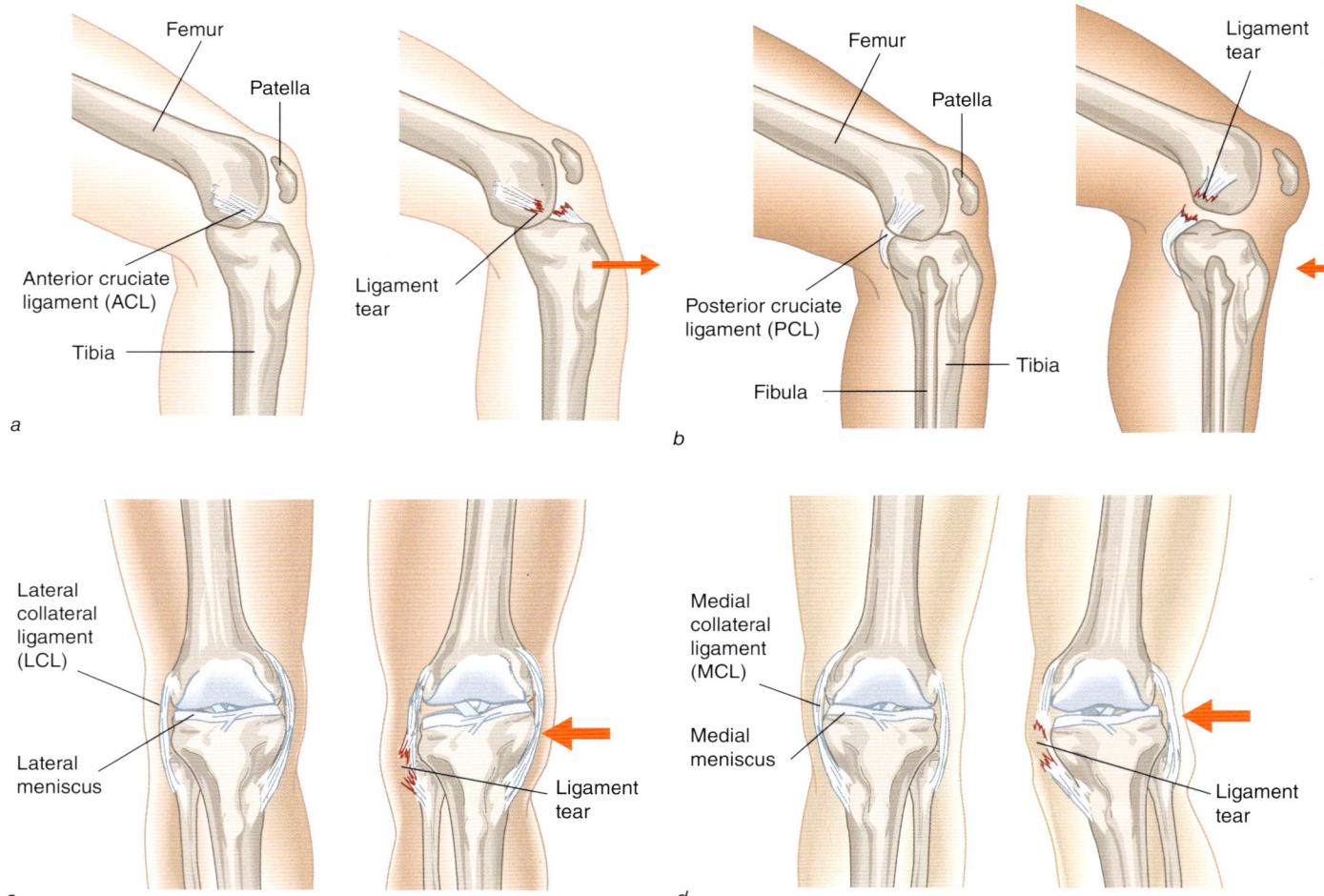

**Figure 13.10** Knee sprains of the *(a)* anterior cruciate ligament (ACL), *(b)* posterior cruciate ligament (PCL), *(c)* lateral collateral ligament (LCL), and *(d)* medial collateral ligament (MCL).

## Signs and Symptoms

### Grade I

- Slight point tenderness
- Mild pain when straightening or bending the knee

## Grades II and III

- Moderate to severe point tenderness
- Moderate to severe pain when straightening or bending the knee
- Feeling of looseness or instability
- Hearing or feeling a pop
- Swelling
- Limping

## FIRST AID

### Grade I

1. Rest the athlete from painful activities.
2. Apply ice to the injury for 15 minutes.
3. Refer the athlete to the appropriate health care provider if symptoms and signs worsen (or occur more often, especially with daily activities such as walking) or do not subside within a few days.

### Grades II and III

1. Rest the athlete from all activities.
2. Prevent the athlete from walking on the injured leg.
3. Monitor the athlete, treat them for shock if needed, and send for emergency medical assistance if shock occurs.
4. Send for emergency medical assistance if you see any symptoms or signs of nerve injury (tingling or numbness in lower leg, foot, or toes) or of disrupted blood supply (bluish foot, toes, or toenails).
5. Apply ice to the injury for 15 minutes, and send the athlete to the appropriate health care provider (if emergency medical assistance is not sent for).

### Playing Status

- For a Grade I knee sprain, the athlete can return to activity if signs and symptoms subside; the knee is free of pain; and they have full range of motion in the knee, and full strength and flexibility in the quadriceps, hamstrings, and calf. If the athlete is sent to a health care provider, they cannot return to activity until examined and released by the health care provider.
- For a Grade II or Grade III knee sprain, the athlete cannot return to activity until examined and released by a health care provider; the knee is free of pain; and they have full range of motion in the knee, and full strength and flexibility in the quadriceps, hamstrings, and calf.

## PREVENTION

- Preseason exercises to strengthen and stretch the hip, quadriceps, hamstrings, and calf

# PATELLAR DISLOCATION OR SUBLUXATION

In a patellar dislocation, the kneecap (patella) slips out of the groove on the femur (see figure 13.11). In a patellar subluxation, the patella slips out of the groove on the femur and then spontaneously shifts back into the groove. Causes of these injuries include compression to the inside of the patella, forceful contraction of the outside quadriceps muscles, torsion of the knee joint, or a weak inside quadriceps muscle.

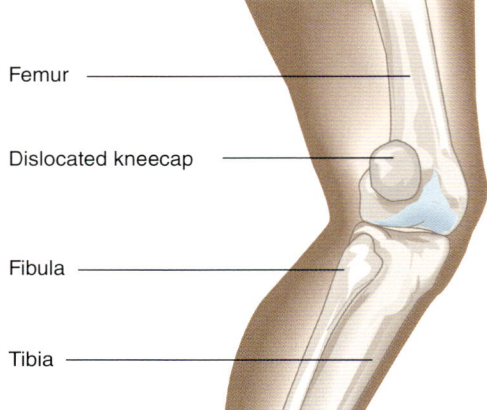

Femur

Dislocated kneecap

Fibula

Tibia

**Figure 13.11**   Dislocated kneecap (patella).

## Signs and Symptoms

### Subluxation

- Point tenderness along the inside of the patella
- Pain when bending or straightening the knee
- Feeling of the kneecap going out of place
- Pain along the inside of the knee
- Hearing or feeling a pop
- Grating sensation
- Swelling
- Limping

### Dislocation

- Severe point tenderness along the inside of the patella
- Obvious deformity (the patella displaced to the outside of the knee)
- Inability to bend or straighten the knee

- Feeling of the kneecap going out of place
- Pain along the inside of the knee
- Hearing or feeling a pop
- Swelling

## FIRST AID

### Subluxation

1. Rest the athlete from all activity.
2. Prevent the athlete from walking on the injured leg.
3. Monitor the athlete, treat them for shock if needed, and send for emergency medical assistance if shock occurs.
4. Apply ice to the injury for 15 minutes, and send the athlete to the appropriate health care provider (if shock does not occur).

### Dislocation

1. Send for emergency medical assistance.
2. Do not try to put the patella back into place.
3. Monitor and treat for shock as needed.
4. Prevent the athlete from moving the leg.
5. Apply ice for 15 minutes (if tolerated by the athlete).

### Playing Status

The athlete cannot return to activity until examined and released by a health care provider; the knee is free of pain; and they have full range of motion in the knee, and full strength and flexibility in the quadriceps, hamstrings, and calf.

## PREVENTION

- Preseason exercises to strengthen and stretch the quadriceps, hamstrings, and calf

# PATELLAR TENDINITIS

Patellar tendinitis is inflammation of the patellar tendon, which attaches the kneecap to the lower leg bone (tibia). It is caused by forceful contraction of the quadriceps muscles, or weak quadriceps muscles and inflexible quadriceps, hamstrings, and calf muscles (see figure 13.12).

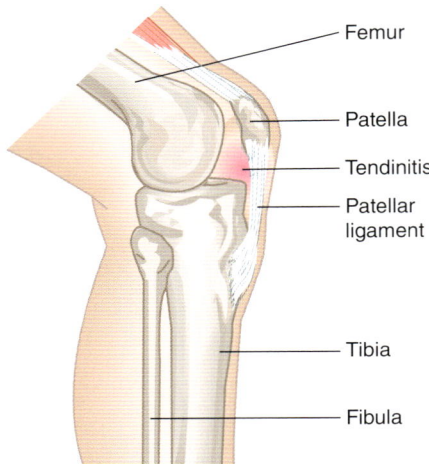

**Figure 13.12**   Patellar tendinitis is inflammation of the tendon that attaches the kneecap to the tibia.

## Signs and Symptoms

### Mild

- Mild pain from the bottom of the patella to the top of the tibia
- Slight point tenderness between the patella and the upper tibia
- Mild pain with running and jumping activities
- Mild pain when forcefully straightening the knee

### Moderate to Severe

- Moderate to severe pain from the bottom of the patella to the top of the tibia
- Moderate to severe point tenderness between the patella and the upper tibia
- Decreased ability or inability to forcefully straighten the knee, especially when jumping, lifting weights, and running
- Moderate to severe pain with running and jumping activities
- Moderate to severe pain when forcefully straightening the knee
- Thickening of the patellar tendon
- Localized swelling
- Limping

## FIRST AID

### Mild

1. Rest the athlete from painful activities.
2. Apply ice to the injury for 15 minutes.
3. Refer the athlete to the appropriate health care provider if symptoms and signs worsen (or occur more often, especially with daily activities) or do not subside within a few days.

### Moderate to Severe

1. Rest the athlete from all activities.
2. Monitor the athlete, treat them for shock if needed, and send for emergency medical assistance if shock occurs.
3. Prevent the athlete from walking on the injured leg.
4. Apply ice to the injury for 15 minutes, and send the athlete to the appropriate health care provider (if shock does not occur).

### Playing Status

- For mild patellar tendinitis, the athlete can return to activity if signs and symptoms subside; the knee is free of pain; they have full knee range of motion and quadriceps strength; and they have full quadriceps, hamstring, and calf flexibility. If the athlete is sent to a health care provider, they cannot return to activity until examined and released by the health care provider. When returning to activity, the athlete may benefit from wearing a neoprene (rubberized) knee sleeve (to keep the tendon warm during activity) and from stretching the hamstring, quadriceps, and calf muscles daily.

- For moderate to severe patellar tendinitis, the athlete cannot return to activity until examined and released by a health care provider; the knee is free of pain; they have full knee range of motion and quadriceps strength; and they have full quadriceps, hamstring, and calf flexibility. When returning to activity, the athlete may benefit from wearing a neoprene (rubberized) knee sleeve (to keep the tendon warm during activity) and from stretching the hamstring, quadriceps, and calf muscles daily.

## PREVENTION

- Preseason exercises to strengthen the core, gluteal, and quadriceps muscles and stretch the quadriceps, hamstring, and calf muscles
- Adequate aerobic warm-up before activity

# ANTERIOR KNEE PAIN

Anterior knee pain is irritation between the patella and femur (see figure 13.13). Typically occurring over time, this injury is caused by compression to the top of the patella; inability of the patella to properly track in the groove in the femur; repeated episodes of patellar dislocation and subluxation; or weak quadriceps and gluteal muscles, or inflexible quadriceps, hamstring, and calf muscles.

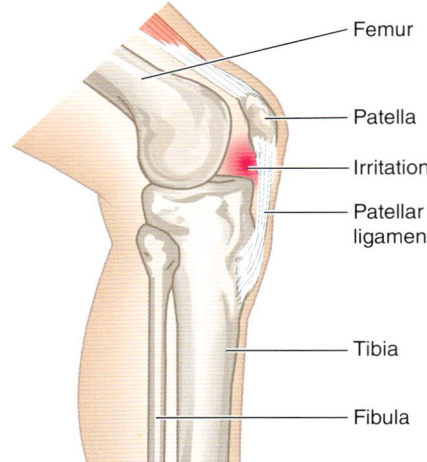

Labels: Femur, Patella, Irritation, Patellar ligament, Tibia, Fibula

**Figure 13.13**   Anterior knee pain is irritation between the patella and femur.

## Signs and Symptoms

### Mild

- Mild pain when running, jumping, or using stairs
- Mild point tenderness underneath the patella
- Mild pain behind the patella
- Grating feeling behind the patella
- Mild achiness while sitting for extended periods

### Moderate to Severe

- Moderate to severe pain when running, jumping, or using stairs
- Moderate to severe point tenderness underneath the patella
- Moderate to severe pain behind the patella
- Decreased ability or inability to forcefully straighten the knee, especially when jumping, lifting weights, and running
- Grating feeling behind the patella
- Moderate to severe achiness while sitting for extended periods
- Limping

## FIRST AID

### Mild

1. Rest the athlete from painful activities.
2. Apply ice to the injury for 15 minutes.
3. Refer the athlete to the appropriate health care provider if symptoms and signs worsen (or occur more often, especially with daily activities) or do not subside within a few days.

### Moderate to Severe

1. Rest the athlete from all activities.
2. Monitor the athlete, treat them for shock if needed, and send for emergency medical assistance if shock occurs.
3. Prevent the athlete from walking on the injured leg.
4. Apply ice to the injury for 15 minutes, and send the athlete to the appropriate health care provider (if shock does not occur).

### Playing Status

- For mild anterior knee pain, the athlete can return to activity if signs and symptoms subside; the knee is free of pain; they have full knee range of motion and quadriceps strength; and they have full quadriceps, hamstring, and calf flexibility. If the athlete is sent to a health care provider, they cannot return to activity until examined and released by the health care provider. When returning to activity, the athlete should stretch the hamstring, quadriceps, and calf muscles daily.

- For moderate to severe anterior knee pain, the athlete cannot return to activity until examined and released by a health care provider; the knee is free of pain; they have full knee range of motion and quadriceps strength; and they have full quadriceps, hamstring, and calf flexibility. When returning to activity, the athlete should stretch the hamstring, quadriceps, and calf muscles daily.

## PREVENTION

- Preseason exercises to strengthen the core, gluteal, and quadriceps muscles and stretch the quadriceps, hamstring, and calf muscles
- Adequate aerobic warm-up before activity

# ILIOTIBIAL (IT) BAND STRAIN

Iliotibial (IT) band strain is a stretch or irritation of the connective tissue along the outside of the thigh (see figure 13.14). IT band strain typically occurs over time. It is caused by forceful stretch of the connective tissue that attaches to the outside of the knee, weak or inflexible thigh muscles, running the same direction on a track or running on the sloped edge of a road, or weak or inflexible hip muscles.

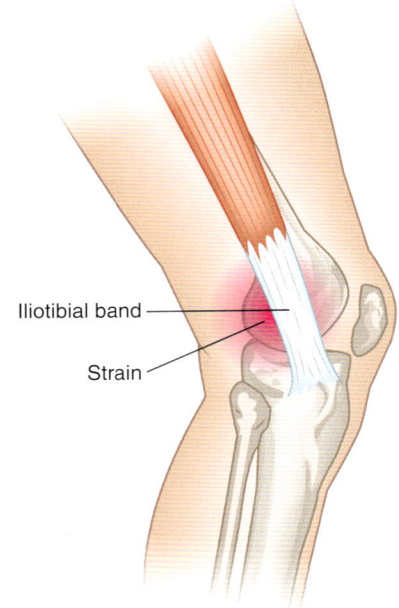

Iliotibial band
Strain

**Figure 13.14**   Iliotibial (IT) band strain.

## Signs and Symptoms

### Grade I

- Mild pain or point tenderness along the outside of the knee
- Mild pain with running, jumping, biking, or using stairs

### Grades II and III

- Moderate to severe pain or point tenderness along the outside of the knee
- Moderate to severe pain when running, jumping, biking, or using stairs
- Swelling
- Limping

## FIRST AID

### Grade I

1. Rest the athlete from painful activities.
2. Apply ice to the injury for 15 minutes.
3. Refer the athlete to the appropriate health care provider if symptoms and signs worsen (or occur more often, especially with daily activities) or do not subside within a few days.

### Grades II and III

1. Rest the athlete from all activities.
2. Monitor the athlete, treat them for shock if needed, and send for emergency medical assistance if shock occurs.
3. Prevent the athlete from walking on the injured leg.
4. Apply ice to the injury for 15 minutes, and send the athlete to the appropriate health care provider (if shock does not occur).

### Playing Status

- For a Grade I IT band strain, the athlete can return to activity if the knee is free of pain; they have full knee range of motion and gluteal muscle strength; and they have full IT band, quadriceps, and hamstring flexibility. If the athlete is sent to a health care provider, they cannot return to activity until examined and released by the health care provider. When returning to activity, the athlete may benefit from wearing a neoprene (rubberized) knee sleeve (to keep the IT band warm during activity) and from stretching the hamstrings and quadriceps daily.

- For a Grade II or Grade III IT band strain, the athlete cannot return to activity until examined and released by a health care provider; the knee is free of pain; they have full knee range of motion and gluteal muscle strength; and they have full IT band, quadriceps, and hamstring flexibility. When returning to activity, the athlete may benefit from wearing a neoprene (rubberized) knee sleeve (to keep the IT band warm during activity) and from stretching the hamstrings and quadriceps daily.

## PREVENTION

- Preseason exercises to strengthen the core and gluteal muscles and stretch the IT band, quadriceps, hamstrings, and calf
- Adequate aerobic warm-up before activity
- Avoid running the same direction on a track or on a sloped edge of a road

# KNEE CARTILAGE TEAR

A knee cartilage tear is a tear of the cartilage on top of the tibia. It is caused by compression; torsion, especially while the knee is bent and the foot is planted; or when the knee is bent to an extreme while the foot is planted (see figure 13.15).

## Signs and Symptoms

- Decreased ability or inability to completely bend or straighten the knee
- Feeling that the knee locks or won't move (can't bend or straighten)
- Feeling of the knee giving out
- Feeling of looseness or instability
- Pain at the injury site, especially along the joint line between the femur and tibia
- Feeling or hearing a pop
- Delayed swelling (cartilage injury alone) or immediate swelling (cartilage injury and ligament sprain)
- Walking with the knee bent or foot pointed
- Limping

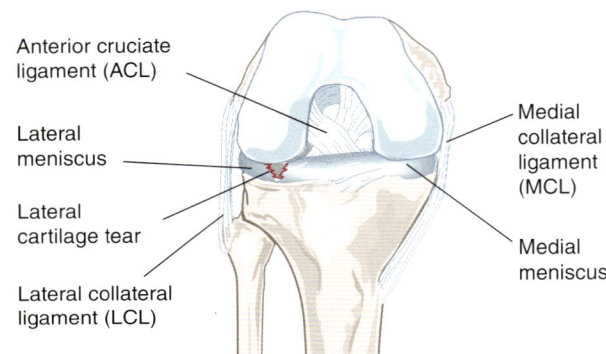

**Figure 13.15**  Knee cartilage tear.

---

### FIRST AID

1. Rest the athlete from activity.
2. Prevent the athlete from walking on the injured leg.
3. Monitor the athlete, treat them for shock if needed, and send for emergency medical assistance if shock occurs.
4. Apply ice to the injury for 15 minutes, and send the athlete to the appropriate health care provider (if shock does not occur).

## Playing Status

The athlete cannot return to activity until examined and released by a health care provider; the knee is free of pain; and they have full range of motion in the knee, and full strength and flexibility in the quadriceps, hamstrings, and calf.

---

### PREVENTION

- Preseason exercises to strengthen and stretch the hip, quadriceps, hamstrings, and calf

# LOWER LEG FRACTURE

A lower leg fracture is a break in one or both lower leg bones (tibia and fibula). It is caused by a direct blow, a compression injury (such as landing from an apparatus), or torsion.

## Signs and Symptoms

- Pain at the injury site when gently squeezed above and then below it
- Numbness or tingling in the lower leg or foot (if the fracture injures nerves)
- Lack of sensation in the lower leg, foot, or toes (if the displaced bone injures nerves)
- Inability to bend or straighten the knee (if the fracture is near the knee)
- Inability to flex the foot up or point it down (if the fracture is near the ankle)
- Inability to walk on the injured leg
- Grating sensation
- Hearing or feeling a pop or snap
- Severe pain with any movement
- Deformity
- Bluish lower leg, foot, or toes (if the displaced bone injures blood supply)
- Swelling

## FIRST AID

1. Send for emergency medical assistance.
2. Prevent the athlete from moving the entire leg.
3. Monitor the athlete, and treat them for shock if needed.

## Playing Status

The athlete cannot return to activity until examined and released by a health care provider; and they have full knee and ankle range of motion, and full quadriceps, hamstring, and lower leg muscle strength and flexibility. The athlete should wear a protective pad over the injury site when returning to activity.

## PREVENTION

- Wearing required protective padding if applicable to the sport

# CALF STRAIN

A calf strain is a stretch or tear of the calf muscles. It is caused by forceful contraction of the calf muscles, forced stretch of the calf muscles (moving the toes up toward the knee), weak or inflexible calf muscles, or explosive jumping or sprinting (see figure 13.16).

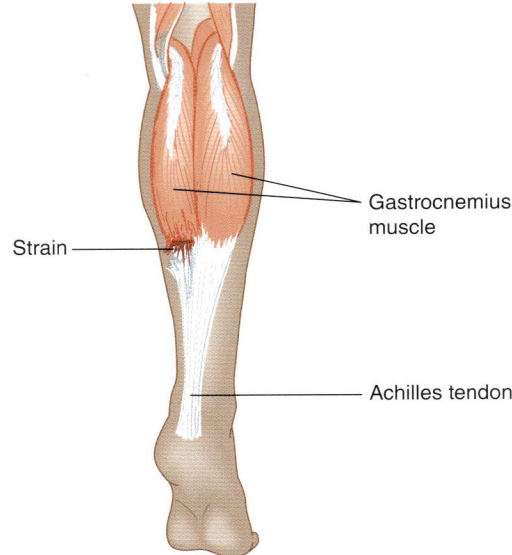

**Figure 13.16**    Calf strain.

## Signs and Symptoms

### Grade I

- Mild calf pain
- Slight point tenderness
- Mild pain when pointing the foot down
- Mild pain when flexing the foot up toward the shin
- Mild pain when jumping and running

### Grades II and III

- Moderate to severe calf pain
- Moderate to severe point tenderness
- Moderate to severe pain when pointing the foot down
- Moderate to severe pain when flexing the foot up toward the shin
- Moderate to severe pain when jumping and running
- Swelling
- Lump or indentation where the muscle is torn
- Decreased ability or inability to point the foot down

- Decreased ability or inability to jump or run
- Bruising down the back of the lower leg, ankle, or foot (appears a day or two after initial injury)
- Limping

## FIRST AID

### Grade I

1. Rest the athlete from painful activities.
2. Apply a compression wrap if available.
3. Apply ice to the injury for 15 minutes.
4. Refer the athlete to the appropriate health care provider if symptoms and signs worsen (or occur more often, especially with daily activities) or do not subside within a few days.

### Grades II and III

1. Rest the athlete from all activities.
2. Monitor the athlete, treat them for shock as needed, and send for emergency medical assistance if shock occurs.
3. Send for emergency medical assistance if the muscle is completely torn (rolled up).
4. Prevent the athlete from walking on the injured leg.
5. Apply a compression wrap and ice the injury for 15 minutes, and send the athlete to the appropriate health care provider (if emergency medical assistance is not sent for).

### Playing Status

- For a Grade I calf strain, the athlete can return to activity if the calf is free of pain; and they have full range of motion in the knee and ankle, and full strength and flexibility in the calf. If the athlete is sent to a health care provider, they cannot return to activity until examined and released by the health care provider. When returning to activity, the athlete may benefit from wearing an elastic wrap or neoprene (rubberized) calf sleeve (to support the calf) and from stretching the calf and Achilles tendon daily.
- For a Grade II or Grade III calf strain, the athlete cannot return to activity until examined and released by a health care provider; the calf is free of pain; and they have full range of motion in the knee and ankle, and full strength and flexibility in the calf. When returning to activity, the athlete may benefit from wearing an elastic wrap or neoprene (rubberized) calf sleeve (to support the calf) and from stretching the calf and Achilles tendon daily.

## PREVENTION

- Preseason exercises to strengthen the calf and stretch the calf and Achilles tendon
- Adequate aerobic warm-up before activity

# ANKLE SPRAIN

An ankle sprain is a stretch or tear of the ligaments holding the ankle bones together. It is caused by compression or torsion of the ankle joint. In an inversion sprain, the foot rolls in, damaging the outside ankle ligaments and sometimes the inside ligaments (figure 13.17). Inversion is the most common type of sprain, occurring in about 80 percent of all ankle sprains. In an eversion sprain, the foot rolls out, damaging the inside ankle ligaments and sometimes the outside ligaments.

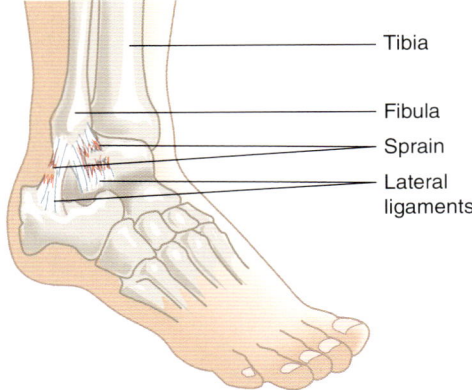

**Figure 13.17**   In an inversion sprain, the outside ankle ligaments are damaged.

## Signs and Symptoms

### Grade I

- Mild pain around the inside or outside ankle bones
- Mild pain when flexing the foot up or pointing it down
- Slight point tenderness just below the outside or inside ankle bones (tibia and fibula)

### Grades II and III

- Moderate to severe pain around the inside or outside ankle bones
- Moderate to severe pain when flexing the foot up or pointing it down
- Moderate to severe point tenderness just below the outside or inside ankle bones (tibia and fibula)
- Feeling of looseness or instability
- Hearing or feeling a pop
- Swelling
- Inability to bear weight, or limping when walking

## FIRST AID

### Grade I

1. Rest the athlete from painful activities.
2. Apply ice to the injury for 15 minutes, then apply a compression wrap.
3. Refer the athlete to the appropriate health care provider if symptoms and signs worsen (or occur more often, especially with daily activities such as walking) or do not subside within a few days.

### Grades II and III

1. Rest the athlete from all activities that require use of the leg.
2. Prevent the athlete from walking on the injured leg.
3. Monitor the athlete, treat them for shock if needed, and send for emergency medical assistance if shock occurs.
4. Send for emergency medical assistance if you notice signs of fracture (obvious deformity or pain at the site of the injury when the tibia and fibula are gently squeezed above or below the injury, or pain along the midline of the lower third of the tibia or fibula); symptoms and signs of nerve compression (tingling and numbness); or symptoms and signs of disrupted blood supply (bluish toes and toenails).
5. Apply ice to the injury for 15 minutes, and send the athlete to the appropriate health care provider (if emergency medical assistance is not sent for).

### Playing Status

- For a Grade I ankle sprain, the athlete can return to activity if signs and symptoms subside; the ankle is free of pain; and they have full ankle range of motion, lower leg strength, and calf and Achilles tendon flexibility. If the athlete is sent to a health care provider, they cannot return to activity until examined and released by the health care provider. When returning to activity, the athlete should wear a protective brace.
- For a Grade II or Grade III ankle sprain, the athlete cannot return to activity until examined and released by a health care provider; the ankle is free of pain; and they have full ankle range of motion, lower leg strength, and calf and Achilles tendon flexibility. When returning to activity, the athlete should wear a protective brace.

## PREVENTION

- Preseason exercises to strengthen the lower leg, calf and Achilles tendon stretching, and balance training

# HEEL CONTUSION

A heel contusion is a bruise to the bone or soft tissues of the heel. It is caused by wearing shoes with little heel cushioning; exercising on hard surfaces, such as concrete; landing flat on the foot; or compression (see figure 13.18).

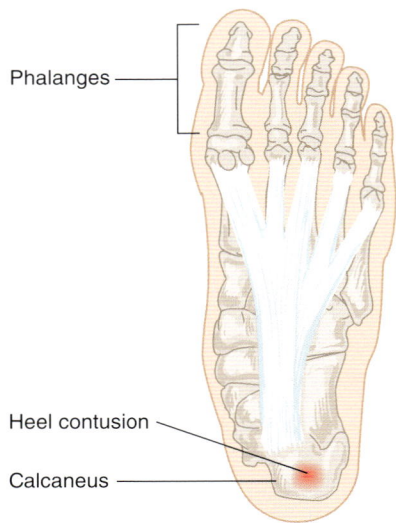

**Figure 13.18**   Heel contusion.

## Signs and Symptoms

### Mild

- Mild pain or point tenderness under the heel
- Mild pain when jumping and running

### Moderate to Severe

- Moderate to severe pain or point tenderness under the heel
- Pain when walking
- Decreased ability or inability to land or walk on the heel
- Moderate to severe pain when jumping and running
- Swelling on the bottom of the foot
- Decreased ability or inability to jump or run
- Bruising (appears a day or two after initial injury)
- Limping

## FIRST AID

### Mild

1. Rest the athlete from painful activities.
2. Apply ice to the injury for 15 minutes.
3. Refer the athlete to the appropriate health care provider if symptoms and signs worsen (or occur more often, especially with daily activities) or do not subside within a few days.

### Moderate to Severe

1. Rest the athlete from all activities.
2. Monitor the athlete, treat them for shock if needed, and send for emergency medical assistance if shock occurs.
3. Send for emergency medical assistance if you notice signs of fracture (obvious deformity or pain when the heel is gently tapped above or below the injury), symptoms and signs of nerve compression (tingling or numbness in the foot or toes), or symptoms and signs of disrupted blood supply (bluish foot or toes).
4. Prevent the athlete from walking on the injured foot.
5. Apply ice to the injury for 15 minutes, and send the athlete to the appropriate health care provider (if emergency medical assistance is not sent for).

### Playing Status

- For a mild heel contusion, the athlete can return to activity if the heel and foot are free of pain; and they have full range of motion in the ankle and foot, and full flexibility in the calf and Achilles tendon. If the athlete is sent to a health care provider, they cannot return to activity until examined and released by the health care provider. When returning to activity, the athlete would benefit from wearing a shock-absorbing heel pad or cushion in both shoes and from stretching the calf and Achilles tendon daily.
- For a moderate to severe heel contusion, the athlete cannot return to activity until examined and released by a health care provider; the heel and foot are free of pain; and they have full ankle range of motion as well as full calf and Achilles tendon flexibility. When returning to activity, the athlete would benefit from wearing a shock-absorbing heel pad or cushion in both shoes and from stretching the calf and Achilles tendon daily.

## PREVENTION

- Shoes with heel cushioning

# TURF TOE

Turf toe is a hyperextension of the great (big) toe. It is caused by forced extension (pushing off) of the big toe (see figure 13.19).

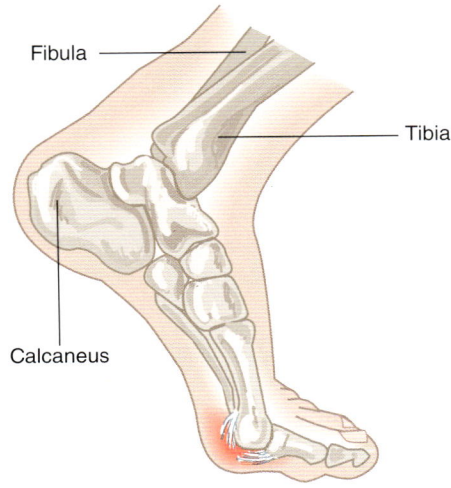

Fibula

Tibia

Calcaneus

**Figure 13.19**    Turf toe occurs when the great (big) toe is hyperextended.

### Signs and Symptoms

### Grade I

- Mild pain underneath the big toe
- Mild pain when bending or extending the big toe
- Mild pain when walking, running, or jumping, particularly when toeing off
- Slight point tenderness over the joint between the big toe and the foot

### Grades II and III

- Moderate to severe pain underneath the big toe
- Moderate to severe pain when bending or extending the big toe
- Moderate to severe pain with walking, running, or jumping, particularly when toeing off
- Moderate to severe point tenderness over the joint between the big toe and the foot
- Decreased ability or inability to land on the ball of the foot or walk on the toes
- Swelling
- Decreased ability or inability to jump or run
- Limping

## FIRST AID

### Grade I

1. Rest the athlete from all activities causing pain.
2. Apply ice to the injury for 15 minutes.
3. Refer the athlete to the appropriate health care provider if symptoms and signs worsen (or occur more often, especially with daily activities) or do not subside within a few days.

### Grades II and III

1. Rest the athlete from all activities.
2. Monitor the athlete, treat them for shock if needed, and send for emergency medical assistance if shock occurs.
3. Prevent the athlete from walking on the injured foot.
4. Apply ice to the injury for 15 minutes, and send the athlete to the appropriate health care provider (if shock does not occur).

### Playing Status

- For Grade I turf toe, the athlete can return to activity if signs and symptoms subside; the toe is free of pain; and they have full strength, flexibility, and range of motion in the toe. If the athlete is sent to a health care provider, they cannot return to activity until examined and released by the health care provider.
- For Grade II or Grade III turf toe, the athlete cannot return to activity until examined and released by a health care provider; the toe is free of pain; and they have full strength, flexibility, and range of motion in the toe.

## PREVENTION

- Shoes with stiffer forefoot bend, particularly in football, soccer, baseball, and softball

# SHIN SPLINTS

Shin splints refers to a stretch, tear, or irritation of the shin muscles, tendons, or bone covering (see figure 13.20). Causes include forceful contraction or stretch of shin muscles, suddenly increasing the intensity of the sport or conditioning program, repeatedly running on an uneven or unyielding surface, a tight Achilles tendon or tight calf muscles, weak or inflexible shin muscles, faulty foot mechanics that fail to absorb shock and allow shock to be transmitted up the lower leg bone, or shoes that are worn out or have inadequate arch support.

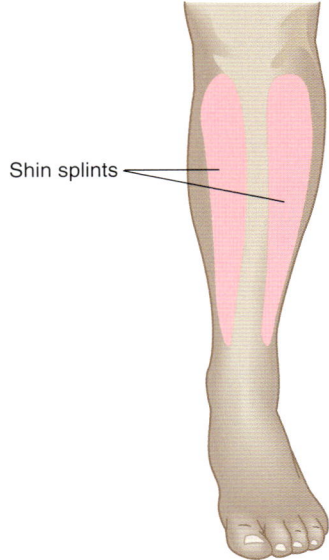

Shin splints

**Figure 13.20**   Areas of pain in shin splints.

## Signs and Symptoms

### Grade I

- Mild pain just to the inside or outside of the tibia
- Mild pain with running and jumping activities
- Pain that decreases with rest
- Slight point tenderness over the site of the injury

### Grades II and III

- Moderate to severe pain just to the inside or outside of the tibia
- Pain with walking
- Pain at rest
- Moderate to severe pain with running and jumping activities
- Moderate to severe point tenderness over the site of the injury
- Swelling
- Decreased ability or inability to run or jump

## FIRST AID

### Grade I

1. Rest the athlete from all activities causing pain.
2. Apply ice to the injury for 15 minutes.
3. Refer the athlete to the appropriate health care provider if symptoms and signs worsen (or occur more often, especially with daily activities) or do not subside within a few days.

### Grades II and III

1. Rest the athlete from all activities.
2. Monitor the athlete, treat them for shock if needed, and send for emergency medical assistance if shock occurs.
3. Send for emergency medical assistance if you notice signs of fracture (obvious deformity, or pain at the site of the injury when compressing the tibia or fibula above, then below the site of the injury), symptoms and signs of compression to nerves (tingling or numbness in the foot or toes), or symptoms and signs of disrupted blood supply (bluish foot or toes that are cold to the touch).
4. Prevent the athlete from walking on the injured leg.
5. Apply ice to the injury for 15 minutes, and send the athlete to the appropriate health care provider (if emergency medical assistance is not sent for).

### Playing Status

- For Grade I shin splints, the athlete can return to activity if signs and symptoms subside; the shin is free of pain; and they have full ankle range of motion, lower leg strength, and calf and Achilles tendon flexibility. If the athlete is sent to a health care provider, they cannot return to activity until examined and released by the health care provider. When returning to activity, the athlete would benefit from wearing shoes with firm arch support and from stretching the calf and Achilles tendon daily.
- For Grade II or Grade III shin splints, the athlete cannot return to activity until examined and released by a health care provider; the shin is free of pain; and they have full ankle range of motion, lower leg strength, and calf and Achilles tendon flexibility. When returning to activity, the athlete would benefit from wearing shoes with firm arch support and from stretching the calf and Achilles tendon daily.

## PREVENTION

- Preseason exercises to strengthen the lower leg and stretch the calf and Achilles tendon
- Adequate aerobic warm-up before activity
- No greater than 10-percent increase in training intensity per week
- Shoes with firm arch support

# TIBIAL STRESS FRACTURE

A tibial stress fracture is a break or crack in the tibia that occurs over time. Causes for this injury include suddenly increasing the intensity of a sport or conditioning program (more than 10% per week); repeatedly running or jumping on an uneven or unyielding surface; faulty foot mechanics that fail to absorb shock, allowing shock to be transmitted up the lower leg bone; shoes that are worn out or have inadequate arch support; or amenorrhea (lack of menstrual period, sometimes caused by anorexia).

Signs and symptoms of a tibial stress fracture may include pain along the front of the shin, pain with walking, pain at rest, moderate to severe pain with running and jumping activities, moderate to severe point tenderness over the site of the injury, pain at the site of the injury when the tibia is pressed above or below the injury, swelling, decreased ability or inability to run or jump, or limping.

First aid for tibial stress fractures should include resting the athlete from all activities that require use of the leg and preventing the athlete from walking on the injured leg. Monitor the athlete, treat them for shock if needed, and send for emergency medical assistance if it occurs. Send for emergency medical assistance if the following are present: obvious deformity, symptoms and signs of nerve compression (tingling or numbness in foot or toes), or symptoms and signs of disrupted blood supply (foot or toes appear bluish and are cold to the touch). If emergency medical assistance was not needed, apply ice to the injury for 15 minutes, and send the athlete to the appropriate health care provider.

The athlete cannot return to activity until examined and released by a health care provider; the shin is free of pain; and they have full ankle range of motion, lower leg strength, and calf and Achilles tendon flexibility. When returning to activity, the athlete should wear shoes with firm arch support. To help prevent tibial stress fractures, use appropriate increments for increasing training intensity no greater than 10 percent per week. Instruct athletes to wear shoes with firm arch support and to run on shock-absorbing and even surfaces such as wood or grass.

# EXERTIONAL COMPARTMENT SYNDROME

Exertional compartment syndrome is an increase in pressure, typically in front of the lower leg, that constricts blood flow to the lower leg and foot (see figure 13.21). Although the cause is not known for certain, it is possibly a result of tight fascia (tissue) surrounding muscles, tendons, nerves, and arteries of the lower leg. Signs and symptoms of exertional compartment syndrome could include burning, aching, or cramping in the front of the lower leg during activity that may continue after activity, tingling in the foot or toes during activity or at rest, feeling of fullness or tightness that may worsen as activity progresses, slight swelling and tightness to the touch, pain that typically begins after starting exercise or after reaching a certain intensity level, and pain that is relieved with rest and recurs upon resuming activity. The athlete may also exhibit redness or warmth to the touch, and inability to hold the toes up while walking.

First aid for exertional compartment syndrome should include resting the athlete from all activities and preventing the athlete from walking on the injured leg. If an athlete complains of numbness, tingling, or weakness in the lower leg, foot, or toes, you should avoid applying a compression wrap; the added compression can worsen the condition by further restricting blood flow to the area or by compressing the nerves to the foot. Monitor the athlete, treat them for shock if needed, and send for emergency medical assistance if shock occurs. If shock does not occur, instruct the athlete to elevate the leg, and send them to the appropriate health care provider.

The athlete cannot return to activity until examined and released by a health care provider; the leg is free of pain; and they have full ankle range of motion, lower leg and toe strength, and calf and Achilles tendon flexibility.

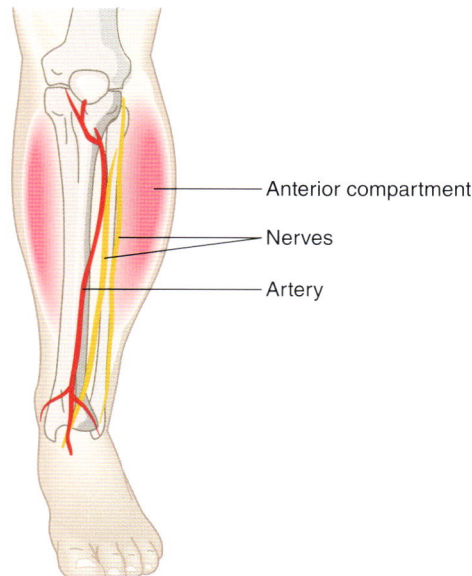

Anterior compartment

Nerves

Artery

**Figure 13.21**   Exertional compartment syndrome.

# ACHILLES TENDINITIS

Achilles tendinitis is a stretch, tear, or irritation to the tendon that attaches the calf muscles to the heel. It is caused by repeated forceful contraction or stretching of the calf muscles; or participating in repetitive, stressful activity that requires going up on the toes, such as gymnastics, basketball, or volleyball (see figure 13.22).

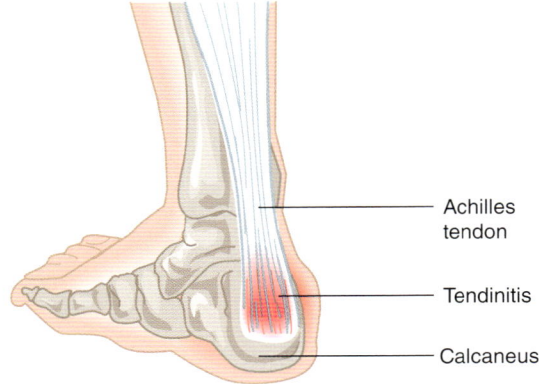

Achilles tendon

Tendinitis

Calcaneus

**Figure 13.22** Achilles tendinitis.

### Signs and Symptoms

### Mild

- Mild pain between the heel and lower calf
- Mild pain when running and jumping
- Mild pain when pointing the foot down
- Mild pain when flexing the foot up toward the shin
- Slight point tenderness

### Moderate to Severe

- Moderate to severe pain between the heel and lower calf
- Moderate to severe pain when pointing the foot down
- Moderate to severe pain when flexing the foot up toward the shin
- Moderate to severe pain when jumping and running
- Moderate to severe point tenderness
- Swelling
- Thickening of the tendon
- Decreased ability or inability to point the foot down or rise up on the toes
- Decreased ability or inability to jump or run
- Limping

## FIRST AID

### Mild

1. Rest the athlete from painful activities.
2. Apply ice for 15 minutes.
3. Refer the athlete to the appropriate health care provider if symptoms and signs worsen (or occur more often, especially with daily activities) or do not subside within a few days.

### Moderate to Severe

1. Rest the athlete from all activities.
2. Monitor the athlete, treat them for shock if needed, and send for emergency medical assistance if it occurs.
3. Prevent the athlete from walking on the injured leg.
4. Apply ice to the injury for 15 minutes, and send the athlete to the appropriate health care provider (if shock does not occur).

### Playing Status

- For mild Achilles tendinitis, the athlete can return to activity if the Achilles tendon is free of pain; and they have full range of motion in the ankle, and full strength and flexibility in the Achilles tendon and calf. If the athlete is sent to a health care provider, they cannot return to activity until examined and released by the health care provider. When returning to activity, the athlete should stretch the Achilles tendon and calf daily.

- For moderate to severe Achilles tendinitis, the athlete cannot return to activity until examined and released by a health care provider; the Achilles tendon is free of pain; and they have full range of motion in the ankle, and full strength and flexibility in the Achilles and calf. When returning to activity, the athlete should stretch the Achilles tendon and calf daily.

## PREVENTION

- Preseason exercises to strengthen and stretch the Achilles tendon and calf
- Adequate aerobic warm-up before activity

# PLANTAR FASCIITIS

Plantar fasciitis is stretching or inflammation of the fascia (connective tissue) that connects to the heel and toes (see figure 13.23). Causes include flat feet, high arches, wearing shoes with inadequate arch support, tight calf muscles, or increasing running intensity too soon (more than 10% per week). Signs and symptoms of plantar fasciitis may include mild pain along the arch or near the bottom of the heel, mild pain when running or jumping, slight point tenderness, moderate to severe pain along the arch or near the bottom of the heel, feeling of muscle tightness or weakness, pain with walking, moderate to severe pain with running or jumping, moderate to severe point tenderness, flattened arch, decreased ability or inability to push off with the foot or point the foot down, swelling, and limping.

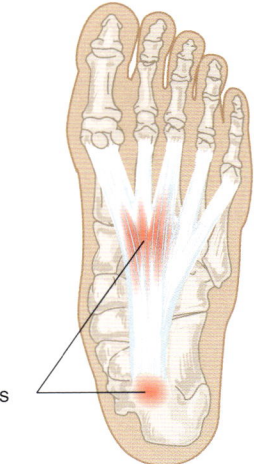

Plantar fasciitis

**Figure 13.23**    Plantar fasciitis.

First aid for plantar fasciitis should include resting the athlete from all activities and preventing the athlete from walking on the injured leg. Monitor the athlete, treat them for shock if needed, and send for emergency medical assistance if shock occurs. Apply ice to the injury for 15 minutes, and send the athlete to the appropriate health care provider (if shock does not occur).

The athlete cannot return to activity until examined and released by a health care provider, the plantar fascia is free of pain, and they have full calf and Achilles tendon flexibility. When returning to activity, the athlete would benefit from wearing shoes with adequate heel cushioning and firm arch support; and stretching the calf, Achilles tendon, and plantar fascia daily. To help prevent plantar fasciitis, encourage athletes to do preseason exercises that stretch the calf, Achilles tendon, and plantar fascia. In addition, make sure they perform an adequate aerobic warm-up before activity. Use appropriate increments for increasing training intensity (no more than 10% increase per week). Instruct athletes to wear shoes with adequate heel cushioning and firm arch support.

## Chapter 13 Recap

❑ What are the signs of hip dislocation?

❑ What is a hip pointer?

❑ What can happen if a thigh contusion is repeatedly subjected to direct blows?

❑ What is the most obvious sign of a dislocated patella?

❑ Turf toe is an injury to which toe?

❑ How can you differentiate between shin splints and a tibial stress fracture?

❑ What are the symptoms and signs of moderate to severe exertional compartment syndrome?

# SCALP, FACIAL, EYE, AND MOUTH INJURIES

## IN THIS CHAPTER, YOU WILL LEARN THE FOLLOWING:

- How to identify serious scalp, facial, eye, and mouth injuries
- How to provide appropriate first aid care for scalp, facial, eye, and mouth injuries
- Ways to prevent scalp, facial, mouth, and eye injuries
- How to determine when a face or scalp laceration requires medical attention

## INJURIES IN THIS CHAPTER

Sports can be tough on the scalp, face, eyes, and mouth. One quick jab of an elbow or an unexpected bounce of a ball on the court can quickly lead to an athlete sitting in an ophthalmologist's or oral surgeon's chair. Consider this scenario: An athlete takes a blow to the face area that results in bleeding from the mouth and nose. What are the steps you follow to ensure the health and safety of the athlete?

Of all injuries reported in each sport during the 2020 to 2021 high school season, scalp, face, eye, and mouth injuries were most prevalent in softball (33.1%), boys' soccer (20.9%), girls' soccer (20.1%), boys' basketball (19.8%), and football (18.9%); girls' volleyball, wrestling, and girls' basketball came in shortly behind (Collins, Robison, and Burus 2022). Because these injuries involve vital sensory organs such as the eyes, nose, mouth, and ears as well as an athlete's appearance, great care should be taken when evaluating and providing first aid care. Before discussing the details of each injury, here is an overview of the common injuries of the face, eyes, and mouth:

- Since an extensive network of blood vessels supply the area, injuries to the scalp, face, eye, and mouth tend to bleed heavily and can seem intimidating. However, their appearance is often worse than the actual injury. Sport-related facial injuries account for 8 percent of all facial soft-tissue injuries, and approximately 11 to 40 percent of all sport injuries involve the face (Collins, Robison, and Burus 2022). Injuries are most often caused by direct hits with a ball or by contact between athletes. For first aid protocols related to lacerations of the face and scalp, see the Face or Scalp Laceration flowchart in the appendix.

- Sports can put the eyes at risk for devastating injuries. For instance, softball and baseball pitchers have been clocked at over 90 miles per hour (145 km/h); tennis, lacrosse, basketball, ice hockey, field hockey, and badminton come with similar risks. Wearing protective eyewear or face guards can significantly reduce the risk of eye injury and the American Academy of Ophthalmology (2024) suggests this can

prevent 90 percent of eye injuries. For first aid procedures related to the eyes, see the Direct Blow to the Eye and Eye Abrasion flowcharts in the appendix.

- A variety of tooth injuries occur in sports, including dislocation, displacement, fracture, and chipping. Basketball, football, hockey, martial arts, and boxing carry the highest risk of these injuries. However, noncontact sports carry risk as well (Young, Macias, and Stephens 2015). Wearing custom-fitted mouth guards can prevent most of these injuries. In fact, an analysis of multiple studies investigating the effectiveness of mouth guards reducing orofacial injuries found that using a mouth guard reduced the overall risk of orofacial injuries (Knapik et al. 2019).

- The external ear is vulnerable to contusions, lacerations, and avulsions. Fortunately, these injuries are easily prevented with protective headgear and rules forbidding jewelry during practices and competitions.

Also, be aware that in some cases of injury to the scalp, face, eyes, and mouth, a concussion may occur. If an athlete has an injury to these areas, you should check for signs and symptoms of a concussion. Please consult chapter 8 for more information on concussion and concussion management.

---

**SAFETY MEASURE**

**With Eye Abrasions and Facial Fractures**

- If an athlete has an eye abrasion,

  - do not rub or wash the eye,
  - do not remove embedded objects or glass, and
  - do not remove contact lenses.

- If an athlete has a nose, face, or jaw fracture,

  - the athlete needs a quick evaluation (because these injuries can affect breathing passages) and
  - use a light touch when feeling for deformities (to avoid causing further damage).

# FACE OR SCALP LACERATION

A face or scalp laceration is a cut, usually around the eyebrow (see figure 14.1), chin, forehead, nose, or scalp. It is caused by a direct blow or contact with an object such as a ball, elbow, or racket.

## Signs and Symptoms

- Pain
- Rapid bleeding
- Swelling
- Possible bruising

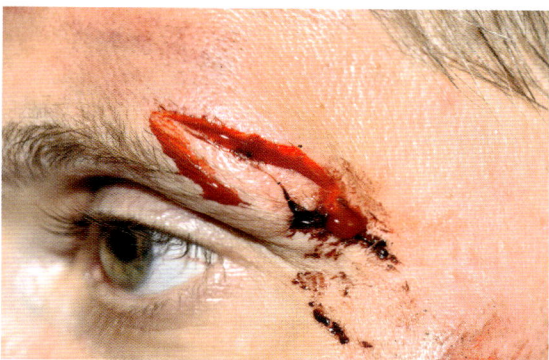

**Figure 14.1**   Face laceration.

DR P. MARAZZI / Science Source

## FIRST AID

If the athlete doesn't have an obvious deformity at the site of the injury, or exhibit signs of brain, spine, or other serious injury, do the following:

1. Place the athlete in a seated position.
2. Cover the injury with sterile gauze, and apply pressure.
3. After the bleeding stops, cover the injury with sterile gauze or a bandage.
4. Send the athlete to the appropriate health care provider if the edges of the wound gape apart (they don't touch), if you're unable to completely clean all debris out of the wound, or if a foreign body is embedded in the wound.
5. If bleeding does not stop, the athlete is experiencing breathing problems, or the athlete exhibits signs of spine, head, or other unstable or serious injuries, send for emergency medical assistance; monitor the athlete's breathing and for signs of shock; and provide CPR and treat them for shock if needed.

## Playing Status

If the edges of the wound gape open, there is concern about disfigurement, or the athlete was sent to a health care provider, the athlete cannot return to activity until examined and released by the health care provider. If bleeding stops, the edges of the wound are touching, and the athlete and parent or guardian are not concerned about disfigurement, the athlete can return to activity (the wound must be covered).

## PREVENTION

- Wearing sport-appropriate protective equipment such as face masks, headgear, helmets, protective eyewear, and mouth guards

# EYE CONTUSION

An eye contusion is a bruise to the structures of the eye. It is caused by a direct blow, such as with an elbow or a ball.

## Signs and Symptoms

- Blood pooling in the white of the eye or the iris (figure 14.2a)
- Restricted eye motion
- Irregularly shaped iris or pupil (figure 14.2b)
- Abrasion or cut to the cornea (figure 14.2c)
- Blind spot
- Double vision
- Floating spots in vision
- Persistent blurred vision
- Pain
- Perception of flashing light
- Dark tissue sticking out of the cornea or sclera
- Pupil inequality (reaction to light, size, tracking)
- Inability to open the eye
- Loss of peripheral vision
- Palpable defect of bones around the eye
- Sensitivity to light
- Pupils misaligned (one higher than other)

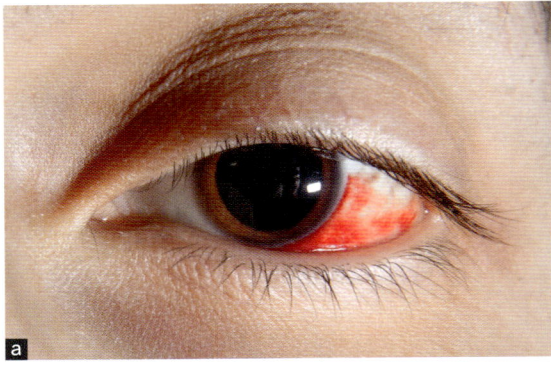

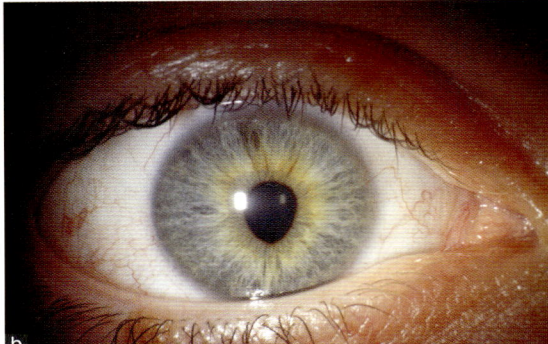

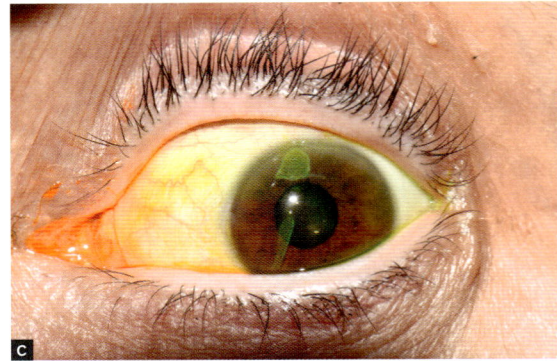

**Figure 14.2** Signs of eye injury: *(a)* blood pooling in the eye, *(b)* irregular pupil, and *(c)* corneal abrasion.

(a) JohnAlexander/iStock/Getty Images; (b) Sue Ford / Science Source; (c) DR P. MARAZZI / Science Source

## FIRST AID

1. Call for emergency medical assistance.
2. Seat the athlete in an upright or semireclining position (45°).
3. If emergency assistance is delayed more than 15 minutes, loosely apply an eye patch over both eyes (to limit motion).
4. Monitor the athlete's breathing, and provide CPR if needed.
5. Monitor the athlete, and treat them for shock if needed.

### Playing Status

The athlete cannot return to activity until examined and released by a health care provider.

## PREVENTION

- Wearing protective glasses, goggles, or face shields designed for sports

# OBJECT EMBEDDED IN EYE

An object embedded in the eye is something that has penetrated the eye tissue and sits firmly in it. It is usually caused by a splinter or other object. In sports, there are many circumstances that may lead to an object being embedded in the eye and objects could be very small. Whenever an athlete complains of any of the signs and symptoms listed next, be sure to follow the first aid steps detailed in this section.

## Signs and Symptoms

- Pain
- Burning
- Blood pooling in the white of the eye or the iris
- Irregularly shaped iris or pupil
- Cut to the cornea
- Dark tissue sticking out of the cornea or sclera
- Embedded object

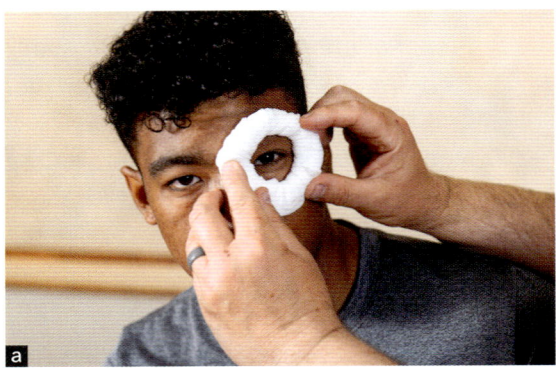
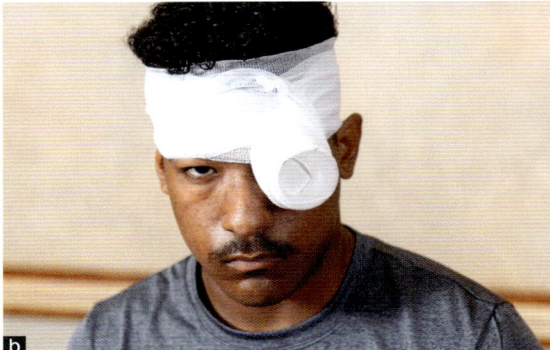

**Figure 14.3**   First aid care for an embedded object in the eye includes *(a)* loosely applying donut-shaped gauze padding around the eye and *(b)* placing a paper cup securely with roller gauze and tape.

## FIRST AID

1. Call for emergency medical assistance.
2. Seat the athlete in an upright position.
3. If emergency assistance is delayed more than 15 minutes, loosely apply a shield over the embedded object to prevent it from moving (see figure 14.3 for two types of eye shields).
4. Monitor breathing, and provide CPR if needed.
5. Monitor the athlete, and treat them for shock if needed.

## Playing Status

The athlete cannot return to activity until examined and released by a health care provider.

## PREVENTION

- Wearing protective glasses, goggles, or face shields designed for sports

# FRACTURED EYE SOCKET

A fractured eye socket is a break in the bony socket surrounding the eye. This injury is caused by a direct blow. Signs and symptoms may include pain, altered sensation beneath the eye, eyelid swelling, double vision, restricted eye movement, deformity, misaligned pupils (one higher than the other), discoloration, or bleeding in the white of the eye.

If you suspect a fractured eye socket, do the following: Seat the athlete in an upright or semireclining position (45°), and send for emergency medical assistance. Monitor the athlete's breathing, and monitor for signs of shock; provide CPR if needed, and treat for shock if needed.

The athlete cannot return to activity until examined and released by a health care provider. Upon return to activity, the athlete should wear protective eye goggles or a face shield. This eyewear must be compliant with your state or sport organization regulations. Additionally, some states require documentation from the health care provider that allows the athlete to wear the protective equipment.

# EYE ABRASION

An eye abrasion is a superficial scratch to the clear part (cornea) covering the eye. It is caused by dirt, sand, or other foreign material entering the eye. In sports, there are many circumstances that may lead to an object entering the eye and objects could be very small. Whenever an athlete complains of any of the signs and symptoms listed next, be sure to follow the first aid steps detailed in this section.

**Signs and Symptoms**

- Pain
- Burning sensation
- Sensation of something in the eye
- Redness
- Tearing
- Foreign object in the eye
- Decreased vision
- Blurred vision
- Sensitivity to light
- Scratch on the eye

## FIRST AID

Unless the object is glass, try to remove any small, irritating particle such as dirt, as shown in figure 14.4. If you are unable to remove the object or decrease the athlete's pain, if the athlete experiences loss or blurring of vision, or if the object is glass, do the following:

1. Seat the athlete in a semireclining position (45°).
2. Loosely apply an eye patch, bandage, or cup over one or both eyes (see figure 14.5). Otherwise, movements of the uninjured eye will cause the injured eye to move.
3. Immediately send the athlete to the appropriate health care provider.

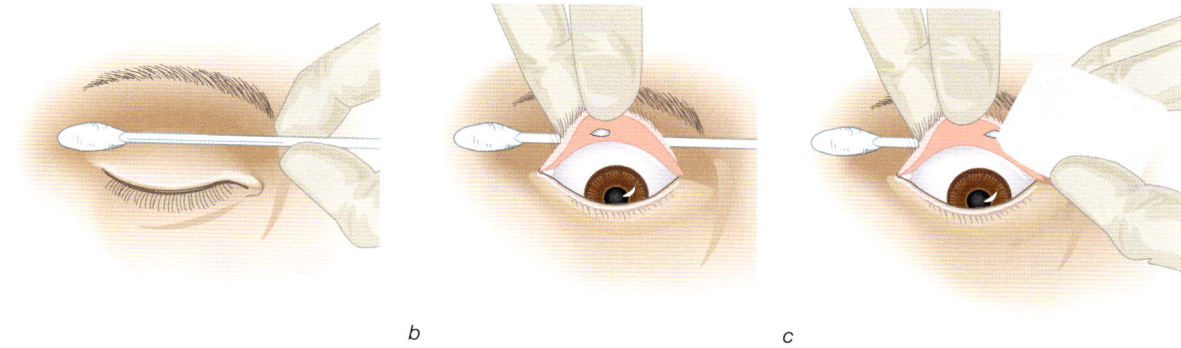

*a*                              *b*                              *c*

**Figure 14.4**   If the object is under the upper eyelid, *(a)* place a cotton-tip applicator over the lid, *(b)* pull the lid up with your fingers, and *(c)* remove the object with sterile gauze. (Be sure to moisten the gauze with sterile saline solution.)

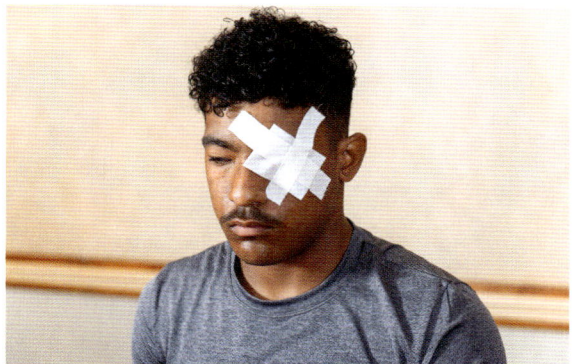

**Figure 14.5**   To cover the eye with a patch, loosely place sterile gauze over the eye and then lightly secure the gauze to the face with tape.

## Playing Status

If the athlete has persistent pain or blurred or decreased vision, they cannot return to activity until examined and released by a health care provider.

### PREVENTION

- Wearing protective eyeglasses, goggles, or face shields designed for sports

# BLOODY NOSE

A bloody nose occurs when a direct blow, head injury, high blood pressure, or dry nasal passages cause the nose to bleed.

**Signs and Symptoms**

- Bleeding from the nose
- Pain (from a direct blow)
- Stuffiness or nasal congestion

## FIRST AID

1. Seat the athlete with their head forward.
2. Using sterile gauze, pinch the nostrils shut for 5 to 10 minutes to apply direct pressure (see figure 14.6).
3. If the bleeding doesn't stop within 15 to 20 minutes, or if it was caused by an injury, send the athlete to the appropriate health care provider.
4. Discourage the athlete from blowing their nose.

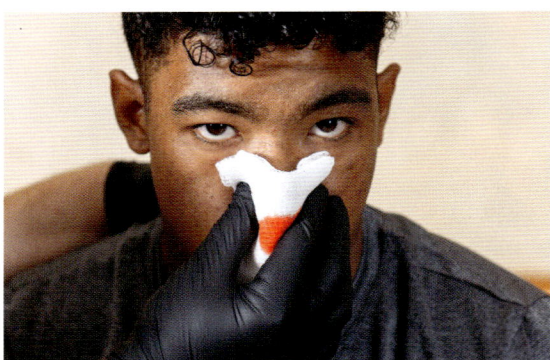

**Figure 14.6**    Direct pressure for bloody nose.

**Playing Status**

The athlete can return to activity once the bleeding has stopped for 5 minutes. If the bleeding was caused by a serious injury, the athlete cannot return to activity until examined and released by a health care provider.

## PREVENTION

- Wearing protective face masks and guards for football, ice hockey, and lacrosse

# FRACTURED NOSE

A fractured (broken) nose is a break in the nose cartilage or bone. It is caused by a direct blow. Signs and symptoms of a broken nose may include pain, a grating sensation, swelling, discoloration, possible deformity, possible bleeding, or the inability to breathe through the nose.

If you suspect a broken nose, seat the athlete with their head forward to allow blood and fluid to drain from the nose, then gently apply ice for 15 minutes. If necessary to stop bleeding, gently pinch the nostrils shut with gauze. Refer the athlete to the appropriate health care provider.

The athlete cannot return to activity until examined and released by a health care provider. When returning to contact activity, the athlete should wear a nose protector (if the health care provider prescribes it as a stipulation for return to play). For prevention, all athletes should wear protective face masks and shields for football, lacrosse, and ice hockey.

# MIDFACE FRACTURE

A midface fracture is a break of the maxilla, the facial bone above the mouth. This injury is caused by a direct blow (see figure 14.7). Signs and symptoms may include pain, numbness, inability to bring the teeth together properly, visual problems, nasal discharge (blood or other fluid), bruising, deformity, and tenderness when the fractured area is touched.

To apply first aid for a midface fracture, do the following: If breathing is impaired or the athlete is experiencing shock, then monitor the athlete, administer CPR or treat for shock if needed, and call for emergency medical assistance. Otherwise, gently apply ice for 15 minutes, and send the athlete to the appropriate health care provider.

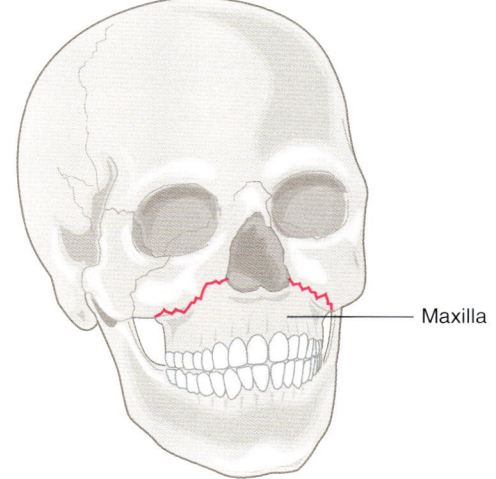

**Figure 14.7**  Midface fracture.

The athlete cannot return to activity until examined and released by a health care provider. When returning to activity, the athlete should wear a protective face shield. This face shield must be compliant with your state or sport organization regulations. Additionally, some states require documentation from the health care provider that allows the athlete to wear it. For prevention, all athletes should wear protective face guards for football, ice hockey, and lacrosse.

# CHEEKBONE FRACTURE

A cheekbone fracture is a break in the zygomatic bone (cheekbone). This injury is caused by a direct blow (see figure 14.8). Signs and symptoms may include pain with jaw movement, altered sensation underneath the eye, pain or numbness in the face or cheeks, a flattened cheek or other deformity, or blood in the side of the eye.

To apply first aid for a cheekbone fracture, do the following: If breathing is impaired or the athlete is experiencing shock, then monitor the athlete, administer CPR or treat for shock if needed, and call for emergency medical assistance. Otherwise, gently apply ice for 15 minutes, and send the athlete to the appropriate health care provider.

The athlete cannot return to activity until examined and released by a health care provider. When returning to activity, the athlete should wear a protective face guard. For prevention, all athletes should wear protective face guards for football, ice hockey, and lacrosse.

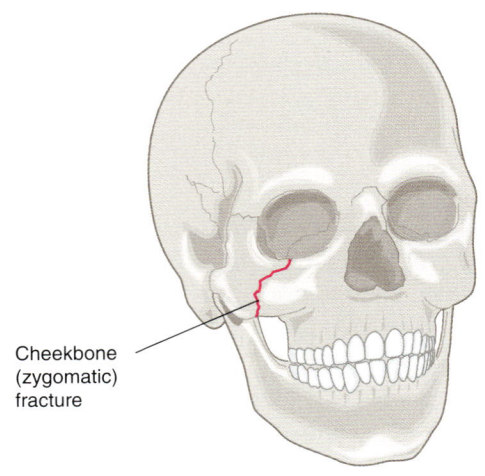

Cheekbone (zygomatic) fracture

**Figure 14.8**   A cheekbone fracture is a break in the zygomatic bone (cheekbone).

# JAW INJURY

A jaw injury could be a fracture, contusion, or dislocation of the mandible (jaw). It is caused by a torsion injury or a direct blow (see figure 14.9).

**Signs and Symptoms**

- Pain
- Popping sensation when opening and closing the mouth
- Deformity
- Discoloration
- Swelling
- Inability to close the mouth
- Jaw out of place
- Occlusion (upper and lower teeth don't line up when jaw is closed)

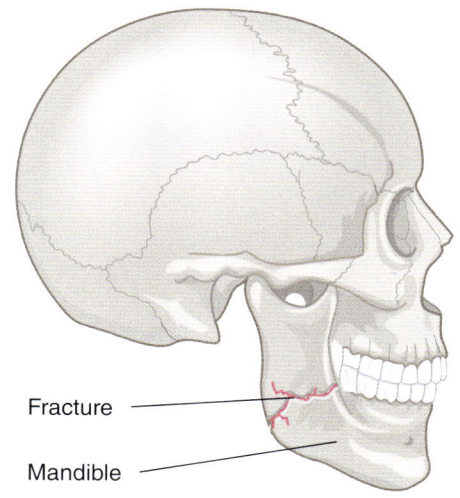

**Figure 14.9**    Fracture of the mandible (jaw).

## FIRST AID

If breathing is impaired, deformity is present, or the athlete is experiencing shock, do the following:

1. Send for emergency medical assistance.
2. Monitor breathing, and administer CPR if needed.
3. If no spine injury is suspected and no signs of shock occur, seat the athlete with the head forward to allow fluid to drain from the mouth. If no spine injury is suspected but the athlete is experiencing shock, then lay the athlete on their side, avoiding pressure to the jaw.

If breathing is not impaired, deformity is not present, and the athlete is not experiencing shock, do the following:

1. Gently apply ice for 15 minutes.
2. Send the athlete to the appropriate health care provider.

**Playing Status**

The athlete cannot return to activity until examined and released by a health care provider.

## PREVENTION

- Wearing helmets, mouth guards, and face masks when appropriate

# DISLOCATED TOOTH

A dislocated tooth occurs when a tooth is knocked out of its socket. This injury is caused by a direct blow. Signs and symptoms may include pain, bleeding, a totally dislodged tooth, or swelling of the gums.

For first aid of a tooth that is dislocated, try to save the tooth and control bleeding. Hold the tooth by the crown (not the root). If the tooth is dirty, rinse (don't scrub) it with saline solution. Water can be used if saline is not available, but it can greatly decrease the chances of a successful reimplantation. Attempt to reimplant the tooth; if the tooth cannot be reimplanted, you can place it in a tooth-preserving kit (if not available, use saliva or cow's milk). Do not store the tooth in tap water.

Seat the athlete with the head forward to allow blood to drain from the mouth, clean bleeding wounds with saline solution or tap water, and have the athlete bite down on a piece of sterile gauze to help soak and slow bleeding. Send the athlete to a dentist immediately. The best chance for successful reimplantation of the tooth is if it is done within 30 minutes of the injury. If the athlete is experiencing breathing difficulties, shock, head or spine injury, compound facial fracture, or other unstable injuries, send for emergency medical assistance while you monitor the athlete and provide CPR or treat for shock if needed.

The athlete cannot return to activity until examined and released by a dentist or oral surgeon. For prevention, athletes should wear mouth guards for contact sports.

# CHIPPED TOOTH

A chipped tooth is a break in a portion of a tooth. It is caused by a direct blow (see figure 14.10).

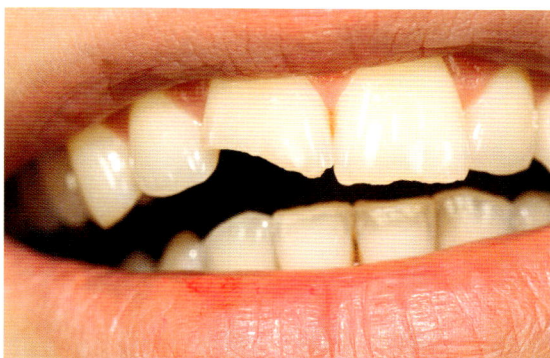

**Figure 14.10**    Chipped tooth.

Dabjola/iStock/Getty Images

## Signs and Symptoms

- Pain (if broken down to the dentin or pulp)
- Sensitivity to heat, cold, or pressure (if broken down to the dentin or pulp)
- Part of the tooth missing
- Bleeding
- Visible crack

## FIRST AID

1. Seat the athlete with the head forward to allow blood to drain from the mouth.
2. Apply pressure with sterile gauze to areas that are bleeding.
3. Send the athlete to a dentist as quickly as possible.

## Playing Status

The athlete cannot return to activity until examined and released by a dentist or oral surgeon.

## PREVENTION

- Wearing mouth guards in contact sports

# EAR CONTUSION (CAULIFLOWER EAR)

An ear contusion (cauliflower ear) is a contusion to the ear. It is caused by a direct blow or repeated rubbing of the ear against a hard surface (see figure 14.11). This condition is common in any activity where significant shearing or impact forces exist, especially wrestling and boxing.

## Signs and Symptoms

- Pain
- Burning feeling
- Swelling of the outer ear
- Discoloration
- Warmth
- Redness
- Deformity

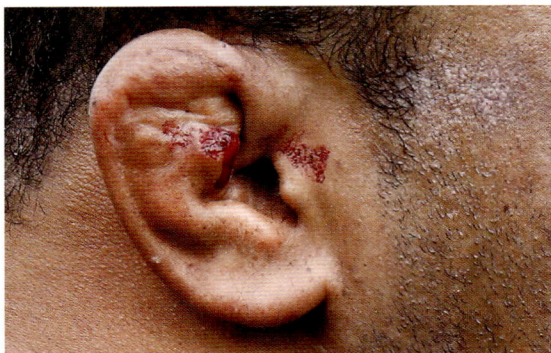

**Figure 14.11** Ear contusion.

Michael Dodge/Getty Images

## FIRST AID

1. Gently apply ice for 5 to 10 minutes.
2. Send the athlete to the appropriate health care provider.

## Playing Status

The athlete cannot return to activity until examined and released by a health care provider.

## PREVENTION

- Wearing sport-appropriate protective headgear or other ear covering

## Chapter 14 Recap

❑ What can athletes do to prevent eye injuries?

❑ Describe the first aid care for a bloody nose.

❑ What are the signs and symptoms of a broken nose?

❑ What are some symptoms and signs of a facial fracture?

❑ What can you do for the best chance of successfully reimplanting a dislocated tooth?

❑ Describe the first aid care for a chipped tooth.

❑ Describe the signs and symptoms of ear contusion.

# SKIN CONDITIONS

## INJURIES AND CONDITIONS IN THIS CHAPTER

A common characteristic of world-class athletes is the ability to concentrate. Even if your athletes are not of such high caliber, concentration can mean the difference between winning and losing. Skin conditions are a common source of distraction. Even worse, they can result in serious infections that can sideline an athlete or spread to other athletes.

Your first aid goal for skin conditions should be to prevent your athletes from being sidelined or distracted by these seemingly minor problems. In this chapter, you'll learn how to recognize and administer first aid for skin disorders, how to determine when a skin disorder requires a health care provider's evaluation, and how to implement skin disorder prevention strategies. Skin disorders can be classified into two categories: noncontagious and contagious. Regardless of contagiousness, you should always wear protective gloves when handling skin conditions.

**SAFETY MEASURE**

**When Cleaning Wounds**
When cleansing and caring for wounds, avoid using iodine. An athlete may have an iodine allergy.

## Noncontagious Skin Conditions

Noncontagious skin conditions are quite common among athletes. Although they tend to be minor problems, it is important to monitor these conditions for signs of serious skin infection, such as pus, fever, and red streaks extending from the area. If any signs of infection occur, refer the athlete to the appropriate health care provider. To learn the first aid protocol for abrasion, see the Abrasion flowchart in the appendix.

# NAIL CONTUSION

A nail contusion is blood between the nail bed and the nail on a finger or toe. It is caused by a direct blow (see figure 15.1).

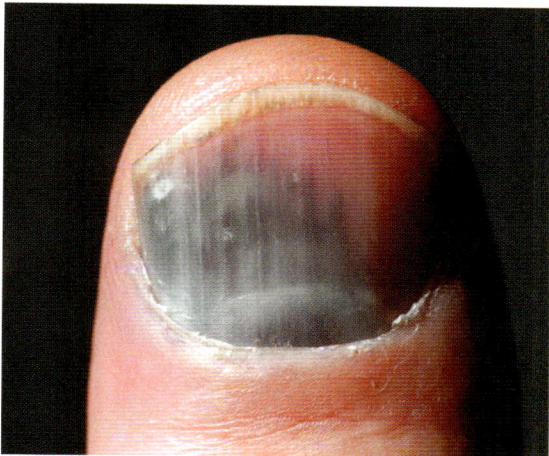

**Figure 15.1**   Contused nail.

Jan Hakan Dahlstrom/Stone/Getty Images

## Signs and Symptoms

- Pain
- Feeling of pressure under the nail
- Blood or bruising under the nail
- Swelling

## FIRST AID

1. Apply ice immediately for 10 to 15 minutes to reduce swelling under the nail.
2. If more than 25 percent of the area of the nail bed is bruised, or if pain is severe, send the athlete to the appropriate health care provider.

## Playing Status

The athlete can return to activity as long as the nail is intact, the athlete is experiencing minimal pain, and there is little risk of further injury. If the athlete is sent to a health care provider, they cannot return to activity until examined and released by the health care provider.

## PREVENTION

- Wearing protective finger padding as appropriate

# INGROWN TOENAIL

An ingrown toenail occurs when the edge of the toenail pushes excessively into the skin. It is caused by trimming nails at an angle, tight shoes or socks, or toenail deformity (see figure 15.2).

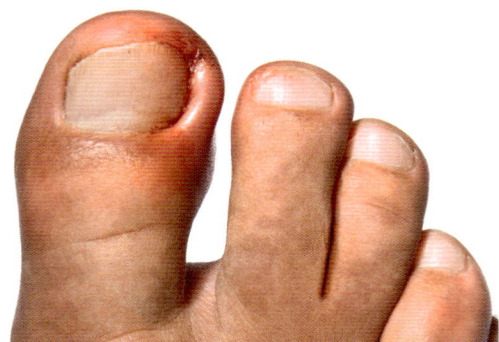

**Figure 15.2**   Ingrown toenail.

apomares/E+/Getty Images

## Signs and Symptoms

- Pain on the sides of the toenail
- Redness
- Warmth
- Swelling
- Pus (severe)

## FIRST AID

1. Soak the foot in warm water.
2. Send the athlete to the appropriate health care provider if there are signs of infection (red streaks extending from the area, fever, pus, or warmth).

## Playing Status

The athlete can return to activity as long as no signs of serious infection (redness, swelling, or fever) are present. If the athlete is sent to a health care provider, they cannot return to activity until examined and released by the health care provider.

## PREVENTION

- Trimming toenails straight across
- Wearing properly fitted shoes

# ABRASION

An abrasion is a scraping injury to the superficial layer of the skin. Also called a turf burn, road rash, or a strawberry, an abrasion is caused by sliding or falling against a rough or hard surface (see figure 15.3).

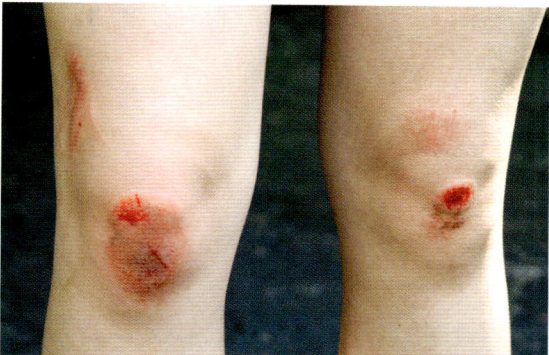

**Figure 15.3**   Abrasion.
iStockphoto.com/Judith Bicking

## Signs and Symptoms

- Pain
- Raw, red patch of skin
- Tightness or pulling sensation over the affected area
- Burning sensation

## FIRST AID

1. Rinse the area with clean running water for 5 minutes or more (use soap if necessary to remove dirt). For superficial abrasions, apply a triple antibiotic ointment or cream. Do not use iodine.
2. If the athlete is returning to activity, cover the abrasion with sterile gauze.
3. To promote healing, instruct the athlete to leave the abrasion uncovered during daily activities.
4. Send the athlete to the appropriate health care provider if you are unable to completely clean debris from the wound, if its edges gape open, or if it shows signs of infection.

## Playing Status

The athlete can return to activity as long as no signs of serious infection (pus, red streaks extending from the area, or fever) are present. If the athlete is sent to a health care provider, they cannot return to activity until examined and released by the health care provider.

## PREVENTION

- Wearing sliding pants or protective padding for the elbows, knees, and hips

# BLISTER

A blister is a fluid-filled pocket between layers of skin. Blisters can be closed or open. In closed blisters, the skin is still intact; in open blisters, the skin is torn (see figure 15.4). One cause of blisters is friction from the skin rubbing against a surface (such as a shoe, bat, or racket handle), which causes layers of skin to separate and fill with fluid.

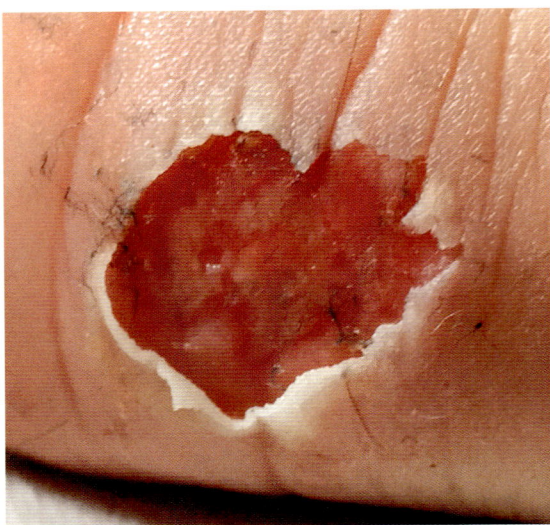

**Figure 15.4** Open blister.

Clem Silverbridge/Istock/Getty Images

## Signs and Symptoms

- Pain
- Burning
- Warmth
- Redness or fluid-filled bump underneath the skin
- Torn skin, open wound, bleeding, or redness

## FIRST AID

### Closed Blisters

1. Leave the blister intact (opening it may cause infection).
2. Adhere a commercial callus, corn, or blister donut pad (see figure 15.5) over the blister to protect against further irritation and to allow healing.
3. Instruct the athlete to keep the area clean.

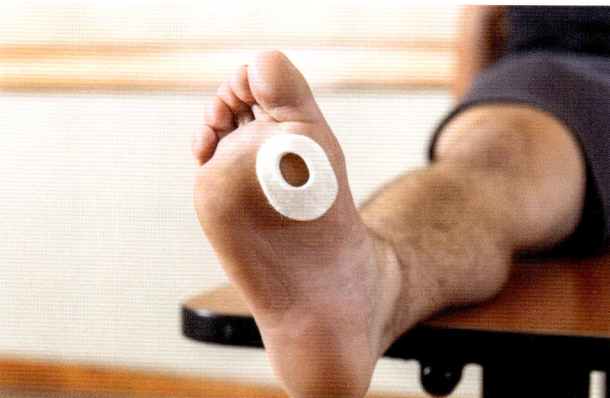

**Figure 15.5**   Blister donut pad.

### Open Blisters

1. Clean the area with antiseptic solution or soap. Do not use iodine.
2. Dry with sterile gauze.
3. Adhere a commercial callus, corn, or blister donut pad (as shown in figure 15.5) over the blister to protect against further irritation and to allow healing.
4. Instruct the athlete to keep the area clean.
5. Instruct the athlete to periodically check for signs of infection (redness, swelling, or warmth that progress to red streaks extending from the wound, pus, or fever).
6. Immediately refer the athlete to the appropriate health care provider if signs of infection are present or if the blister doesn't heal after a week or two of self-care.

### Playing Status

The athlete can return to activity as long as no signs of serious infection are present. If the athlete is sent to a health care provider, they cannot return to activity until examined and released by the health care provider.

## PREVENTION

- Ice application to hot spots (warm, red, and tender skin but not yet a blister)
- Petroleum jelly application to high-friction areas
- Wearing protective gloves and properly fitted shoes specific to the sport

# BOIL

A boil is a large, infected, pus-filled bump on the skin. Boils are caused by a bacterial infection of a hair follicle (see figure 15.6). Signs and symptoms of a boil may include pain, warmth, a red or white bump on the skin, and localized swelling. For first aid, leave the boil intact, and refer the athlete to the appropriate health care provider.

The athlete can return to activity as long as no signs of serious infection (redness, swelling, or fever) are present. If the athlete is sent to a health care provider, they cannot return to activity until examined and released by the health care provider. To prevent boils, encourage athletes to shower after activity and to wear newly laundered athletic clothes for each practice and competition.

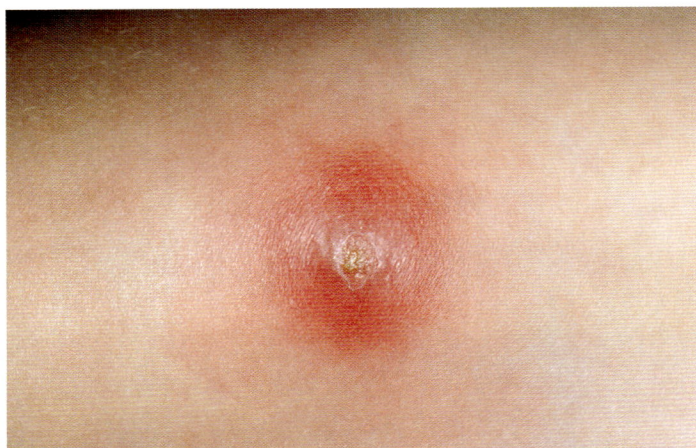

**Figure 15.6**   Boil.

Dr P. Marazzi / Science Source

# POISONOUS PLANT RASH

A poisonous plant rash is a skin reaction to a poisonous plant. Causes include direct contact with poison ivy (figure 15.7a), poison oak (figure 15.7b), or poison sumac (figure 15.7c); contact with animals, clothing, tools, or sports equipment that are contaminated with the plant's oil; or inhalation of or skin exposure to airborne oil particles of burning plants. Signs and symptoms may include burning, itching, redness, rash, swelling, blisters, high fever (if severe), and crusting or scaling of blisters. If the athlete is seen within 5 minutes of exposure, remove all contaminated clothes, and flush the skin with cool, running water. If a rash develops, instruct the athlete to avoid scratching the rash and see the appropriate health care provider.

The athlete can return to activity as long as no signs of serious infection (redness, swelling, or fever) are present and they have been examined and released by a health care provider. To help prevent poisonous plant rashes, teach athletes to identify these plants and wear protective clothing or hire someone else to remove the plants to avoid your own reaction to them.

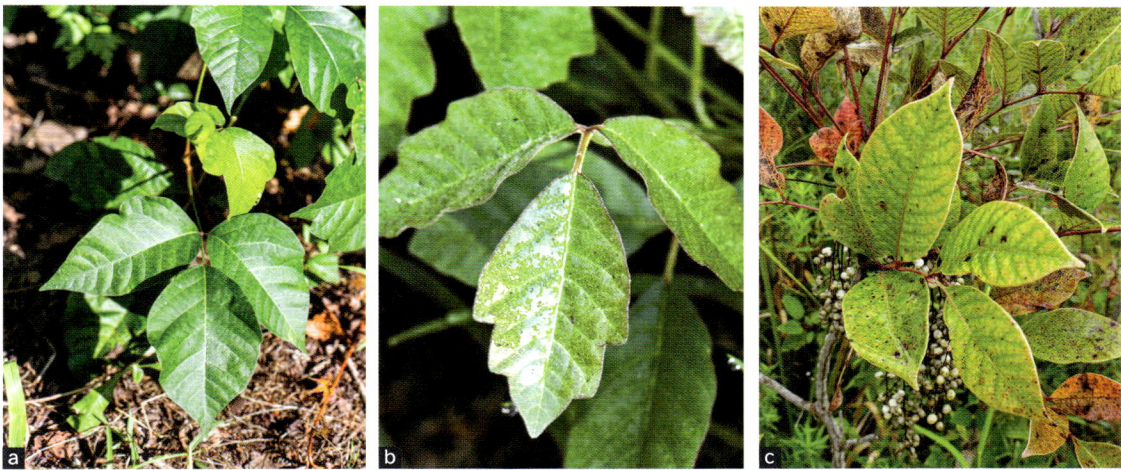

**Figure 15.7**   Poisonous plants: *(a)* poison ivy, *(b)* poison oak, and *(c)* poison sumac.

*(a)* John Greim/LightRocket via Getty Images; *(b)* Ed Reschke/Stone/Getty Images; *(c)* "poison sumac" by Sarah Culliton is licensed under CC BY 4.0. To view a copy of this license, visit http://creativecommons.org/licenses/by/4.0/?ref=openverse

## Contagious Skin Conditions

The following infections are considered contagious. Any athletes exhibiting signs and symptoms of these conditions should be sent to the appropriate health care provider for an evaluation of the condition, appropriate treatment, and release for return to participation.

Your role is to help detect such conditions and prevent infected athletes from coming into direct or indirect contact with others. You can prevent the spread of skin infections by assigning individual towels and water bottles and requiring shower shoes. It may be necessary to withhold athletes from participation until they have been examined and released by a health care provider. For example, the National Federation of State High School Associations (NFHS) prohibits wrestlers with suspected skin infections from participating until they have been examined and released (Hopkins 2023). Regardless of contagiousness, you should always wear protective gloves when handling skin conditions. It is particularly important because of the existence of antibiotic-resistant bacteria that can infect damaged skin.

### SAFETY MEASURE

**With Skin Conditions**

Always wear protective gloves when handling skin conditions, even if you think the condition is not contagious.

# CA-MRSA

Community-associated methicillin-resistant Staphylococcus aureus (CA-MRSA) is a dangerous skin infection that can be transmitted in communal situations through personal contact or by sharing toiletries or equipment.

The Centers for Disease Control and Prevention (CDC) estimates that Staphylococcus aureus, also known as staph, is carried within the nose of about 33 percent of the U.S. population (CDC 2024). Staph is particularly dangerous because it can infect athletes' wounds. The CDC also estimates that about 2 percent of the U.S. population carries MRSA, the particularly dangerous variety that is resistant to methicillin and other related antibiotics (CDC 2024).

Community-associated (CA) MRSA has been found to spread through person-to-person contact, shared towels, shared soaps, and improperly disinfected whirlpools and equipment. CA-MRSA infections typically appear as skin infections, such as pimples or boils (see figure 15.8). The danger is that these infections may spread to other areas of the body and cause pneumonia and blood infections. Signs and symptoms may include fever; localized pain at the site of the wound; or a wound that has redness that spreads, swelling, and pus or fluid drainage. An athlete with suspected CA-MRSA should be immediately referred to the appropriate health care provider.

Playing status of the athlete should be determined by the treating health care provider and the athlete cannot return to activity until examined and released by the health care provider. To help prevent the spread of CA-MRSA, enforce strict hygiene policies as well as regularly clean equipment and facilities. Cover all wounds before allowing an athlete to participate in practices or competitions, and prohibit athletes with open wounds from using shared whirlpools or tubs.

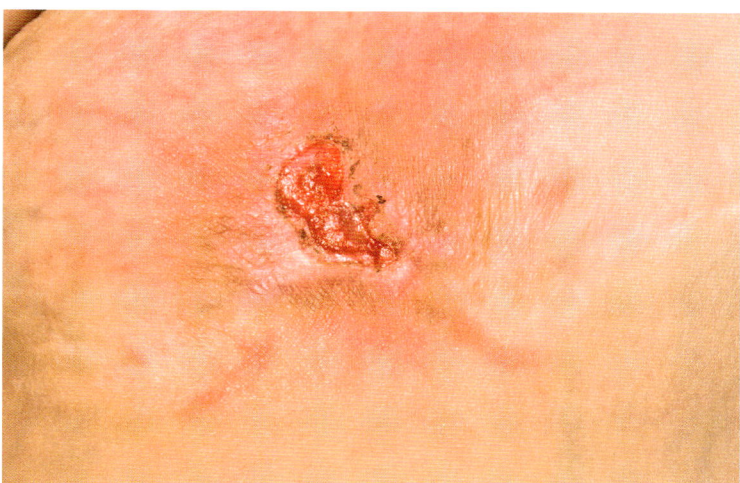

**Figure 15.8**    CA-MRSA infection.

JodiJacobson/E+/Getty Images

# MOLLUSCUM CONTAGIOSUM

Molluscum contagiosum is a skin growth caused by a viral infection in the top layers of the skin, occurring from direct skin contact with the virus (see figure 15.9). It usually occurs at hair follicles or where the skin is broken. Signs and symptoms of molluscum contagiosum may include small, flesh-colored or pink, dome-shaped growths; clusters of growths on the skin of the chest, abdomen, arms, groin, buttocks, face, and eyelids; a shiny appearance; a small indentation in the center of each growth; or red or inflamed appearance. Send the athlete to the appropriate health care provider for accurate diagnosis and appropriate treatment.

Check your organization's rules and regulations regarding participation with molluscum contagiosum. The athlete cannot return to activity until examined and released by a health care provider. To help prevent the spread of molluscum contagiosum, prevent direct contact between an infected athlete and other athletes. In addition, prevent indirect contact with an infected athlete by enforcing strict hygiene policies in showers and locker rooms and by prohibiting the sharing of towels or whirlpools.

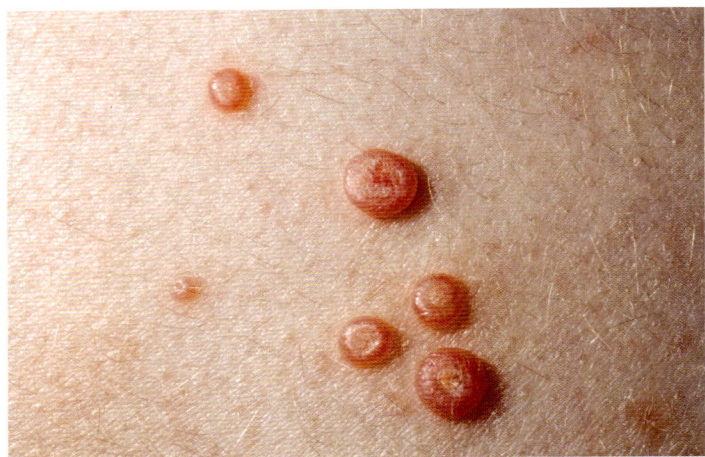

**Figure 15.9**   Molluscum contagiosum.
Dr P. Marazzi / Science Source

# WART

A wart is an abnormal skin growth caused by direct skin contact with the human papillomavirus (HPV), typically occurring where the skin is broken. Two types of warts exist: the common wart (figure 15.10a), which is found on fingers, backs of hands, and nail beds; and the plantar wart (figure 15.10b), which is found on the sole of the foot.

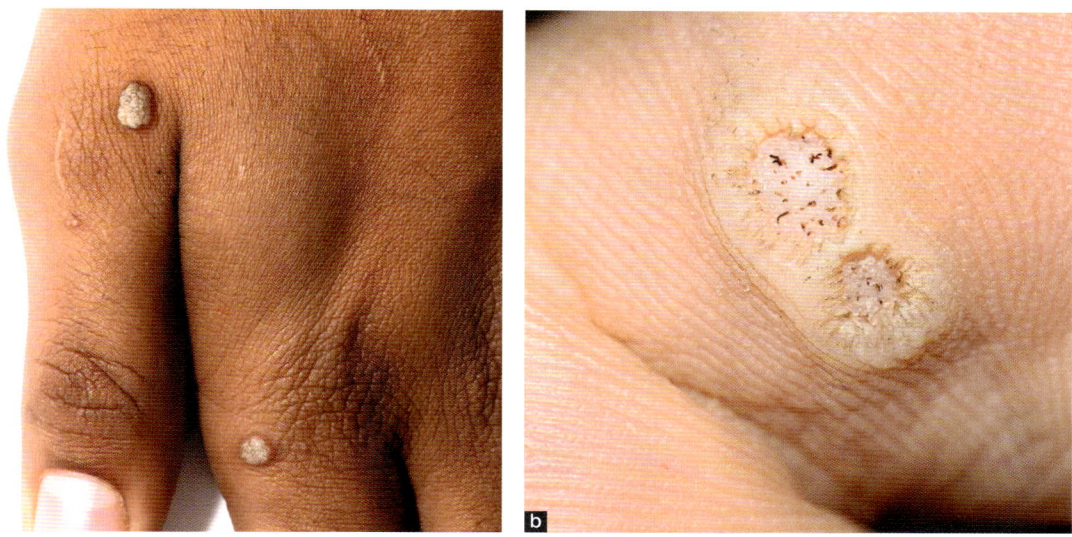

**Figure 15.10**   Types of warts: *(a)* common and *(b)* plantar.

*(a)* SCIENCE PHOTO LIBRARY / Science Source; *(b)* Kagenmi/iStock/Getty Images

## Signs and Symptoms

- Pain
- Localized skin growth
- Black dots in plantar warts caused by blood vessels (called seeds)

## FIRST AID

Send the athlete to the appropriate health care provider for accurate diagnosis and appropriate treatment.

## Playing Status

The athlete can participate in activity if an exposed common wart is covered with sterile gauze. For plantar warts, ensure the athlete wears footwear at all times and sees a health care provider. For athletes, such as swimmers, who cannot wear shoes, seek guidance from the appropriate health care provider. The athlete cannot return to activity until examined and released by the health care provider.

## PREVENTION

- No direct contact between an infected athlete and others
- No indirect contact with an infected athlete through shared towels, showers, and floors

# HERPES SIMPLEX

Herpes simplex is a fever blister or cold sore on the lips, mouth, nose, chin, or cheek. It is caused by contact with the type 1 herpes simplex virus (HSV-1) (see figure 15.11). It usually results from direct contact with an individual who carries the virus.

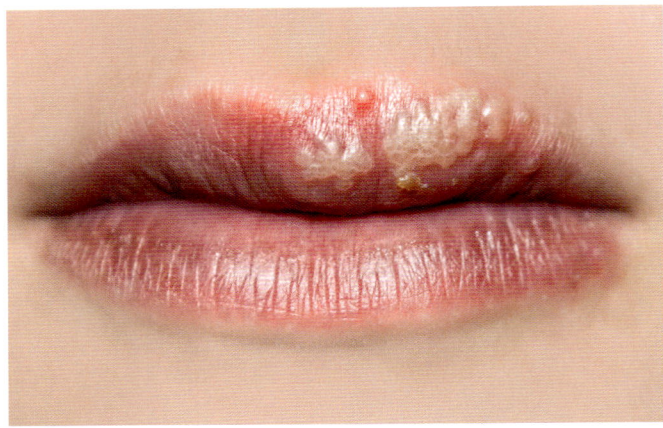

**Figure 15.11**   Herpes simplex (fever blister or cold sore).

Apichsn/iStock/Getty Images

## Signs and Symptoms

- Tiny, fluid-filled blisters
- Clear fluid oozing from broken blisters
- Itching or burning
- Sensitive skin

## FIRST AID

Send the athlete to the appropriate health care provider for accurate diagnosis and appropriate treatment.

### Playing Status

Check your organization's rules and regulations regarding participation with herpes simplex. The athlete cannot return to activity until examined and released by the appropriate health care provider. You may need to provide documentation according to your state or local rules.

## PREVENTION

- No direct contact of an infected athlete with others
- No indirect contact with an infected athlete through shared water bottles, towels, and clothing

# RINGWORM

Ringworm is a fungal infection of the skin. It is usually caused by direct contact with infected humans and animals; a less common cause is contact with infected soil. As healing progresses from the middle of the infected area, the lesion will begin to look like a ring (see figure 15.12).

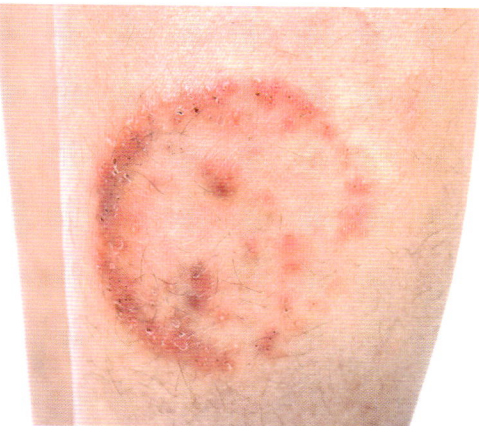

**Figure 15.12**   Ringworm.

Phanasitti/iStock/Getty Images

## Signs and Symptoms

- Red, scaly patches of skin
- Lesion that looks like a ring
- Pain
- Itching
- Burning

## FIRST AID

Send the athlete to the appropriate health care provider for accurate diagnosis and appropriate treatment.

## Playing Status

Check your sport rules for regulations regarding participation with ringworm. The athlete cannot return to activity until examined and released by the appropriate health care provider. You may need to provide documentation according to your state or local rules.

## PREVENTION

- No direct contact of an infected athlete with others
- No indirect contact with an infected athlete through towels and clothing

# ATHLETE'S FOOT

Athlete's foot is a fungal infection that affects the feet. It is caused by prolonged exposure of feet to a sweaty, hot, and poorly ventilated environment (see figure 15.13). An example would be wearing leather shoes with dirty, wet socks.

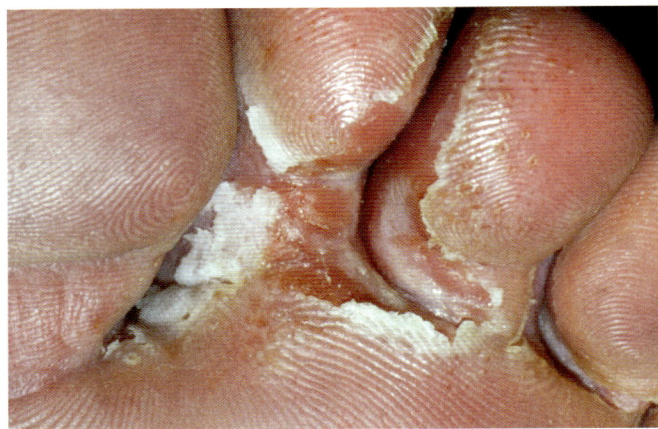

**Figure 15.13**   Athlete's foot.

SPL / Science Source

## Signs and Symptoms

- Red, scaly rash around the toes and other areas of the feet
- Peeling or cracking skin
- Burning
- Itching
- Blisters (severe cases)

## FIRST AID

1. Change socks to keep the feet dry.
2. Wash and thoroughly dry the feet daily.
3. Apply antifungal cream or powder to the area.
4. Send the athlete to the appropriate health care provider if symptoms persist.

## Playing Status

The athlete can participate as long as the infected area is not exposed to other athletes.

## PREVENTION

- Keeping feet clean and dry with proper hygiene, foot powder, and clean socks
- Wearing shower shoes to prevent the spread of fungus

# JOCK ITCH

Jock itch is a fungal infection affecting the genital area. It is caused by prolonged exposure of the skin to a sweaty, hot environment, such as when wearing soiled, damp practice clothes.

## Signs and Symptoms

- Red, scaly patches of skin
- Burning
- Itching

## FIRST AID

1. Have the athlete change into clean, dry clothing.
2. Have the athlete apply antifungal cream or powder to the infected area.
3. Send the athlete to the appropriate health care provider if symptoms persist.

## Playing Status

The athlete can participate in activity as tolerated.

## PREVENTION

- Use of powder to help absorb sweat
- Wearing of clean, dry workout clothes

# Chapter 15 Recap

- ❑ How should you protect yourself when providing first aid care for skin conditions?
- ❑ What are the signs and symptoms of a CA-MRSA infection?
- ❑ What can be applied to blisters to prevent further irritation?
- ❑ When should a nail contusion be evaluated and treated by a health care provider?
- ❑ What first aid technique helps promote healing of abrasions?
- ❑ What first aid technique can be immediately used to reduce the skin reaction caused by poisonous plants such as ivy, oak, and sumac?
- ❑ What substances cause contagious skin infections?
- ❑ Describe the steps that can be taken to reduce the spread of a contagious skin condition among athletes.
- ❑ What can athletes do to help prevent bacterial and fungal skin infections?

# APPENDIX: FIRST AID PROCEDURES

# EMERGENCY ACTION STEPS

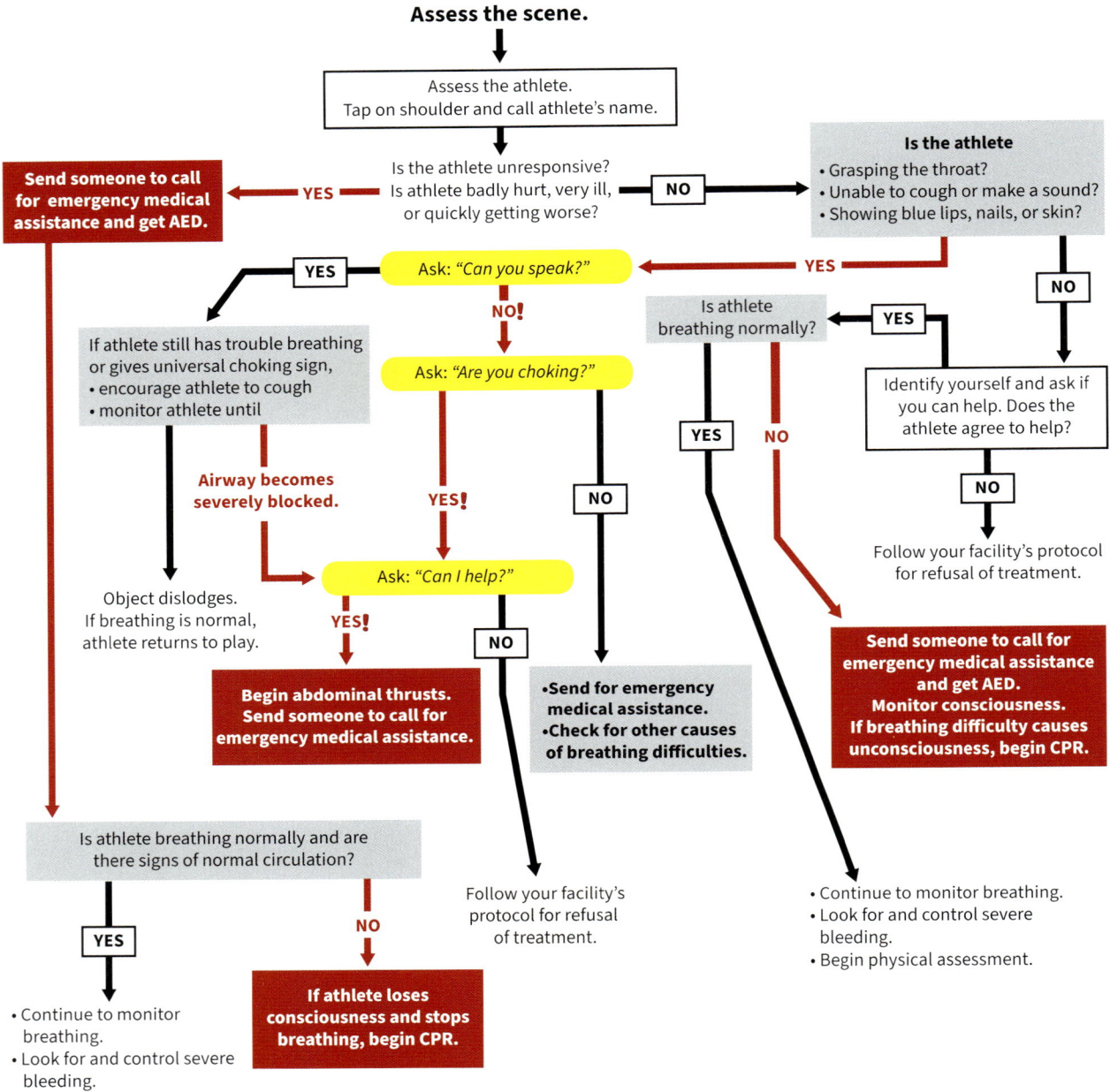

# ATTENDING TO A RESPONSIVE ATHLETE

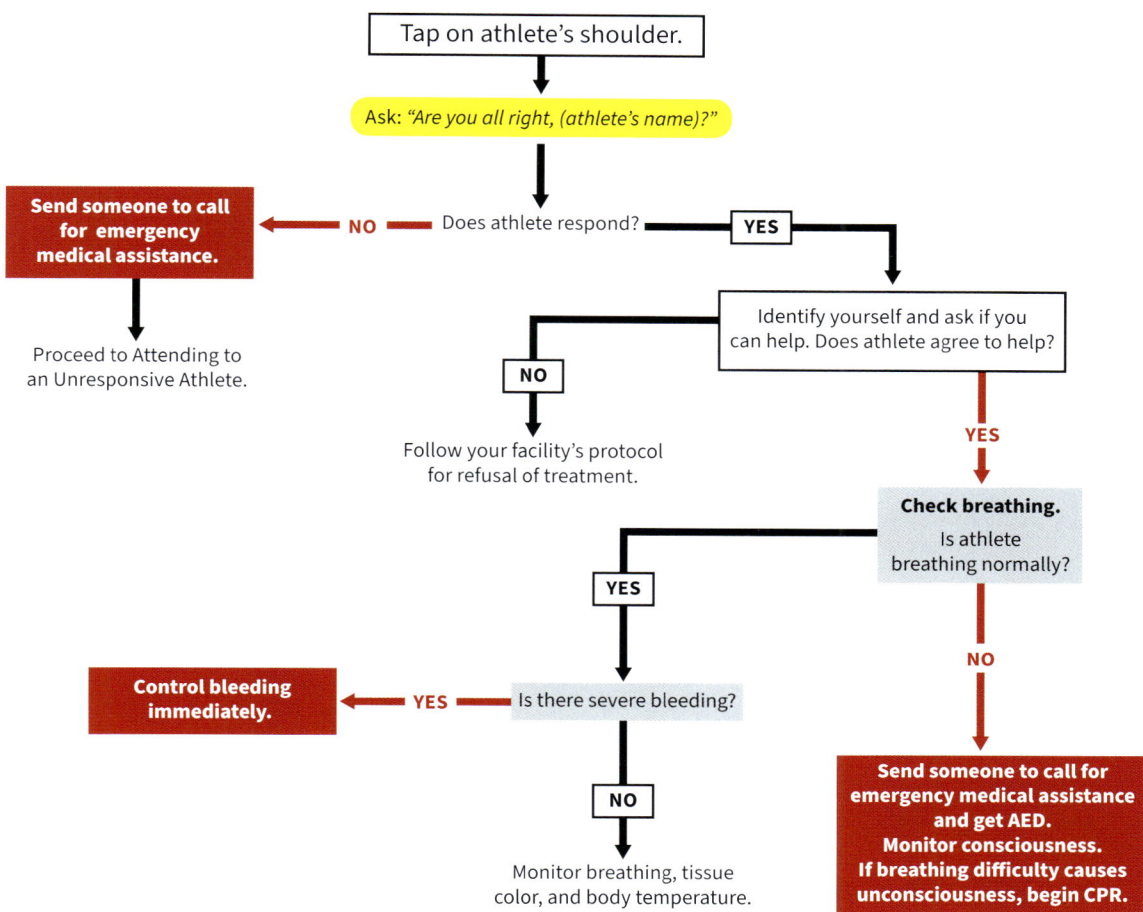

# ATTENDING TO AN UNRESPONSIVE ATHLETE

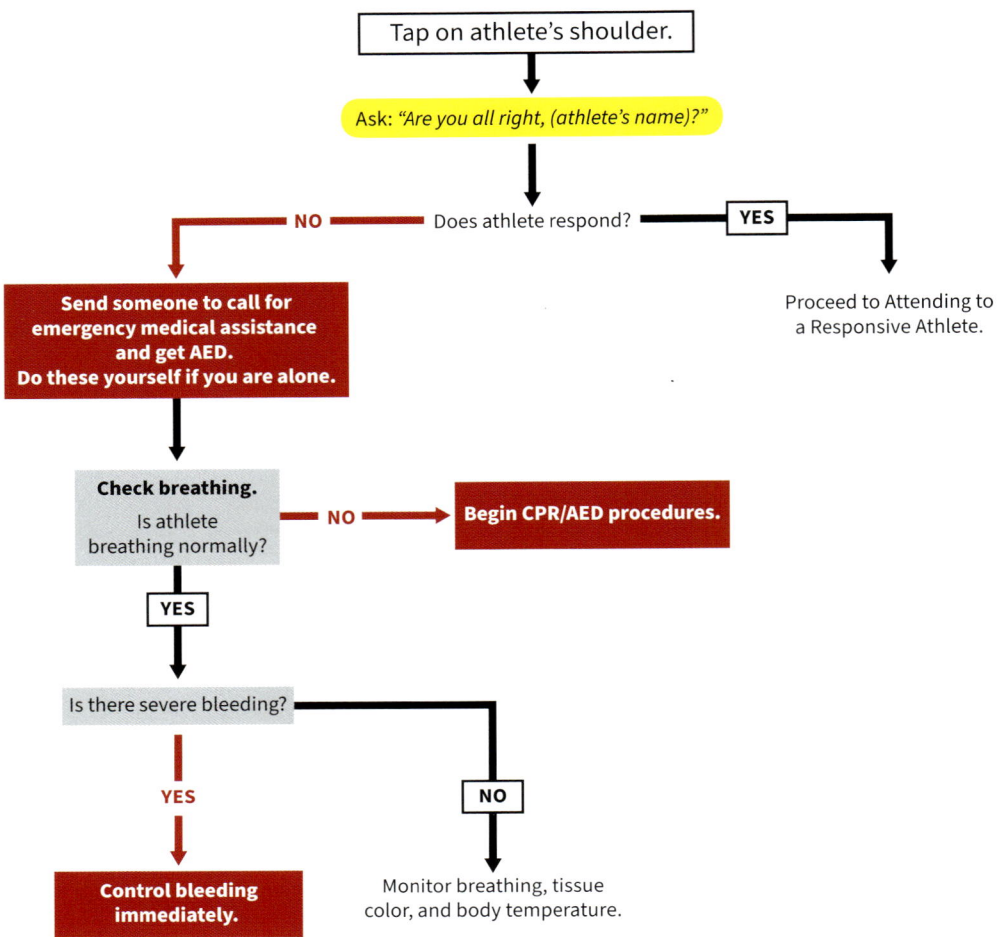

Tap on athlete's shoulder.

Ask: *"Are you all right, (athlete's name)?"*

Does athlete respond?

**NO** → Send someone to call for emergency medical assistance and get AED. Do these yourself if you are alone.

**YES** → Proceed to Attending to a Responsive Athlete.

**Check breathing.** Is athlete breathing normally?

**NO** → Begin CPR/AED procedures.

**YES** → Is there severe bleeding?

**YES** → Control bleeding immediately.

**NO** → Monitor breathing, tissue color, and body temperature.

# AIRWAY BLOCKAGE IN A RESPONSIVE ATHLETE

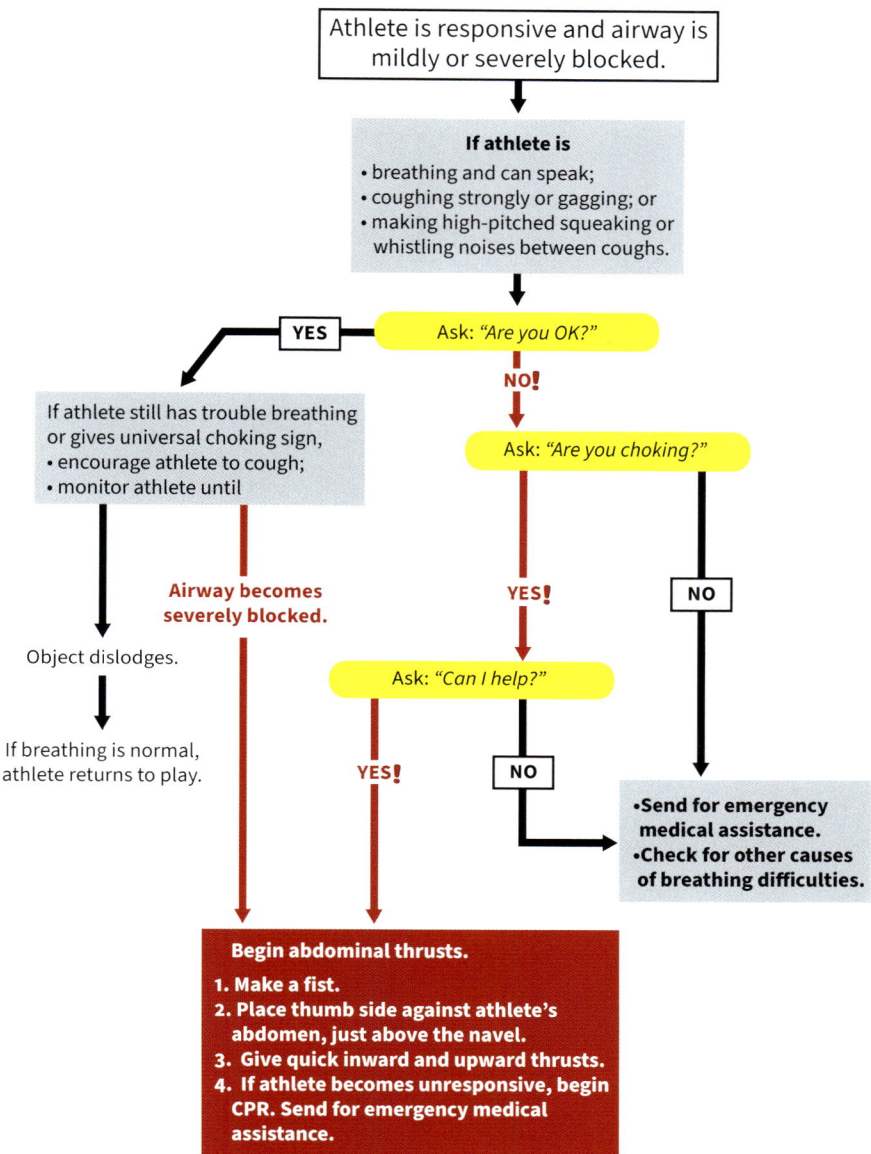

# AIRWAY BLOCKAGE IN AN UNRESPONSIVE ATHLETE

Athlete becomes unresponsive (still not breathing) while you are performing abdominal thrusts.

1. Slowly lower athlete to floor.
2. Have someone call for emergency medical assistance.
3. Place athlete on back.
4. Open mouth and remove object if you see it and make sure tongue is not obstructing the airway. If it is, gently tilt the head back until the tongue moves out of the airway.
5. Begin CPR. Use AED if available.

Continue until
• Athlete starts breathing normally.
• AED arrives. Stop compressions and apply AED; follow AED instructions.
• EMS takes over.

# CPR

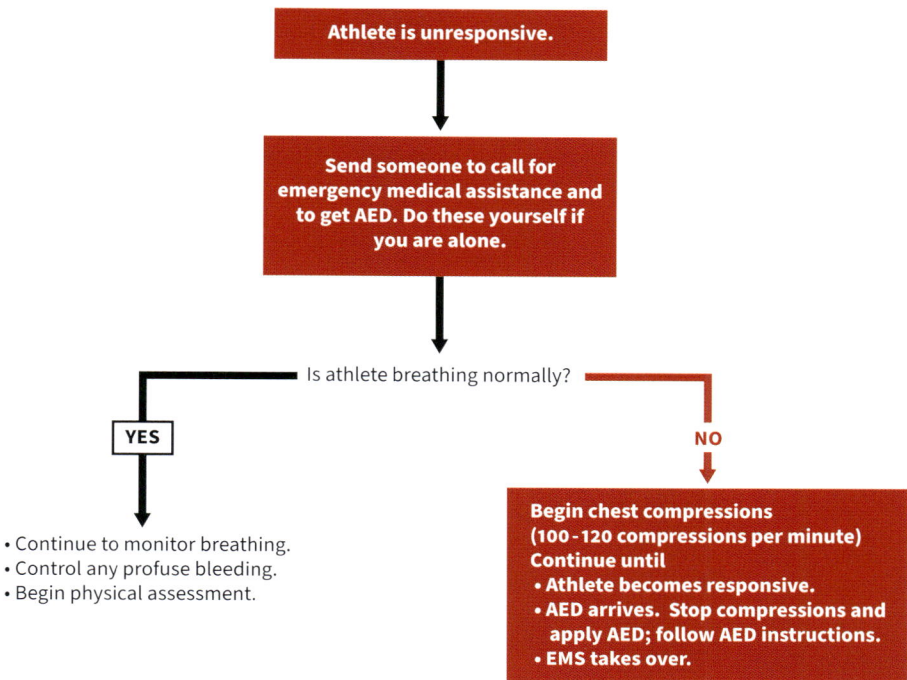

# AED

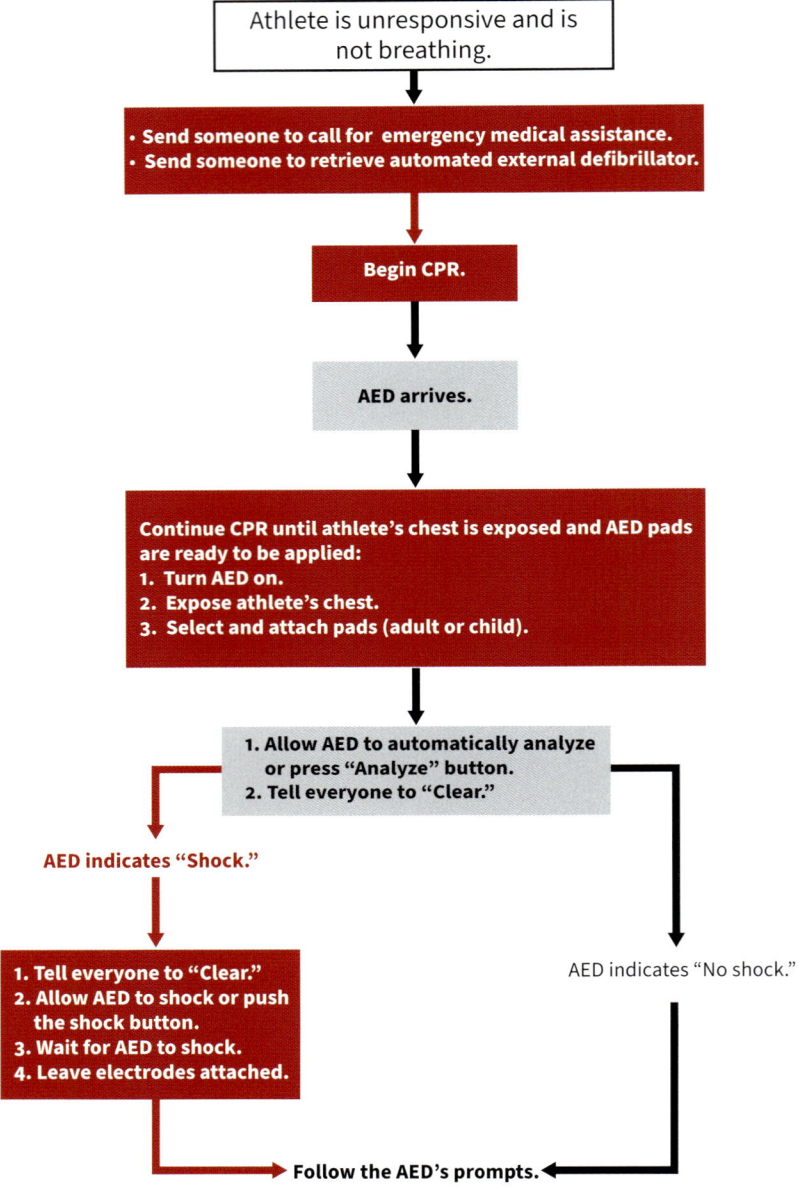

Athlete is unresponsive and is not breathing.

• Send someone to call for emergency medical assistance.
• Send someone to retrieve automated external defibrillator.

Begin CPR.

AED arrives.

Continue CPR until athlete's chest is exposed and AED pads are ready to be applied:
1. Turn AED on.
2. Expose athlete's chest.
3. Select and attach pads (adult or child).

1. Allow AED to automatically analyze or press "Analyze" button.
2. Tell everyone to "Clear."

AED indicates "Shock."

AED indicates "No shock."

1. Tell everyone to "Clear."
2. Allow AED to shock or push the shock button.
3. Wait for AED to shock.
4. Leave electrodes attached.

Follow the AED's prompts.

**Note:** If athlete becomes responsive and is breathing, monitor breathing and do secondary assessment.

# SECONDARY ASSESSMENT

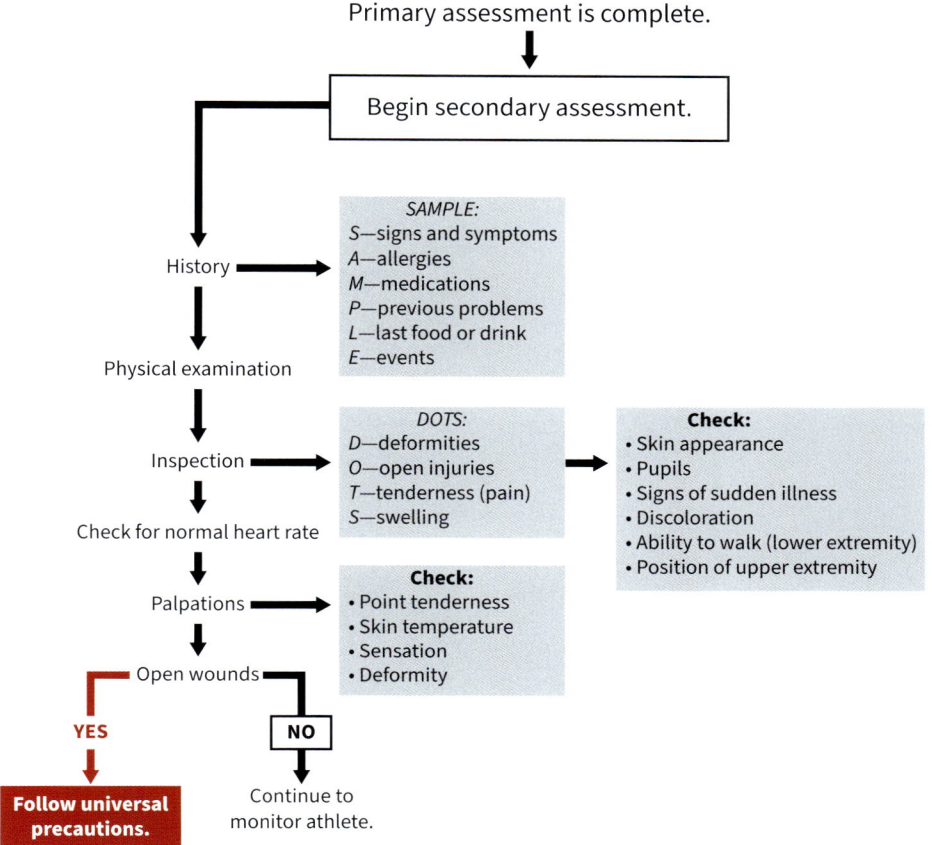

# PROFUSE BLEEDING

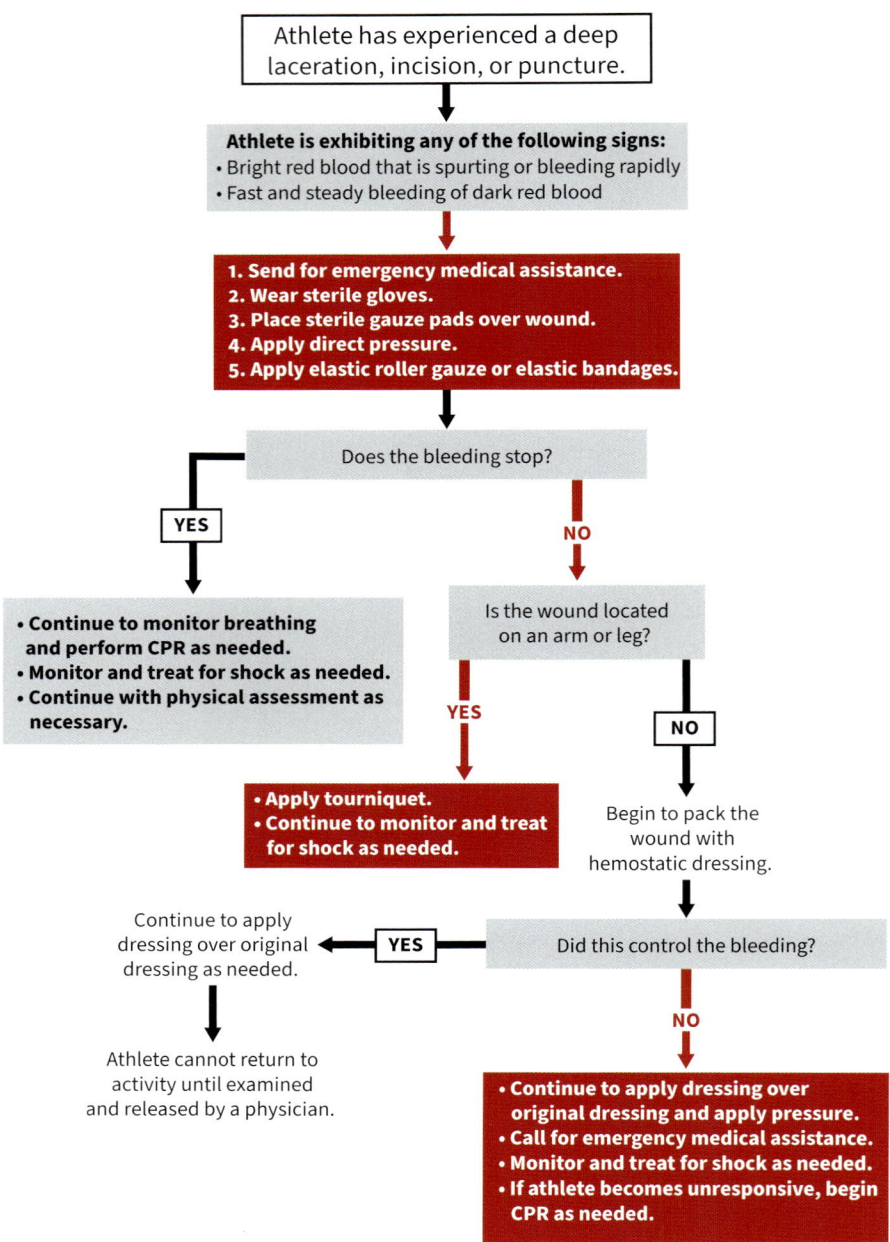

Athlete has experienced a deep laceration, incision, or puncture.

**Athlete is exhibiting any of the following signs:**
• Bright red blood that is spurting or bleeding rapidly
• Fast and steady bleeding of dark red blood

1. **Send for emergency medical assistance.**
2. **Wear sterile gloves.**
3. **Place sterile gauze pads over wound.**
4. **Apply direct pressure.**
5. **Apply elastic roller gauze or elastic bandages.**

Does the bleeding stop?

**YES**

• **Continue to monitor breathing and perform CPR as needed.**
• **Monitor and treat for shock as needed.**
• **Continue with physical assessment as necessary.**

**NO**

Is the wound located on an arm or leg?

**YES**

**NO**

• **Apply tourniquet.**
• **Continue to monitor and treat for shock as needed.**

Begin to pack the wound with hemostatic dressing.

Continue to apply dressing over original dressing as needed.

**YES**

Did this control the bleeding?

**NO**

Athlete cannot return to activity until examined and released by a physician.

• **Continue to apply dressing over original dressing and apply pressure.**
• **Call for emergency medical assistance.**
• **Monitor and treat for shock as needed.**
• **If athlete becomes unresponsive, begin CPR as needed.**

# SPLINTING

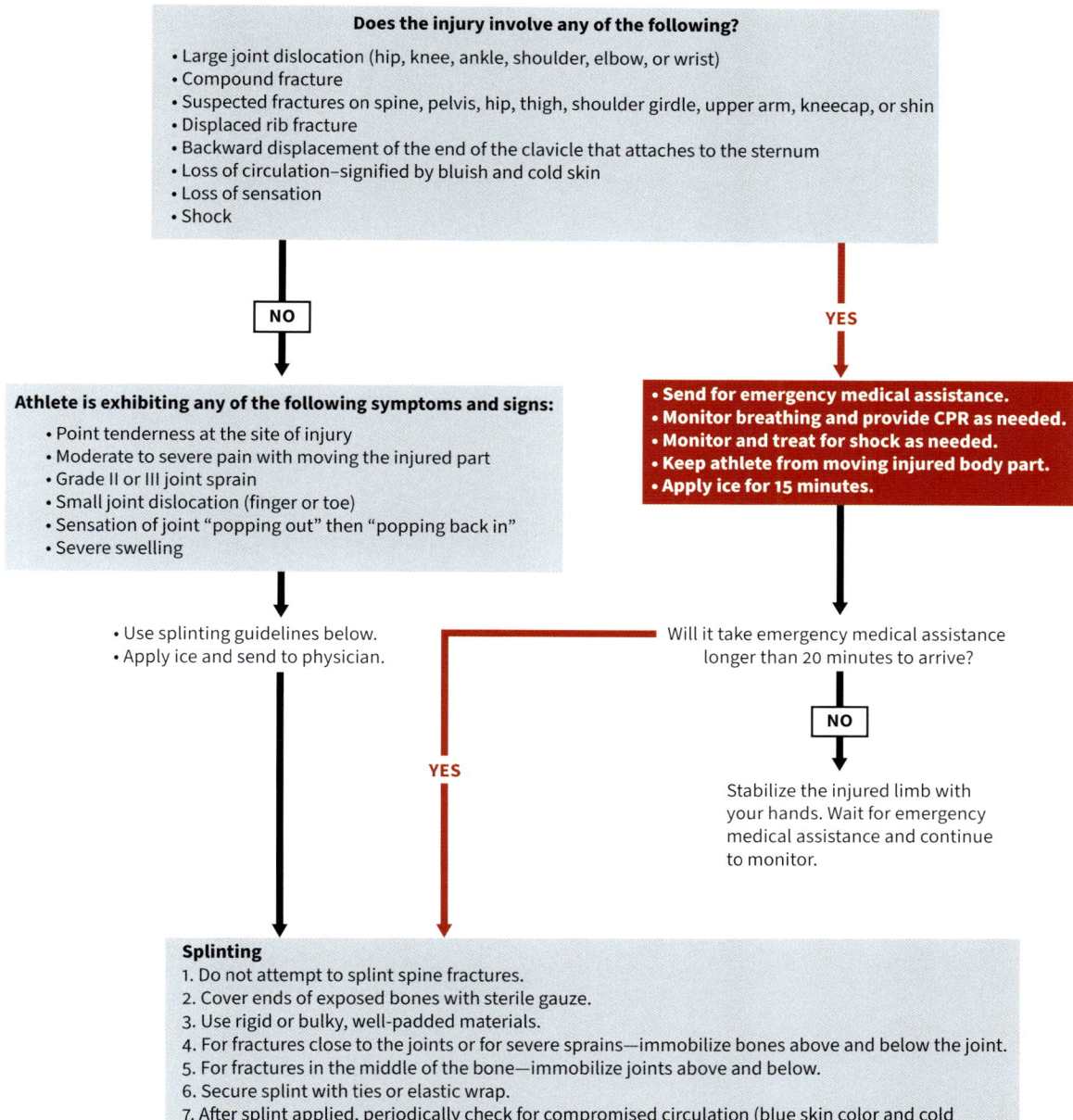

**Does the injury involve any of the following?**

- Large joint dislocation (hip, knee, ankle, shoulder, elbow, or wrist)
- Compound fracture
- Suspected fractures on spine, pelvis, hip, thigh, shoulder girdle, upper arm, kneecap, or shin
- Displaced rib fracture
- Backward displacement of the end of the clavicle that attaches to the sternum
- Loss of circulation–signified by bluish and cold skin
- Loss of sensation
- Shock

**NO**

**YES**

**Athlete is exhibiting any of the following symptoms and signs:**

- Point tenderness at the site of injury
- Moderate to severe pain with moving the injured part
- Grade II or III joint sprain
- Small joint dislocation (finger or toe)
- Sensation of joint "popping out" then "popping back in"
- Severe swelling

- **Send for emergency medical assistance.**
- **Monitor breathing and provide CPR as needed.**
- **Monitor and treat for shock as needed.**
- **Keep athlete from moving injured body part.**
- **Apply ice for 15 minutes.**

- Use splinting guidelines below.
- Apply ice and send to physician.

Will it take emergency medical assistance longer than 20 minutes to arrive?

**YES**

**NO**

Stabilize the injured limb with your hands. Wait for emergency medical assistance and continue to monitor.

**Splinting**

1. Do not attempt to splint spine fractures.
2. Cover ends of exposed bones with sterile gauze.
3. Use rigid or bulky, well-padded materials.
4. For fractures close to the joints or for severe sprains—immobilize bones above and below the joint.
5. For fractures in the middle of the bone—immobilize joints above and below.
6. Secure splint with ties or elastic wrap.
7. After splint applied, periodically check for compromised circulation (blue skin color and cold temperature) caused by splints that are too tight. Loosen ties and resecure as needed.

# MOVING AN INJURED OR SICK ATHLETE

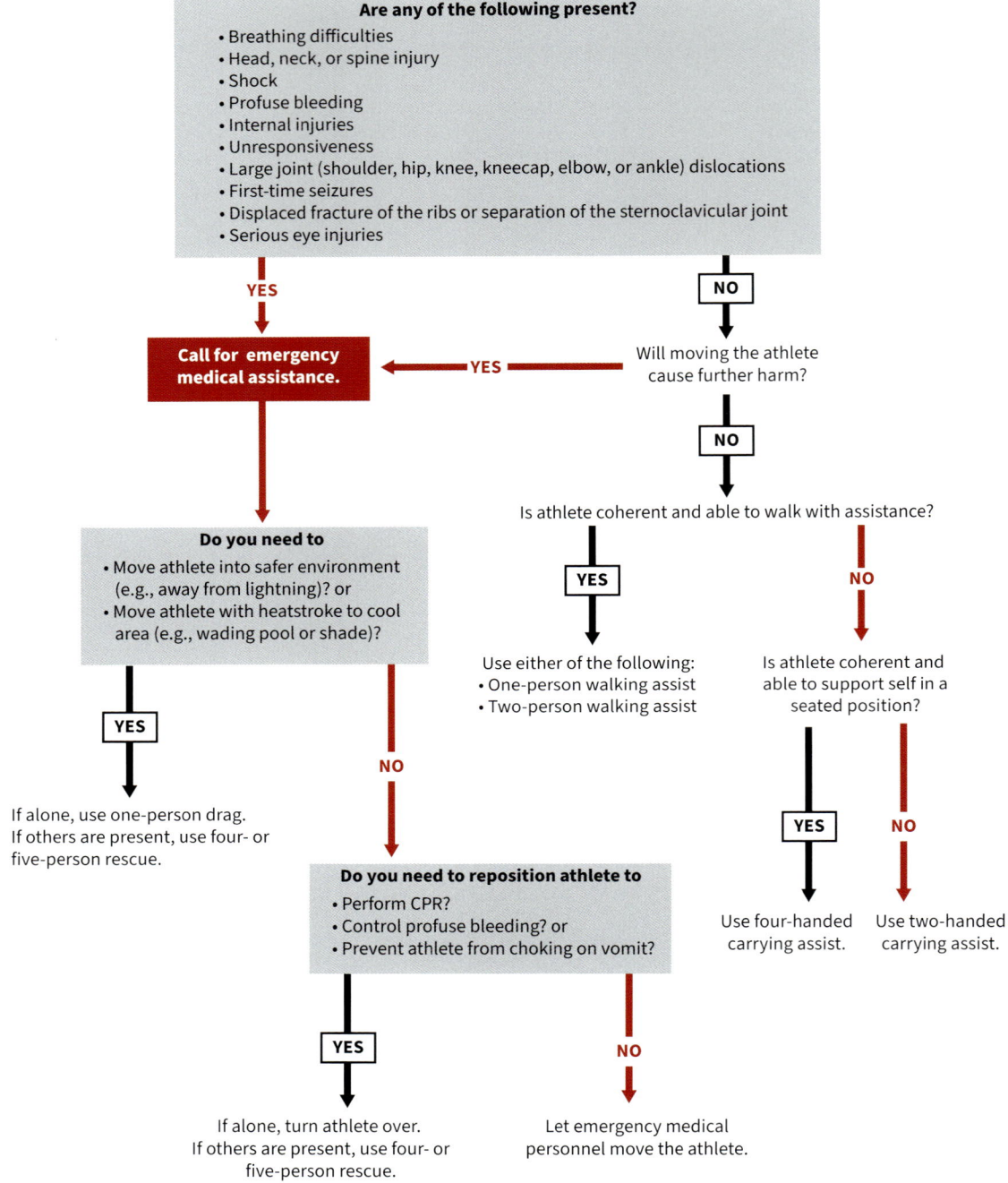

**Are any of the following present?**
- Breathing difficulties
- Head, neck, or spine injury
- Shock
- Profuse bleeding
- Internal injuries
- Unresponsiveness
- Large joint (shoulder, hip, knee, kneecap, elbow, or ankle) dislocations
- First-time seizures
- Displaced fracture of the ribs or separation of the sternoclavicular joint
- Serious eye injuries

**YES** →

**Call for emergency medical assistance.**

← **YES** — **NO** → Will moving the athlete cause further harm?

**NO** → Is athlete coherent and able to walk with assistance?

**Do you need to**
- Move athlete into safer environment (e.g., away from lightning)? or
- Move athlete with heatstroke to cool area (e.g., wading pool or shade)?

**YES** → If alone, use one-person drag. If others are present, use four- or five-person rescue.

**NO** →

**YES** → Use either of the following:
- One-person walking assist
- Two-person walking assist

**NO** → Is athlete coherent and able to support self in a seated position?

**YES** → Use four-handed carrying assist.

**NO** → Use two-handed carrying assist.

**Do you need to reposition athlete to**
- Perform CPR?
- Control profuse bleeding? or
- Prevent athlete from choking on vomit?

**YES** → If alone, turn athlete over. If others are present, use four- or five-person rescue.

**NO** → Let emergency medical personnel move the athlete.

# ANAPHYLACTIC SHOCK

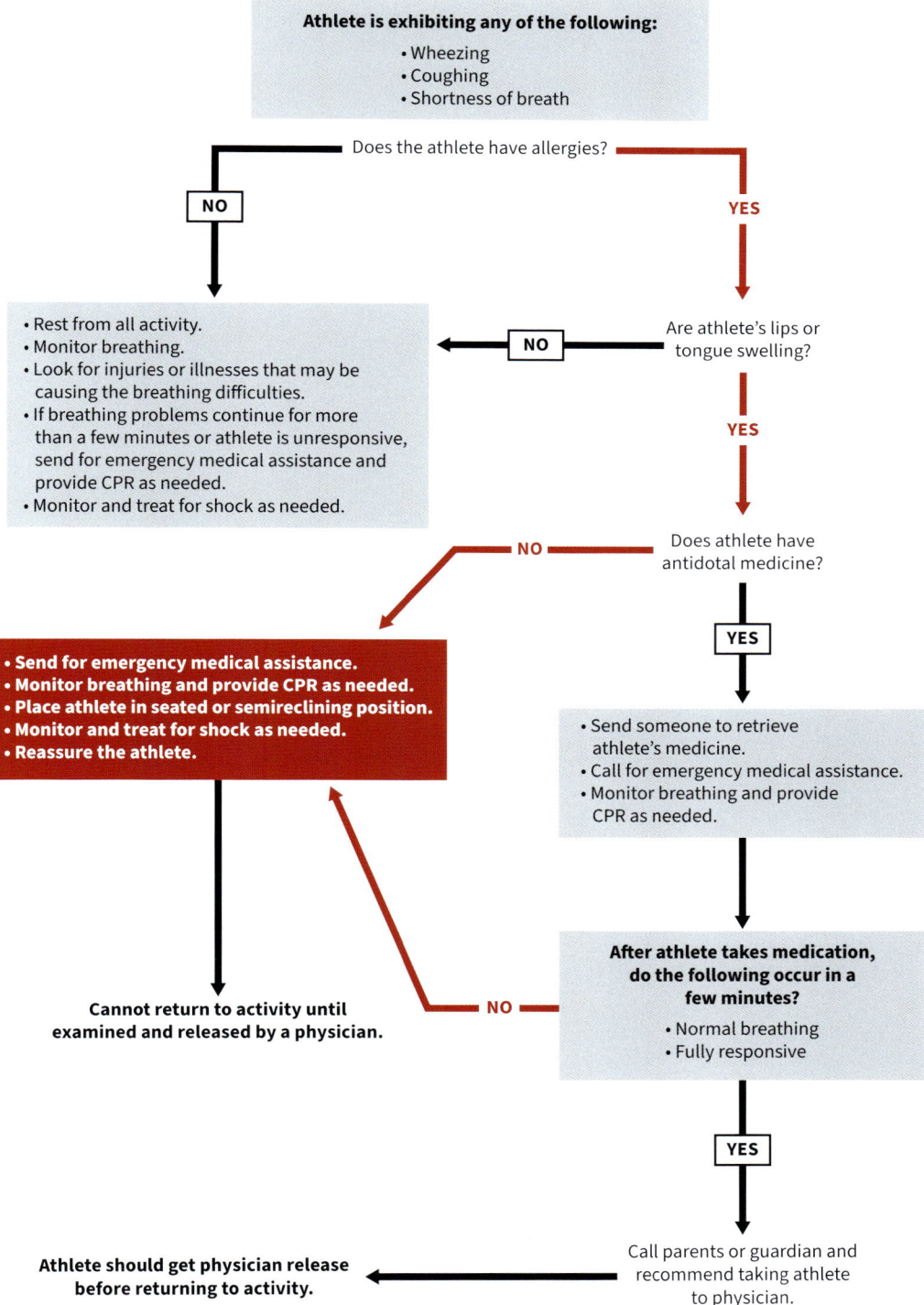

**Athlete is exhibiting any of the following:**

- Wheezing
- Coughing
- Shortness of breath

Does the athlete have allergies?

**NO** → 
- Rest from all activity.
- Monitor breathing.
- Look for injuries or illnesses that may be causing the breathing difficulties.
- If breathing problems continue for more than a few minutes or athlete is unresponsive, send for emergency medical assistance and provide CPR as needed.
- Monitor and treat for shock as needed.

**YES**

Are athlete's lips or tongue swelling?

**NO** →

**YES**

Does athlete have antidotal medicine?

**NO** →

**YES**

- **Send for emergency medical assistance.**
- **Monitor breathing and provide CPR as needed.**
- **Place athlete in seated or semireclining position.**
- **Monitor and treat for shock as needed.**
- **Reassure the athlete.**

- Send someone to retrieve athlete's medicine.
- Call for emergency medical assistance.
- Monitor breathing and provide CPR as needed.

**Cannot return to activity until examined and released by a physician.**

**After athlete takes medication, do the following occur in a few minutes?**

- Normal breathing
- Fully responsive

**NO**

**YES**

Call parents or guardian and recommend taking athlete to physician.

**Athlete should get physician release before returning to activity.**

# ASTHMA

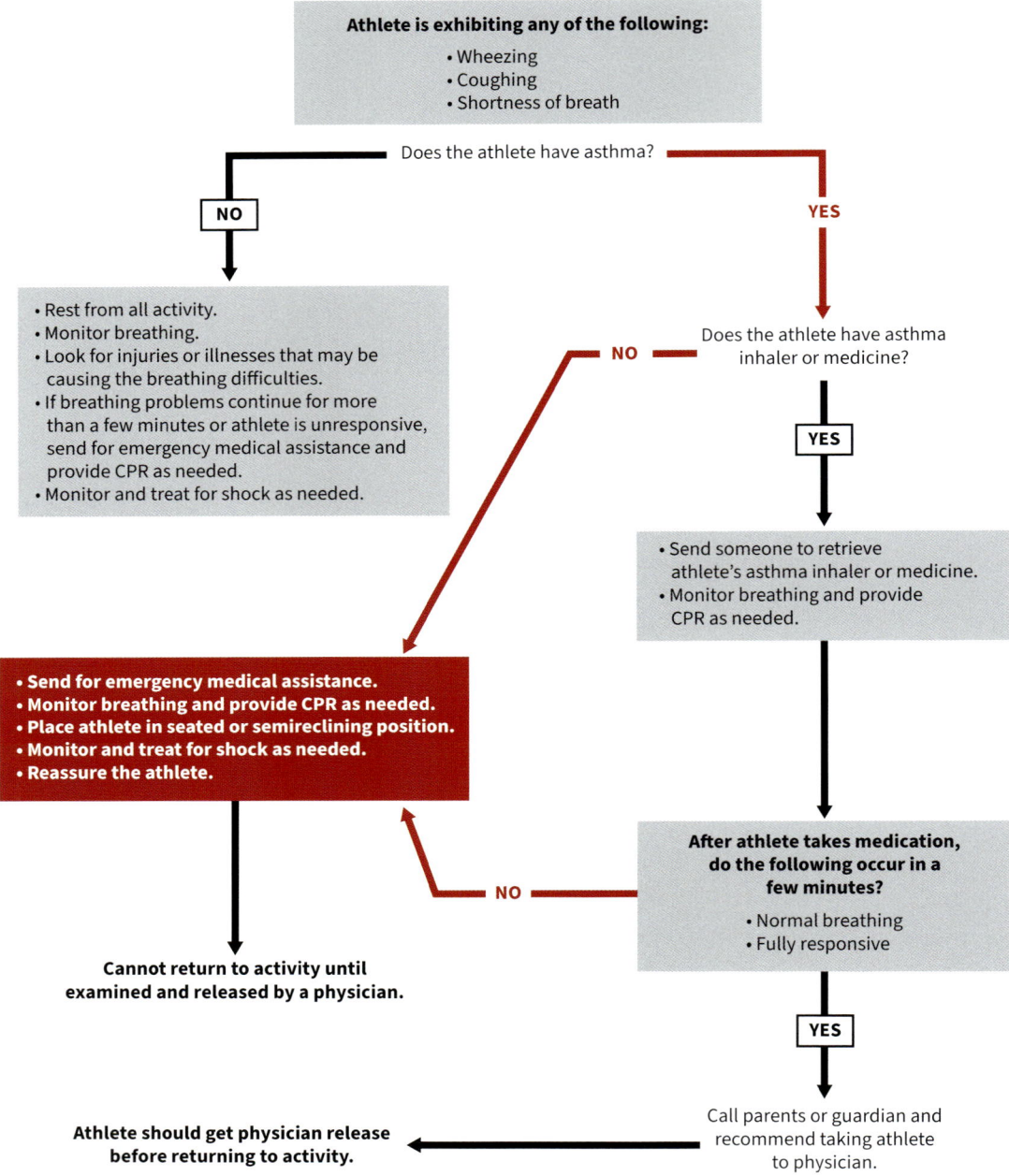

**Athlete is exhibiting any of the following:**

- Wheezing
- Coughing
- Shortness of breath

Does the athlete have asthma?

**NO**

**YES**

- Rest from all activity.
- Monitor breathing.
- Look for injuries or illnesses that may be causing the breathing difficulties.
- If breathing problems continue for more than a few minutes or athlete is unresponsive, send for emergency medical assistance and provide CPR as needed.
- Monitor and treat for shock as needed.

Does the athlete have asthma inhaler or medicine?

**NO**

**YES**

- Send someone to retrieve athlete's asthma inhaler or medicine.
- Monitor breathing and provide CPR as needed.

- **Send for emergency medical assistance.**
- **Monitor breathing and provide CPR as needed.**
- **Place athlete in seated or semireclining position.**
- **Monitor and treat for shock as needed.**
- **Reassure the athlete.**

**After athlete takes medication, do the following occur in a few minutes?**

- Normal breathing
- Fully responsive

**NO**

**Cannot return to activity until examined and released by a physician.**

**YES**

**Athlete should get physician release before returning to activity.**

Call parents or guardian and recommend taking athlete to physician.

# HEAD INJURY

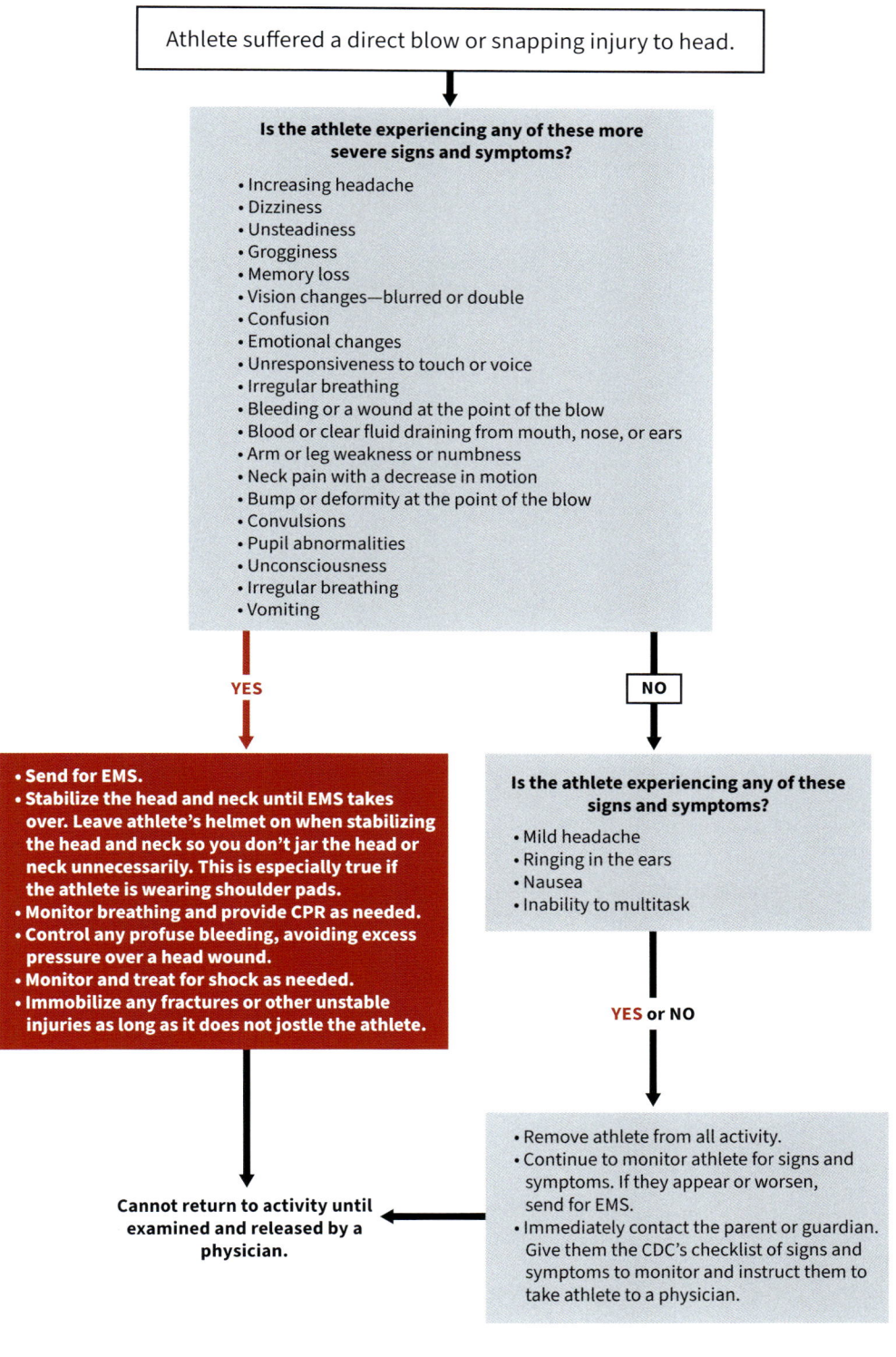

Athlete suffered a direct blow or snapping injury to head.

**Is the athlete experiencing any of these more severe signs and symptoms?**

- Increasing headache
- Dizziness
- Unsteadiness
- Grogginess
- Memory loss
- Vision changes—blurred or double
- Confusion
- Emotional changes
- Unresponsiveness to touch or voice
- Irregular breathing
- Bleeding or a wound at the point of the blow
- Blood or clear fluid draining from mouth, nose, or ears
- Arm or leg weakness or numbness
- Neck pain with a decrease in motion
- Bump or deformity at the point of the blow
- Convulsions
- Pupil abnormalities
- Unconsciousness
- Irregular breathing
- Vomiting

**YES**

**NO**

- **Send for EMS.**
- **Stabilize the head and neck until EMS takes over. Leave athlete's helmet on when stabilizing the head and neck so you don't jar the head or neck unnecessarily. This is especially true if the athlete is wearing shoulder pads.**
- **Monitor breathing and provide CPR as needed.**
- **Control any profuse bleeding, avoiding excess pressure over a head wound.**
- **Monitor and treat for shock as needed.**
- **Immobilize any fractures or other unstable injuries as long as it does not jostle the athlete.**

**Is the athlete experiencing any of these signs and symptoms?**

- Mild headache
- Ringing in the ears
- Nausea
- Inability to multitask

**YES or NO**

**Cannot return to activity until examined and released by a physician.**

- Remove athlete from all activity.
- Continue to monitor athlete for signs and symptoms. If they appear or worsen, send for EMS.
- Immediately contact the parent or guardian. Give them the CDC's checklist of signs and symptoms to monitor and instruct them to take athlete to a physician.

# SPLEEN INJURY

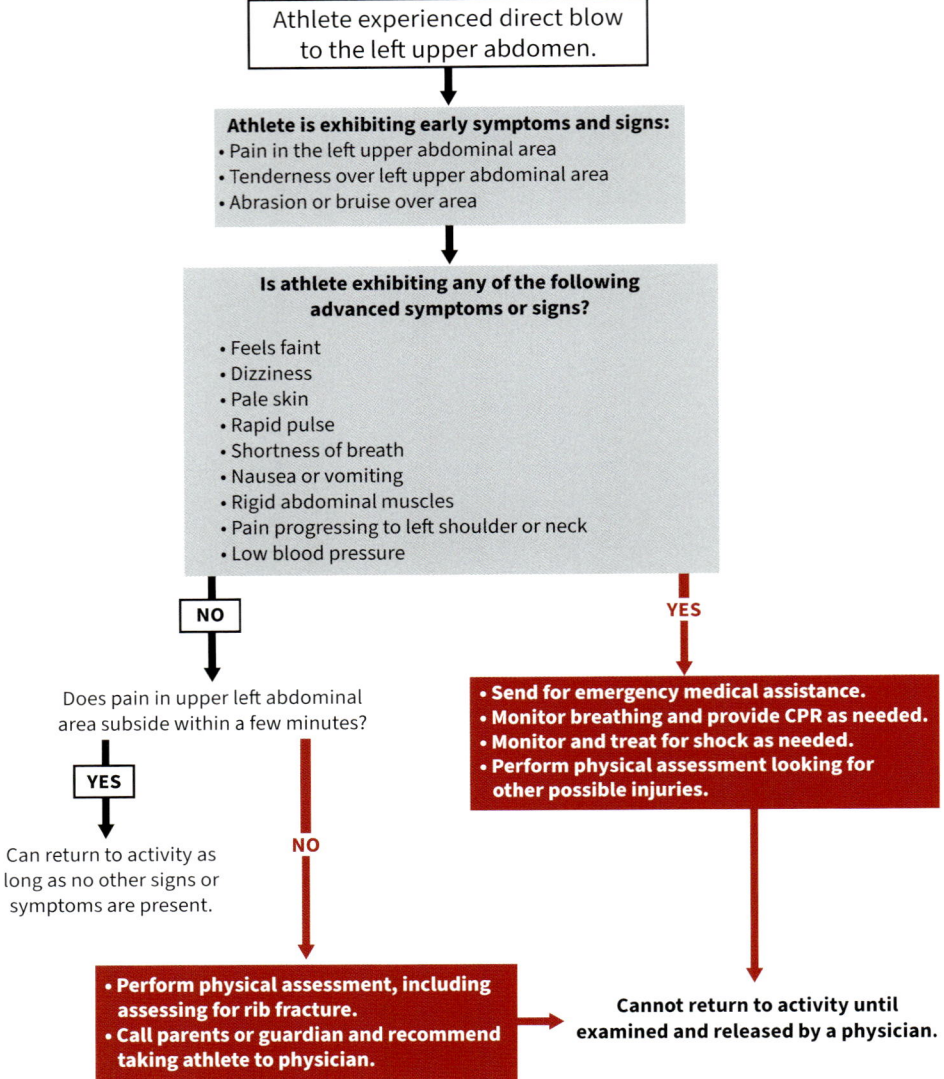

Athlete experienced direct blow to the left upper abdomen.

**Athlete is exhibiting early symptoms and signs:**
- Pain in the left upper abdominal area
- Tenderness over left upper abdominal area
- Abrasion or bruise over area

**Is athlete exhibiting any of the following advanced symptoms or signs?**

- Feels faint
- Dizziness
- Pale skin
- Rapid pulse
- Shortness of breath
- Nausea or vomiting
- Rigid abdominal muscles
- Pain progressing to left shoulder or neck
- Low blood pressure

**NO**

Does pain in upper left abdominal area subside within a few minutes?

**YES**

Can return to activity as long as no other signs or symptoms are present.

**NO**

**YES**

- **Send for emergency medical assistance.**
- **Monitor breathing and provide CPR as needed.**
- **Monitor and treat for shock as needed.**
- **Perform physical assessment looking for other possible injuries.**

- **Perform physical assessment, including assessing for rib fracture.**
- **Call parents or guardian and recommend taking athlete to physician.**

**Cannot return to activity until examined and released by a physician.**

# BRUISED KIDNEY

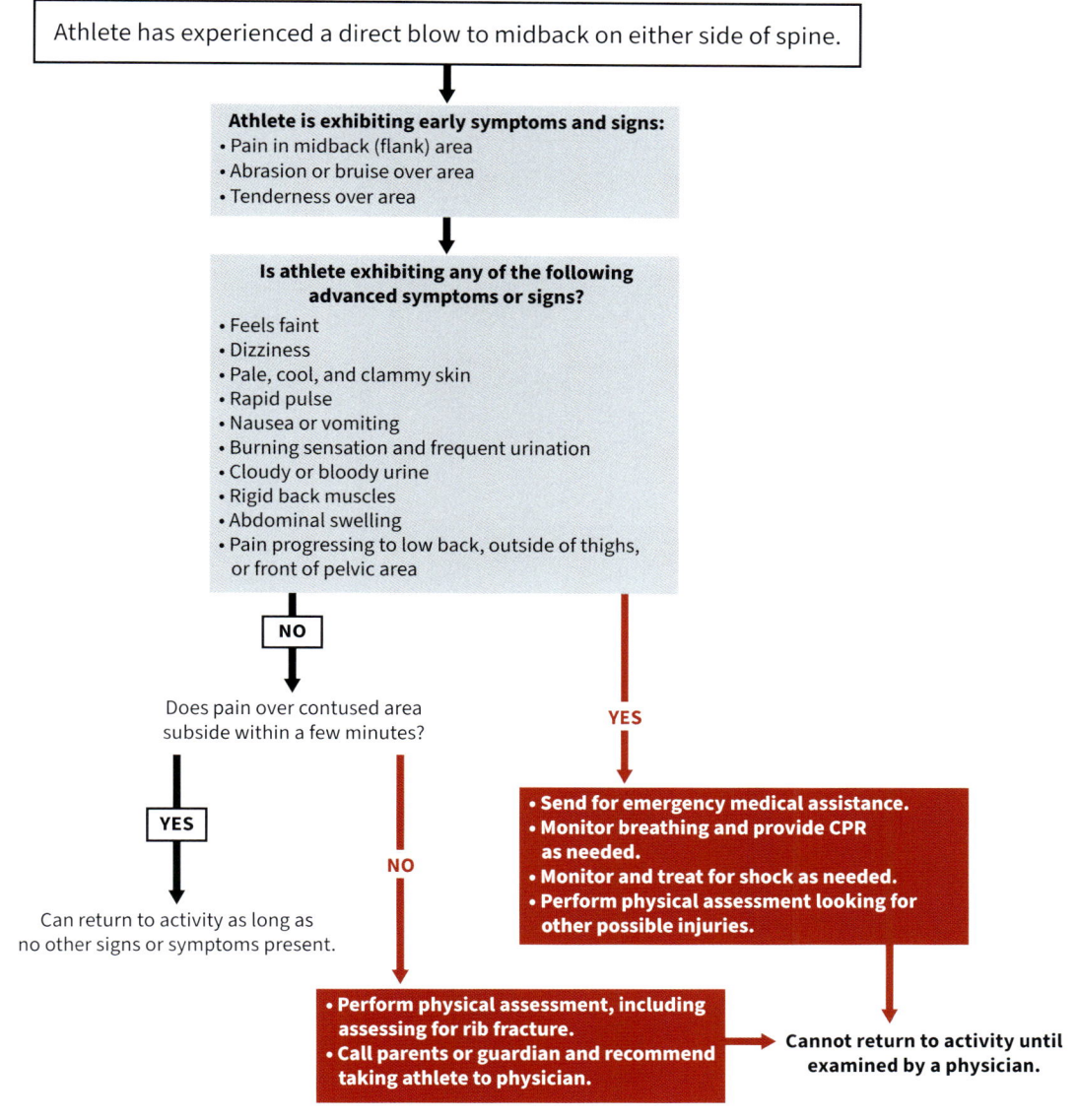

Athlete has experienced a direct blow to midback on either side of spine.

**Athlete is exhibiting early symptoms and signs:**
- Pain in midback (flank) area
- Abrasion or bruise over area
- Tenderness over area

**Is athlete exhibiting any of the following advanced symptoms or signs?**
- Feels faint
- Dizziness
- Pale, cool, and clammy skin
- Rapid pulse
- Nausea or vomiting
- Burning sensation and frequent urination
- Cloudy or bloody urine
- Rigid back muscles
- Abdominal swelling
- Pain progressing to low back, outside of thighs, or front of pelvic area

**NO**

Does pain over contused area subside within a few minutes?

**YES**

**YES**

Can return to activity as long as no other signs or symptoms present.

**NO**

- **Send for emergency medical assistance.**
- **Monitor breathing and provide CPR as needed.**
- **Monitor and treat for shock as needed.**
- **Perform physical assessment looking for other possible injuries.**

- **Perform physical assessment, including assessing for rib fracture.**
- **Call parents or guardian and recommend taking athlete to physician.**

**Cannot return to activity until examined by a physician.**

# TESTICULAR TRAUMA

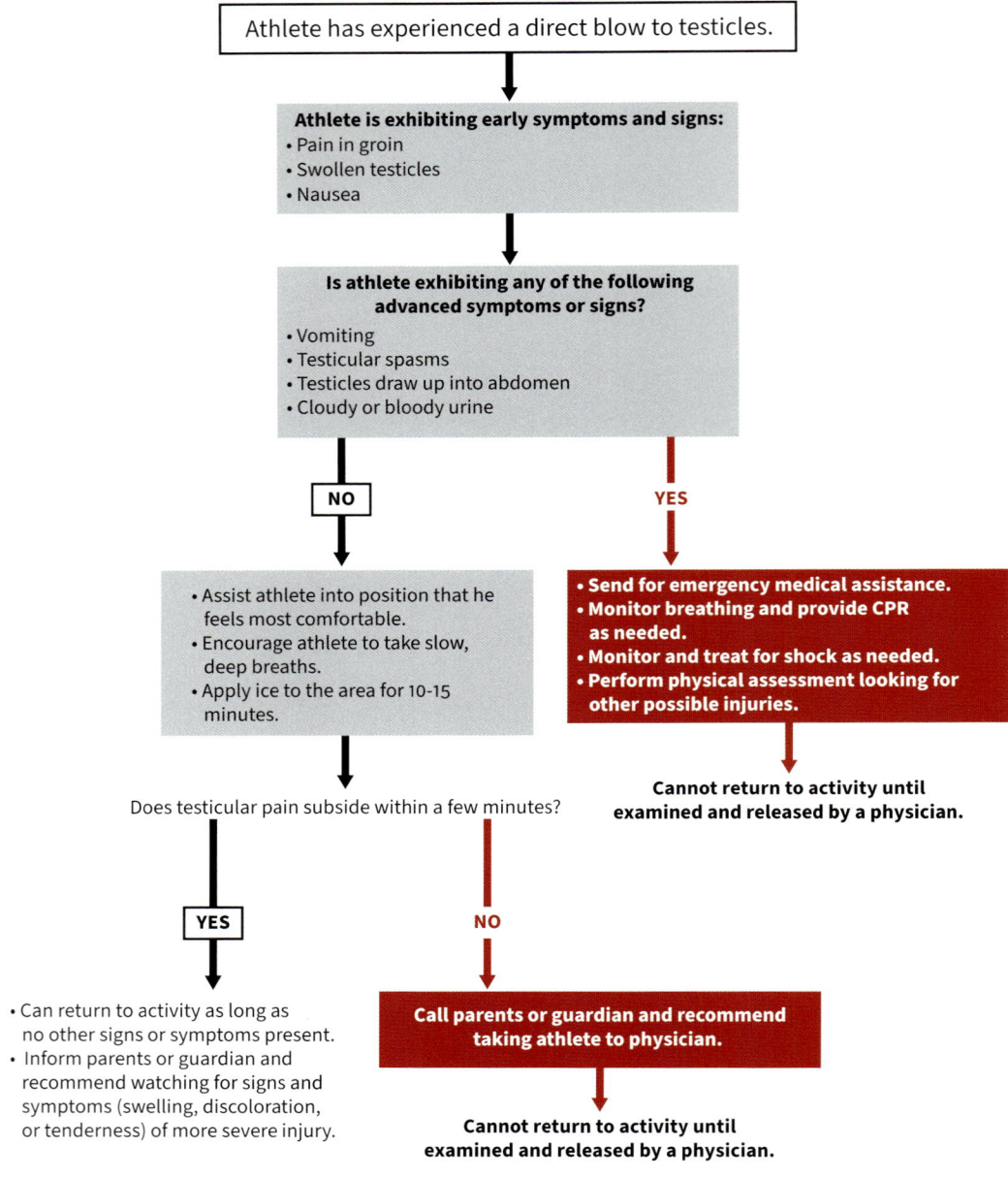

Athlete has experienced a direct blow to testicles.

**Athlete is exhibiting early symptoms and signs:**
- Pain in groin
- Swollen testicles
- Nausea

**Is athlete exhibiting any of the following advanced symptoms or signs?**
- Vomiting
- Testicular spasms
- Testicles draw up into abdomen
- Cloudy or bloody urine

**NO**

**YES**

- Assist athlete into position that he feels most comfortable.
- Encourage athlete to take slow, deep breaths.
- Apply ice to the area for 10-15 minutes.

- **Send for emergency medical assistance.**
- **Monitor breathing and provide CPR as needed.**
- **Monitor and treat for shock as needed.**
- **Perform physical assessment looking for other possible injuries.**

**Cannot return to activity until examined and released by a physician.**

Does testicular pain subside within a few minutes?

**YES**

**NO**

- Can return to activity as long as no other signs or symptoms present.
- Inform parents or guardian and recommend watching for signs and symptoms (swelling, discoloration, or tenderness) of more severe injury.

**Call parents or guardian and recommend taking athlete to physician.**

**Cannot return to activity until examined and released by a physician.**

# HYPOGLYCEMIA IN AN ATHLETE WITH DIABETES

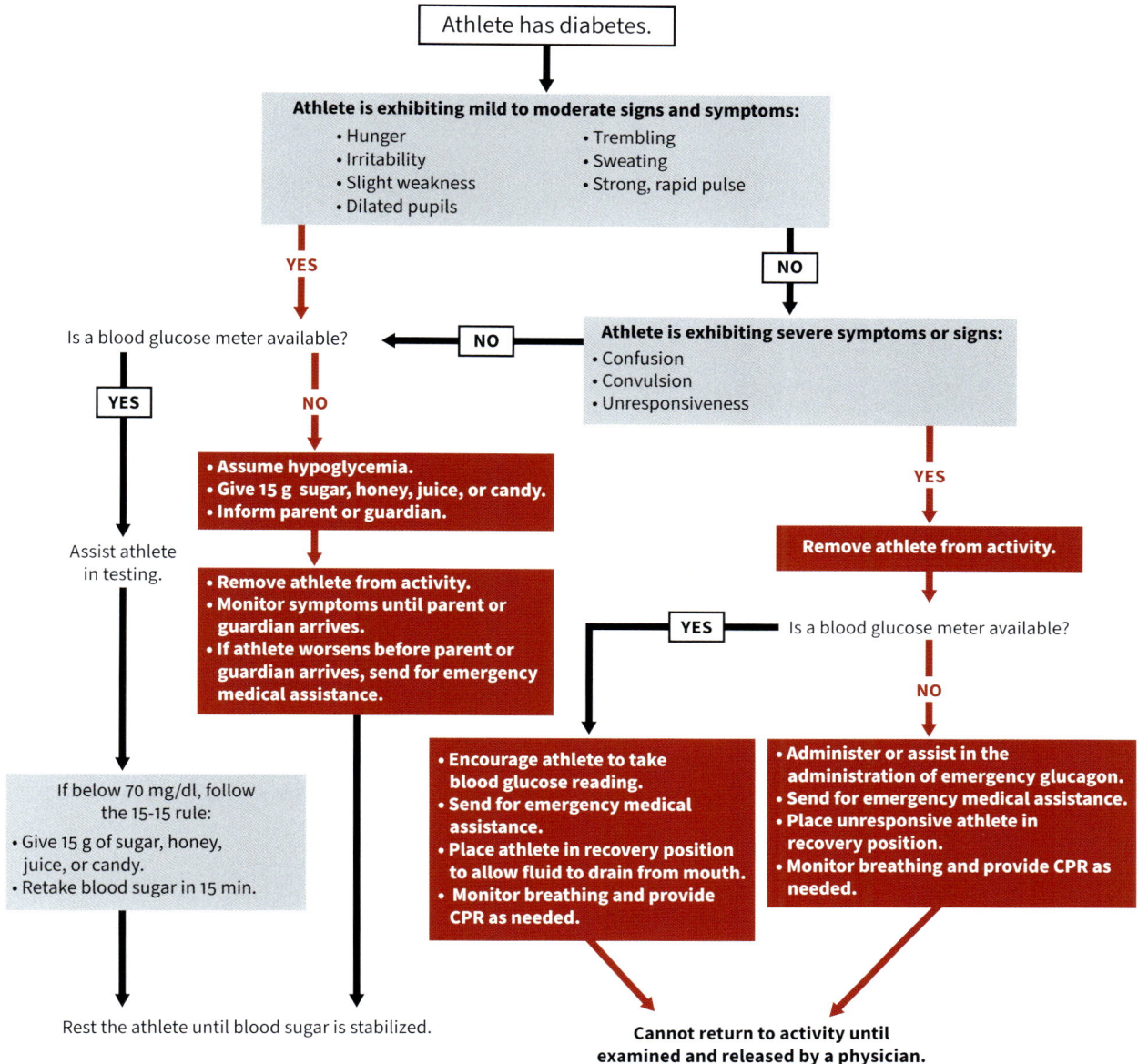

Athlete has diabetes.

**Athlete is exhibiting mild to moderate signs and symptoms:**
- Hunger
- Irritability
- Slight weakness
- Dilated pupils
- Trembling
- Sweating
- Strong, rapid pulse

**YES**

**NO**

Is a blood glucose meter available?  ← **NO** — **Athlete is exhibiting severe symptoms or signs:**
- Confusion
- Convulsion
- Unresponsiveness

**YES**

**NO**

**YES**

- **Assume hypoglycemia.**
- **Give 15 g sugar, honey, juice, or candy.**
- **Inform parent or guardian.**

Assist athlete in testing.

- **Remove athlete from activity.**
- **Monitor symptoms until parent or guardian arrives.**
- **If athlete worsens before parent or guardian arrives, send for emergency medical assistance.**

**Remove athlete from activity.**

**YES**   Is a blood glucose meter available?

**NO**

If below 70 mg/dl, follow the 15-15 rule:
- Give 15 g of sugar, honey, juice, or candy.
- Retake blood sugar in 15 min.

- **Encourage athlete to take blood glucose reading.**
- **Send for emergency medical assistance.**
- **Place athlete in recovery position to allow fluid to drain from mouth.**
- **Monitor breathing and provide CPR as needed.**

- **Administer or assist in the administration of emergency glucagon.**
- **Send for emergency medical assistance.**
- **Place unresponsive athlete in recovery position.**
- **Monitor breathing and provide CPR as needed.**

Rest the athlete until blood sugar is stabilized.

**Cannot return to activity until examined and released by a physician.**

# HYPERGLYCEMIA

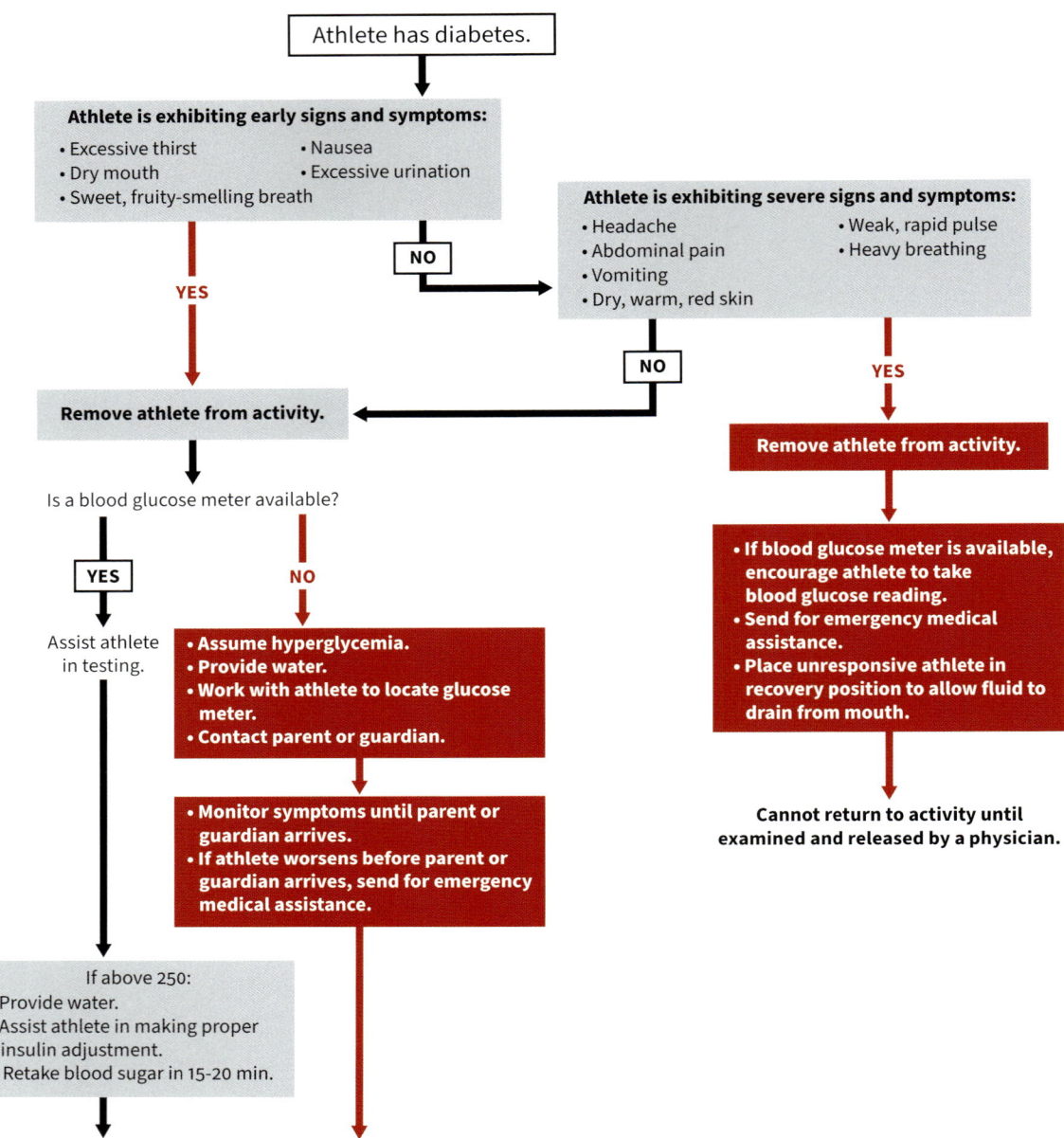

Athlete has diabetes.

**Athlete is exhibiting early signs and symptoms:**
- Excessive thirst
- Dry mouth
- Sweet, fruity-smelling breath
- Nausea
- Excessive urination

**YES**

**NO**

**Athlete is exhibiting severe signs and symptoms:**
- Headache
- Abdominal pain
- Vomiting
- Dry, warm, red skin
- Weak, rapid pulse
- Heavy breathing

**NO**

**YES**

**Remove athlete from activity.**

Is a blood glucose meter available?

**YES**

**NO**

Assist athlete in testing.

- **Assume hyperglycemia.**
- **Provide water.**
- **Work with athlete to locate glucose meter.**
- **Contact parent or guardian.**

- **Monitor symptoms until parent or guardian arrives.**
- **If athlete worsens before parent or guardian arrives, send for emergency medical assistance.**

**Remove athlete from activity.**

- **If blood glucose meter is available, encourage athlete to take blood glucose reading.**
- **Send for emergency medical assistance.**
- **Place unresponsive athlete in recovery position to allow fluid to drain from mouth.**

**Cannot return to activity until examined and released by a physician.**

If above 250:
- Provide water.
- Assist athlete in making proper insulin adjustment.
- Retake blood sugar in 15-20 min.

Rest the athlete until blood sugar is stabilized.

# SEIZURE

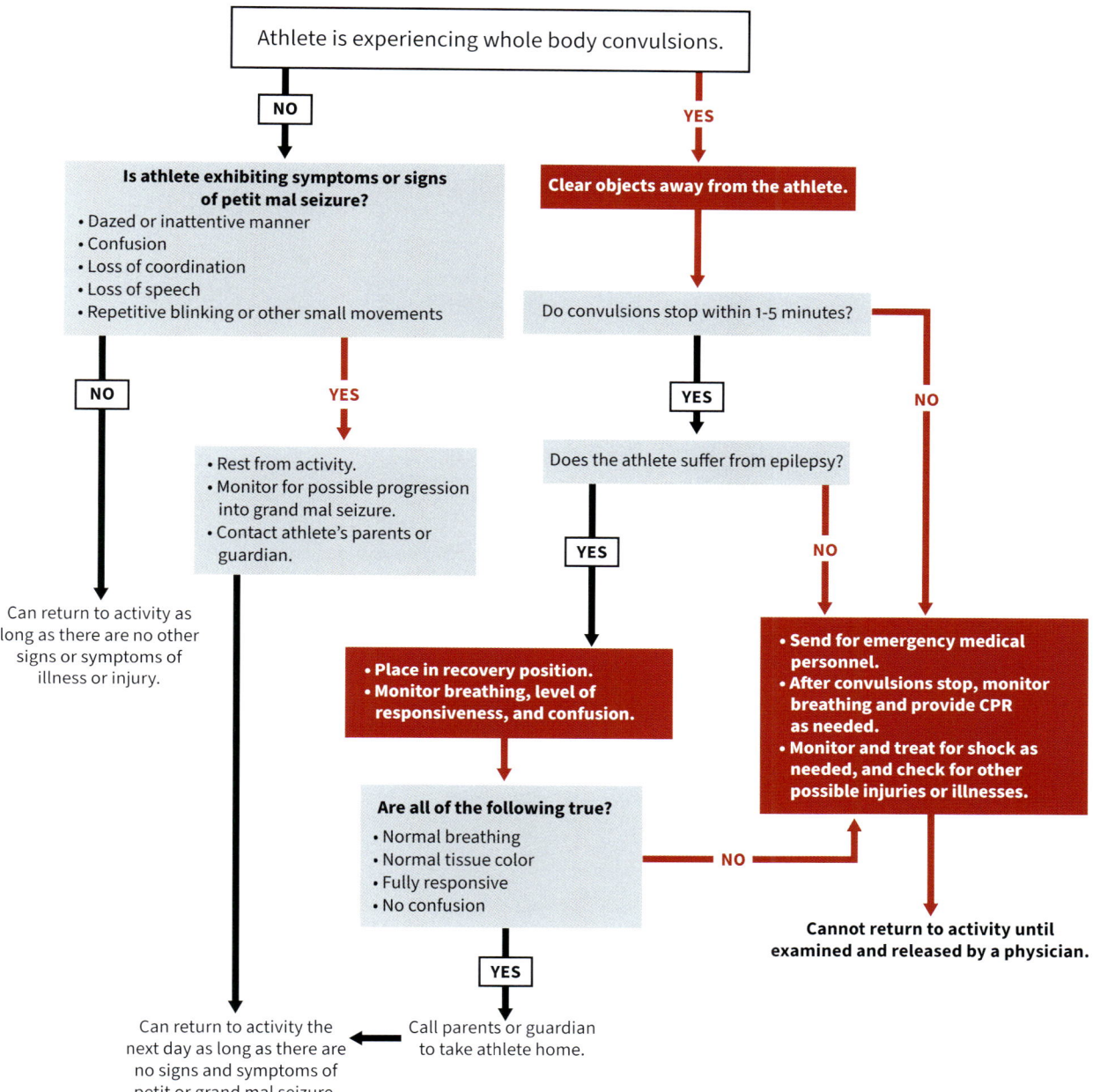

# HEAT CRAMP

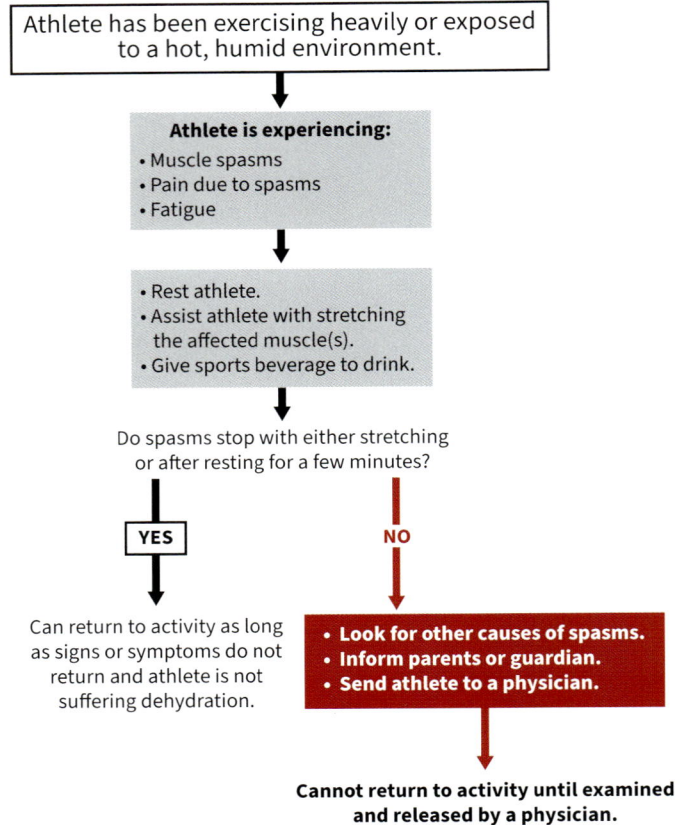

Athlete has been exercising heavily or exposed to a hot, humid environment.

**Athlete is experiencing:**
- Muscle spasms
- Pain due to spasms
- Fatigue

- Rest athlete.
- Assist athlete with stretching the affected muscle(s).
- Give sports beverage to drink.

Do spasms stop with either stretching or after resting for a few minutes?

**YES**

Can return to activity as long as signs or symptoms do not return and athlete is not suffering dehydration.

**NO**

- **Look for other causes of spasms.**
- **Inform parents or guardian.**
- **Send athlete to a physician.**

**Cannot return to activity until examined and released by a physician.**

# HEAT EXHAUSTION

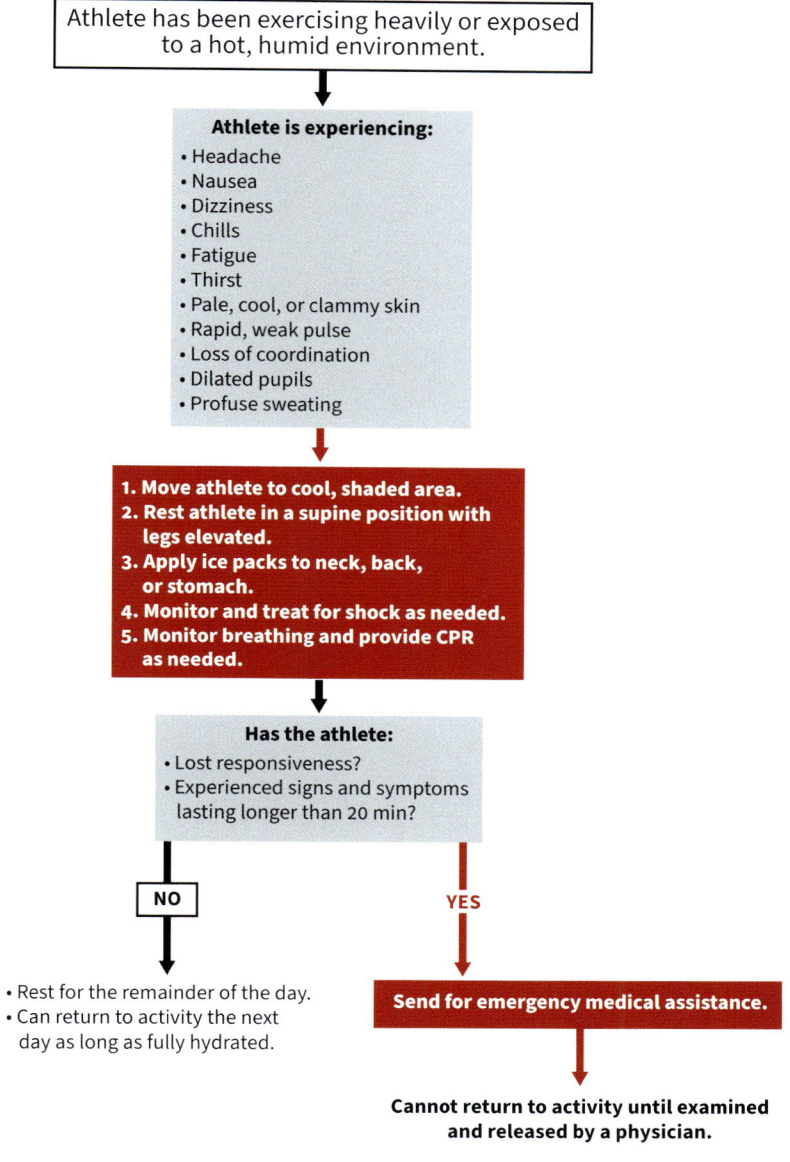

Athlete has been exercising heavily or exposed to a hot, humid environment.

**Athlete is experiencing:**
- Headache
- Nausea
- Dizziness
- Chills
- Fatigue
- Thirst
- Pale, cool, or clammy skin
- Rapid, weak pulse
- Loss of coordination
- Dilated pupils
- Profuse sweating

1. **Move athlete to cool, shaded area.**
2. **Rest athlete in a supine position with legs elevated.**
3. **Apply ice packs to neck, back, or stomach.**
4. **Monitor and treat for shock as needed.**
5. **Monitor breathing and provide CPR as needed.**

**Has the athlete:**
- Lost responsiveness?
- Experienced signs and symptoms lasting longer than 20 min?

**NO**

- Rest for the remainder of the day.
- Can return to activity the next day as long as fully hydrated.

**YES**

**Send for emergency medical assistance.**

**Cannot return to activity until examined and released by a physician.**

# HEATSTROKE

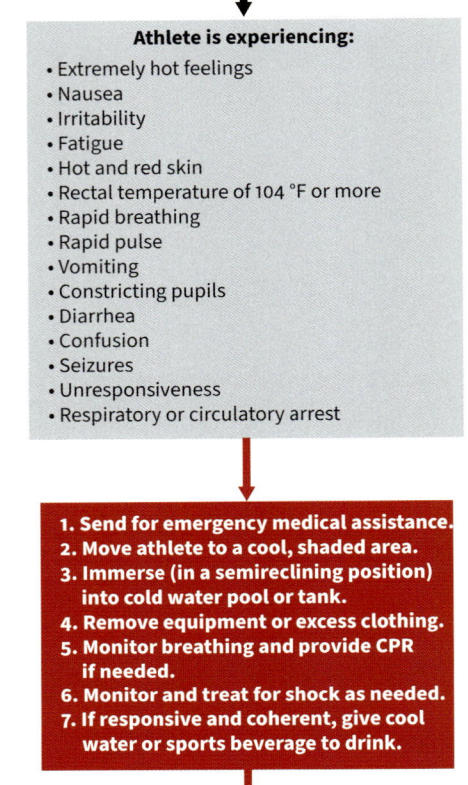

Athlete has been exercising heavily or exposed to a hot, humid environment.

**Athlete is experiencing:**
- Extremely hot feelings
- Nausea
- Irritability
- Fatigue
- Hot and red skin
- Rectal temperature of 104 °F or more
- Rapid breathing
- Rapid pulse
- Vomiting
- Constricting pupils
- Diarrhea
- Confusion
- Seizures
- Unresponsiveness
- Respiratory or circulatory arrest

1. **Send for emergency medical assistance.**
2. **Move athlete to a cool, shaded area.**
3. **Immerse (in a semireclining position) into cold water pool or tank.**
4. **Remove equipment or excess clothing.**
5. **Monitor breathing and provide CPR if needed.**
6. **Monitor and treat for shock as needed.**
7. **If responsive and coherent, give cool water or sports beverage to drink.**

**Cannot return to activity until examined and released by a physician.**

# FROSTBITE

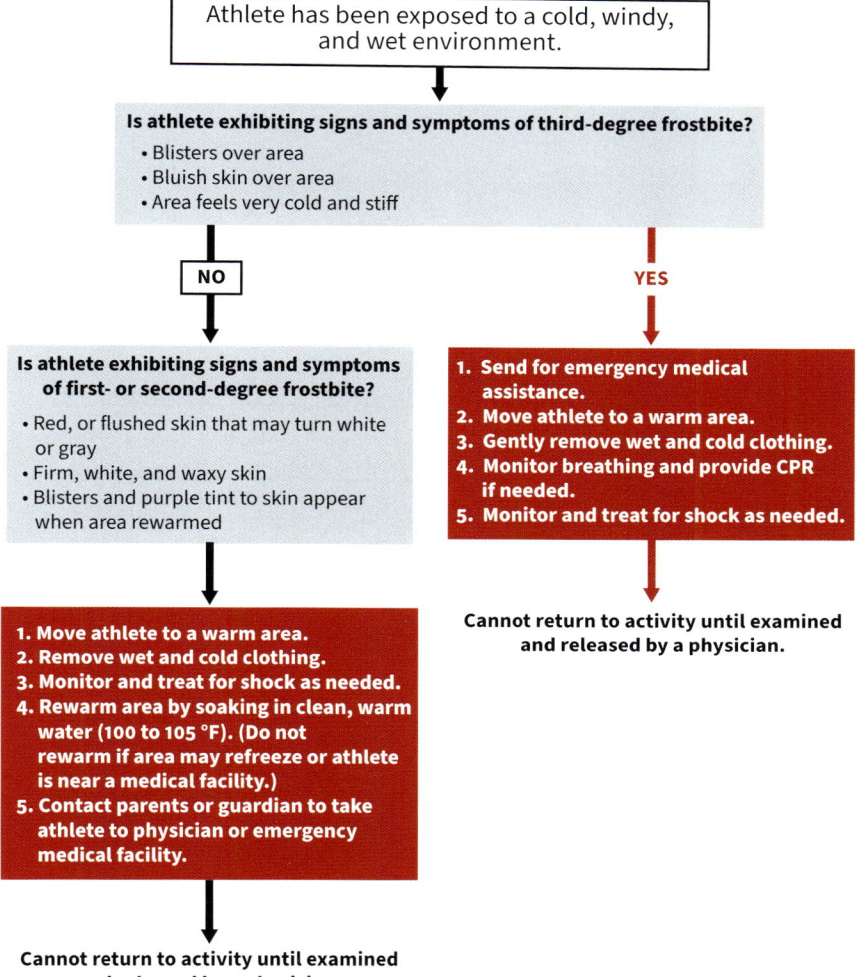

Athlete has been exposed to a cold, windy, and wet environment.

**Is athlete exhibiting signs and symptoms of third-degree frostbite?**
- Blisters over area
- Bluish skin over area
- Area feels very cold and stiff

**NO**

**YES**

**Is athlete exhibiting signs and symptoms of first- or second-degree frostbite?**
- Red, or flushed skin that may turn white or gray
- Firm, white, and waxy skin
- Blisters and purple tint to skin appear when area rewarmed

1. **Send for emergency medical assistance.**
2. **Move athlete to a warm area.**
3. **Gently remove wet and cold clothing.**
4. **Monitor breathing and provide CPR if needed.**
5. **Monitor and treat for shock as needed.**

**Cannot return to activity until examined and released by a physician.**

1. **Move athlete to a warm area.**
2. **Remove wet and cold clothing.**
3. **Monitor and treat for shock as needed.**
4. **Rewarm area by soaking in clean, warm water (100 to 105 °F). (Do not rewarm if area may refreeze or athlete is near a medical facility.)**
5. **Contact parents or guardian to take athlete to physician or emergency medical facility.**

**Cannot return to activity until examined and released by a physician.**

# HYPOTHERMIA

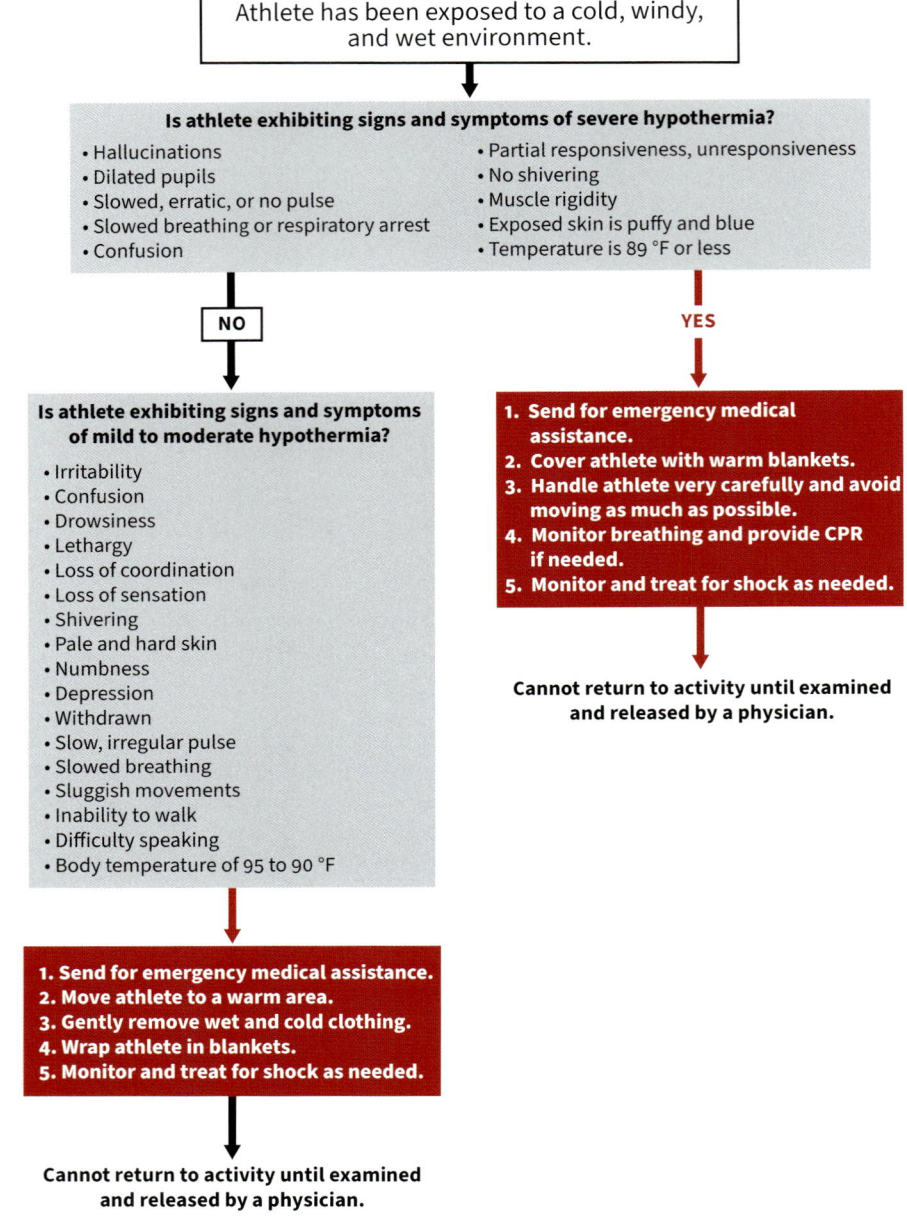

Athlete has been exposed to a cold, windy, and wet environment.

**Is athlete exhibiting signs and symptoms of severe hypothermia?**

- Hallucinations
- Dilated pupils
- Slowed, erratic, or no pulse
- Slowed breathing or respiratory arrest
- Confusion
- Partial responsiveness, unresponsiveness
- No shivering
- Muscle rigidity
- Exposed skin is puffy and blue
- Temperature is 89 °F or less

**NO**

**YES**

**Is athlete exhibiting signs and symptoms of mild to moderate hypothermia?**

- Irritability
- Confusion
- Drowsiness
- Lethargy
- Loss of coordination
- Loss of sensation
- Shivering
- Pale and hard skin
- Numbness
- Depression
- Withdrawn
- Slow, irregular pulse
- Slowed breathing
- Sluggish movements
- Inability to walk
- Difficulty speaking
- Body temperature of 95 to 90 °F

1. **Send for emergency medical assistance.**
2. **Cover athlete with warm blankets.**
3. **Handle athlete very carefully and avoid moving as much as possible.**
4. **Monitor breathing and provide CPR if needed.**
5. **Monitor and treat for shock as needed.**

**Cannot return to activity until examined and released by a physician.**

1. **Send for emergency medical assistance.**
2. **Move athlete to a warm area.**
3. **Gently remove wet and cold clothing.**
4. **Wrap athlete in blankets.**
5. **Monitor and treat for shock as needed.**

**Cannot return to activity until examined and released by a physician.**

# SHOULDER FRACTURE OR SPRAIN

Athlete suffers a direct blow, torsion, or tension injury to shoulder.

**Is athlete exhibiting any of the following symptoms and signs of a severe shoulder injury?**

- Deformity
- Bone protruding through skin
- Dislocated shoulder
- Severe SC joint sprain with clavicle displaced backward
- Bluish appearance of skin on arm, hand, or fingers
- Grating sensation at the site of the injury
- Shock
- Inability to move arm overhead, across body, or to rotate arm
- Loss of sensation in the arm, hand, or fingers

**NO**

**YES**

**Is athlete exhibiting any of the following symptoms and signs of a moderate injury?**

- Point tenderness at the site of the injury
- Moderate to severe pain with moving the arm
- Grade II or III AC joint sprain
- Grade II SC joint sprain with clavicle displaced slightly forward
- Sensation of arm "popping out" then "popping back in"
- Swelling

- **Send for emergency medical assistance.**
- **Monitor breathing and provide CPR as needed.**
- **Monitor and treat for shock as needed.**
- **Keep athlete from moving arm.**

**Cannot return to activity until athlete**

- has been examined and released by a physician; and
- has full shoulder range of motion, flexibility, and strength.

**NO**

**Is athlete exhibiting symptoms and signs of minor injury?**

- Mild pain with certain movements, but full range of motion
- Minimal point tenderness

**YES**

- Apply sling and secure arm to body with an elastic wrap.
- Monitor and treat for shock as needed and send for emergency medical assistance if it occurs.
- Apply ice and send to physician.

- Rest from all activities that cause pain.
- Refer to physician if signs and symptoms worsen or don't improve after a few days.

**Can return to activity if athlete**

- no longer has signs and symptoms;
- has been examined and released by a physician (if sent to one); and
- has full shoulder range of motion, flexibility, and strength.

# SHOULDER STRAIN

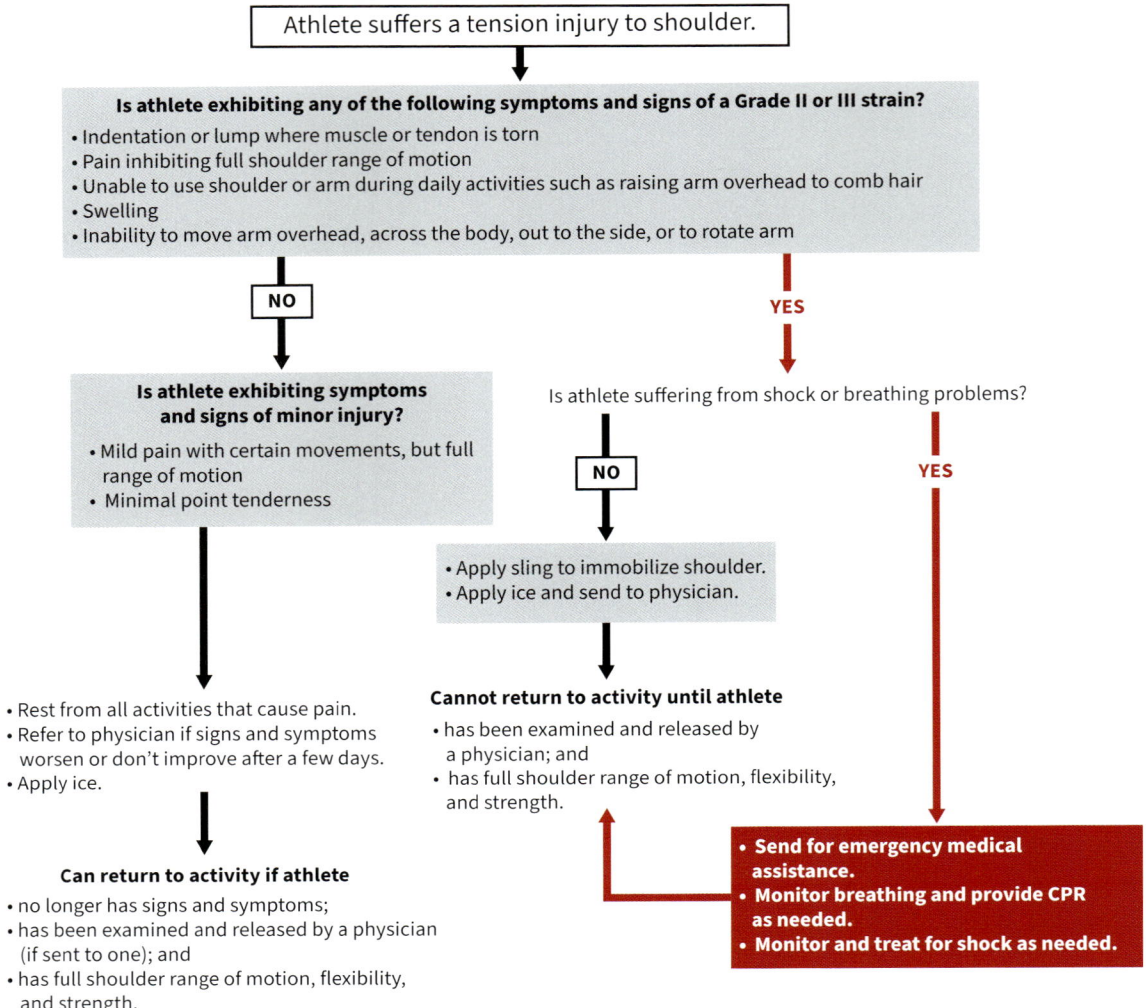

Athlete suffers a tension injury to shoulder.

**Is athlete exhibiting any of the following symptoms and signs of a Grade II or III strain?**
- Indentation or lump where muscle or tendon is torn
- Pain inhibiting full shoulder range of motion
- Unable to use shoulder or arm during daily activities such as raising arm overhead to comb hair
- Swelling
- Inability to move arm overhead, across the body, out to the side, or to rotate arm

**NO**

**YES**

**Is athlete exhibiting symptoms and signs of minor injury?**
- Mild pain with certain movements, but full range of motion
- Minimal point tenderness

Is athlete suffering from shock or breathing problems?

**NO**

**YES**

- Apply sling to immobilize shoulder.
- Apply ice and send to physician.

- Rest from all activities that cause pain.
- Refer to physician if signs and symptoms worsen or don't improve after a few days.
- Apply ice.

**Cannot return to activity until athlete**
- has been examined and released by a physician; and
- has full shoulder range of motion, flexibility, and strength.

**Can return to activity if athlete**
- no longer has signs and symptoms;
- has been examined and released by a physician (if sent to one); and
- has full shoulder range of motion, flexibility, and strength.

- **Send for emergency medical assistance.**
- **Monitor breathing and provide CPR as needed.**
- **Monitor and treat for shock as needed.**

# ACUTE ELBOW INJURY

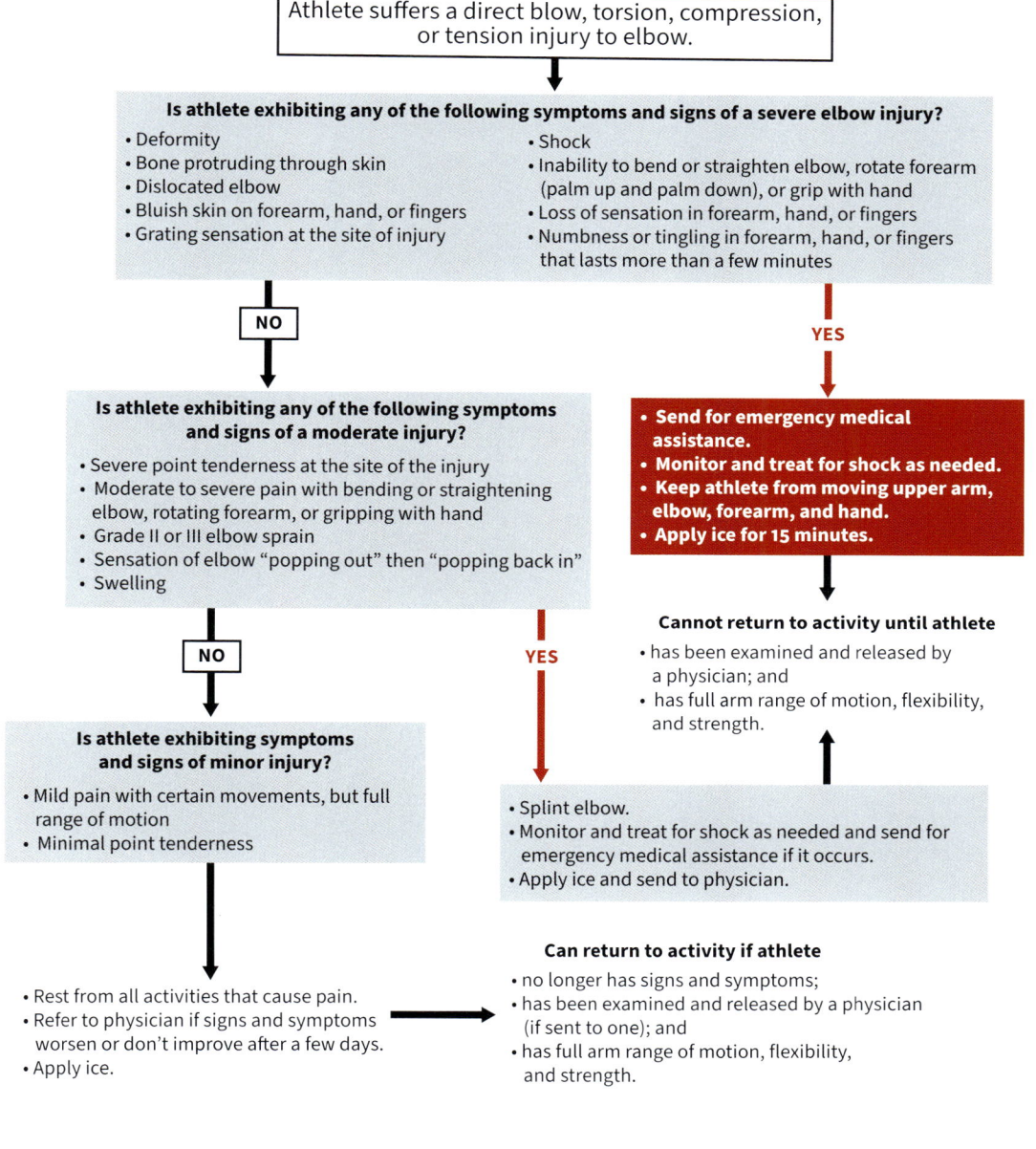

Athlete suffers a direct blow, torsion, compression, or tension injury to elbow.

**Is athlete exhibiting any of the following symptoms and signs of a severe elbow injury?**

- Deformity
- Bone protruding through skin
- Dislocated elbow
- Bluish skin on forearm, hand, or fingers
- Grating sensation at the site of injury

- Shock
- Inability to bend or straighten elbow, rotate forearm (palm up and palm down), or grip with hand
- Loss of sensation in forearm, hand, or fingers
- Numbness or tingling in forearm, hand, or fingers that lasts more than a few minutes

**NO**

**YES**

**Is athlete exhibiting any of the following symptoms and signs of a moderate injury?**

- Severe point tenderness at the site of the injury
- Moderate to severe pain with bending or straightening elbow, rotating forearm, or gripping with hand
- Grade II or III elbow sprain
- Sensation of elbow "popping out" then "popping back in"
- Swelling

- **Send for emergency medical assistance.**
- **Monitor and treat for shock as needed.**
- **Keep athlete from moving upper arm, elbow, forearm, and hand.**
- **Apply ice for 15 minutes.**

**Cannot return to activity until athlete**

- has been examined and released by a physician; and
- has full arm range of motion, flexibility, and strength.

**NO**

**YES**

**Is athlete exhibiting symptoms and signs of minor injury?**

- Mild pain with certain movements, but full range of motion
- Minimal point tenderness

- Splint elbow.
- Monitor and treat for shock as needed and send for emergency medical assistance if it occurs.
- Apply ice and send to physician.

**Can return to activity if athlete**

- no longer has signs and symptoms;
- has been examined and released by a physician (if sent to one); and
- has full arm range of motion, flexibility, and strength.

- Rest from all activities that cause pain.
- Refer to physician if signs and symptoms worsen or don't improve after a few days.
- Apply ice.

# ACUTE FOREARM, WRIST, OR HAND INJURY

Athlete suffers a direct blow, torsion, compression, or tension injury to forearm, wrist, hand, or finger.

**Is athlete exhibiting any of the following symptoms and signs of a severe injury?**

- Deformity
- Bone protruding through skin
- Bluish skin on forearm, hand, or fingers
- Grating sensation at the site of injury
- Shock

- Inability to bend wrist up or down, rotate forearm (palm up and palm down), or grip with hand
- Loss of sensation in forearm, hand, or fingers
- Numbness or tingling in forearm, hand, or fingers that lasts more than a few minutes

**NO**

**YES**

**Is athlete exhibiting any of the following symptoms and signs of a moderate injury?**

- Severe point tenderness at the site of the injury
- Moderate to severe pain with bending wrist up or down, rotating forearm, or gripping with hand
- Grade II or III wrist or finger sprain
- Sensation of finger "popping out" then "popping back in"
- Swelling

- **Send for emergency medical assistance.**
- **Monitor and treat for shock as needed.**
- **Keep athlete from moving upper arm, elbow, forearm, and hand.**
- **Apply ice for 15 minutes (as long as no suspected nerve injury).**

**Cannot return to activity until athlete**

- has been examined and released by a physician; and
- has full forearm, wrist, hand, and finger range of motion, flexibility, and strength.

**NO**

**YES**

**Is athlete exhibiting any of the following symptoms and signs of minor injury?**

- Mild pain with certain movements, but full range of motion
- Minimal point tenderness

- Splint forearm, wrist, and hand; or finger.
- Monitor and treat for shock as needed and send for emergency medical assistance if it occurs.
- Apply ice, elevate, and send to physician.

**Can return to activity if athlete**

- no longer has signs and symptoms;
- has been examined and released by a physician (if sent to one); and
- has full forearm, wrist, hand, and finger range of motion, flexibility, and strength.

- Rest from all activities that cause pain.
- Refer to physician if signs and symptoms worsen or don't improve after a few days.
- Apply ice.

# ABDOMINAL INJURY

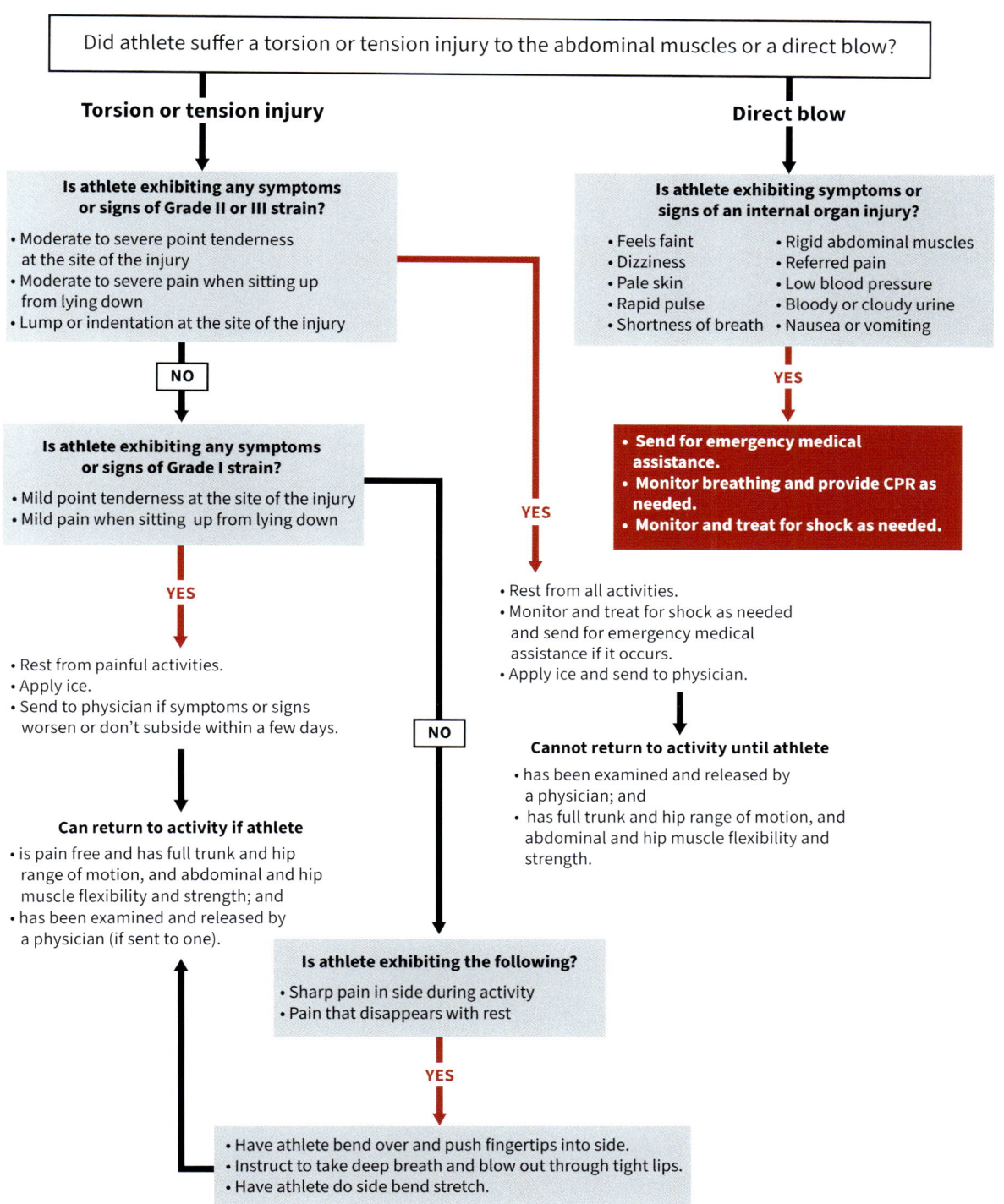

# LOW BACK STRAIN

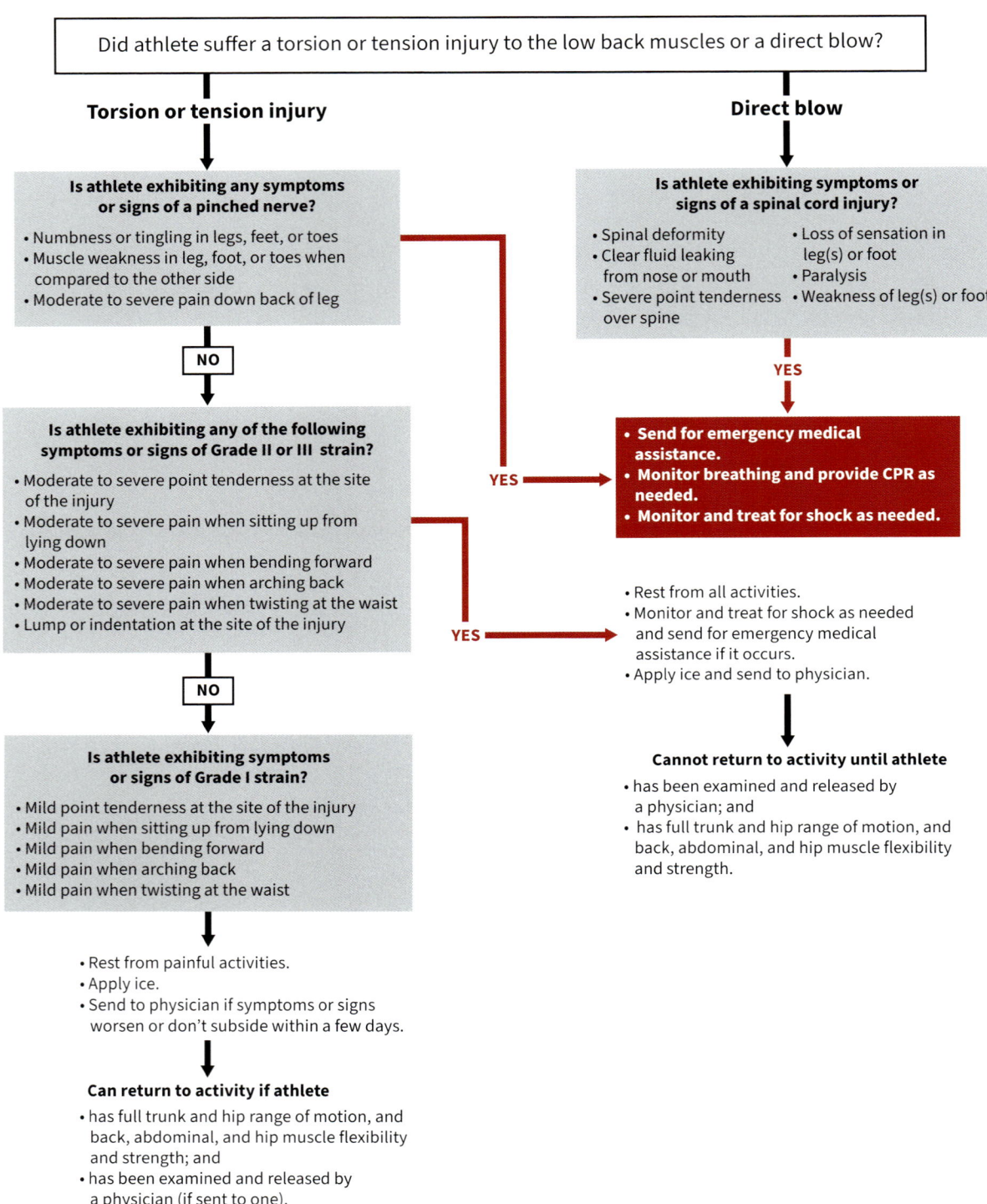

Did athlete suffer a torsion or tension injury to the low back muscles or a direct blow?

**Torsion or tension injury**

**Is athlete exhibiting any symptoms or signs of a pinched nerve?**

• Numbness or tingling in legs, feet, or toes
• Muscle weakness in leg, foot, or toes when compared to the other side
• Moderate to severe pain down back of leg

**NO**

**Is athlete exhibiting any of the following symptoms or signs of Grade II or III strain?**

• Moderate to severe point tenderness at the site of the injury
• Moderate to severe pain when sitting up from lying down
• Moderate to severe pain when bending forward
• Moderate to severe pain when arching back
• Moderate to severe pain when twisting at the waist
• Lump or indentation at the site of the injury

**NO**

**Is athlete exhibiting symptoms or signs of Grade I strain?**

• Mild point tenderness at the site of the injury
• Mild pain when sitting up from lying down
• Mild pain when bending forward
• Mild pain when arching back
• Mild pain when twisting at the waist

• Rest from painful activities.
• Apply ice.
• Send to physician if symptoms or signs worsen or don't subside within a few days.

**Can return to activity if athlete**

• has full trunk and hip range of motion, and back, abdominal, and hip muscle flexibility and strength; and
• has been examined and released by a physician (if sent to one).

**Direct blow**

**Is athlete exhibiting symptoms or signs of a spinal cord injury?**

• Spinal deformity
• Clear fluid leaking from nose or mouth
• Severe point tenderness over spine
• Loss of sensation in leg(s) or foot
• Paralysis
• Weakness of leg(s) or foot

**YES**

• **Send for emergency medical assistance.**
• **Monitor breathing and provide CPR as needed.**
• **Monitor and treat for shock as needed.**

**YES**

**YES**

• Rest from all activities.
• Monitor and treat for shock as needed and send for emergency medical assistance if it occurs.
• Apply ice and send to physician.

**Cannot return to activity until athlete**

• has been examined and released by a physician; and
• has full trunk and hip range of motion, and back, abdominal, and hip muscle flexibility and strength.

# ACUTE HIP INJURY

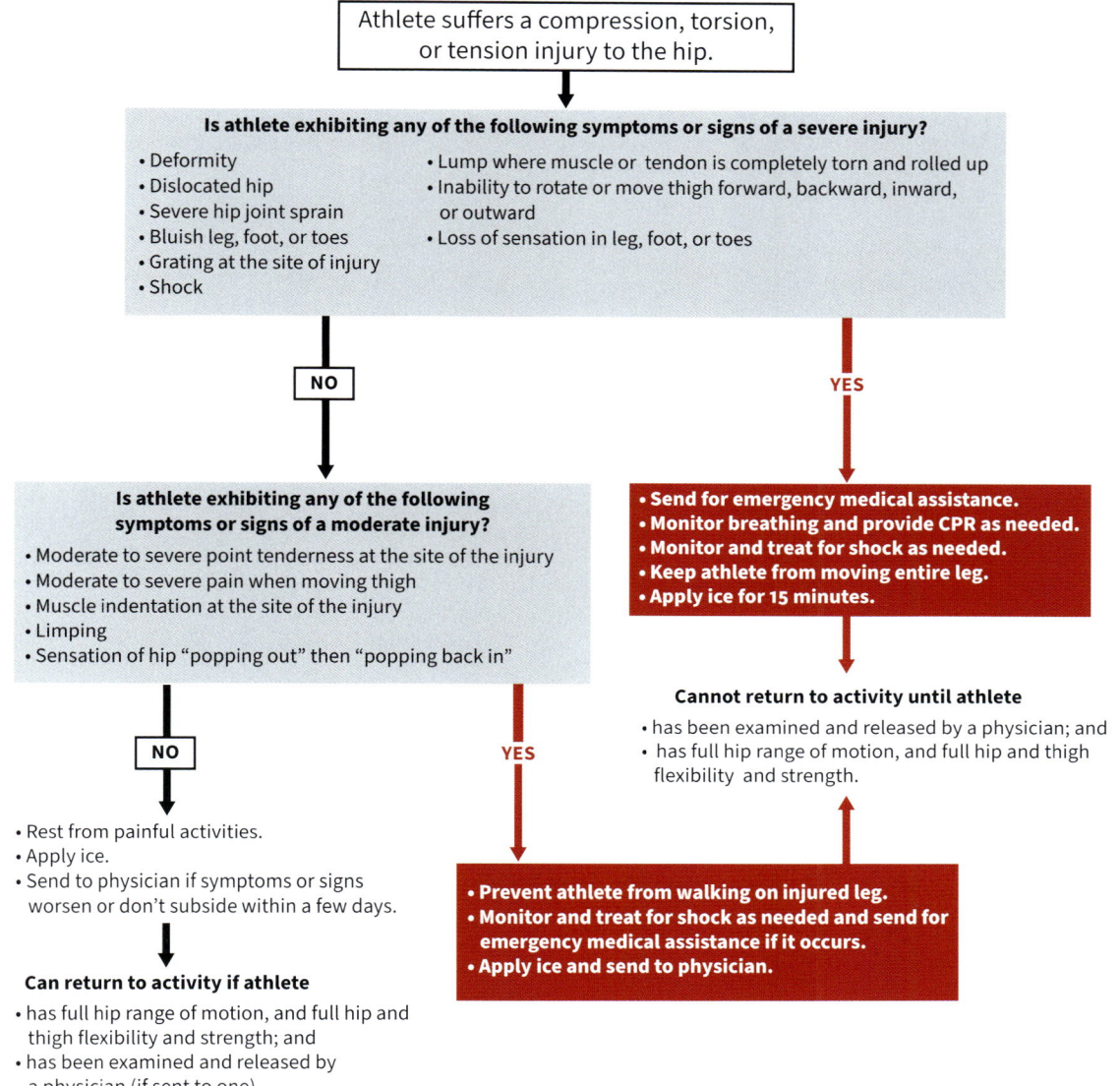

Athlete suffers a compression, torsion, or tension injury to the hip.

**Is athlete exhibiting any of the following symptoms or signs of a severe injury?**

- Deformity
- Dislocated hip
- Severe hip joint sprain
- Bluish leg, foot, or toes
- Grating at the site of injury
- Shock
- Lump where muscle or tendon is completely torn and rolled up
- Inability to rotate or move thigh forward, backward, inward, or outward
- Loss of sensation in leg, foot, or toes

**NO**

**YES**

**Is athlete exhibiting any of the following symptoms or signs of a moderate injury?**

- Moderate to severe point tenderness at the site of the injury
- Moderate to severe pain when moving thigh
- Muscle indentation at the site of the injury
- Limping
- Sensation of hip "popping out" then "popping back in"

- **Send for emergency medical assistance.**
- **Monitor breathing and provide CPR as needed.**
- **Monitor and treat for shock as needed.**
- **Keep athlete from moving entire leg.**
- **Apply ice for 15 minutes.**

**Cannot return to activity until athlete**

- has been examined and released by a physician; and
- has full hip range of motion, and full hip and thigh flexibility and strength.

**NO**

**YES**

- Rest from painful activities.
- Apply ice.
- Send to physician if symptoms or signs worsen or don't subside within a few days.

- **Prevent athlete from walking on injured leg.**
- **Monitor and treat for shock as needed and send for emergency medical assistance if it occurs.**
- **Apply ice and send to physician.**

**Can return to activity if athlete**

- has full hip range of motion, and full hip and thigh flexibility and strength; and
- has been examined and released by a physician (if sent to one).

# ACUTE THIGH INJURY

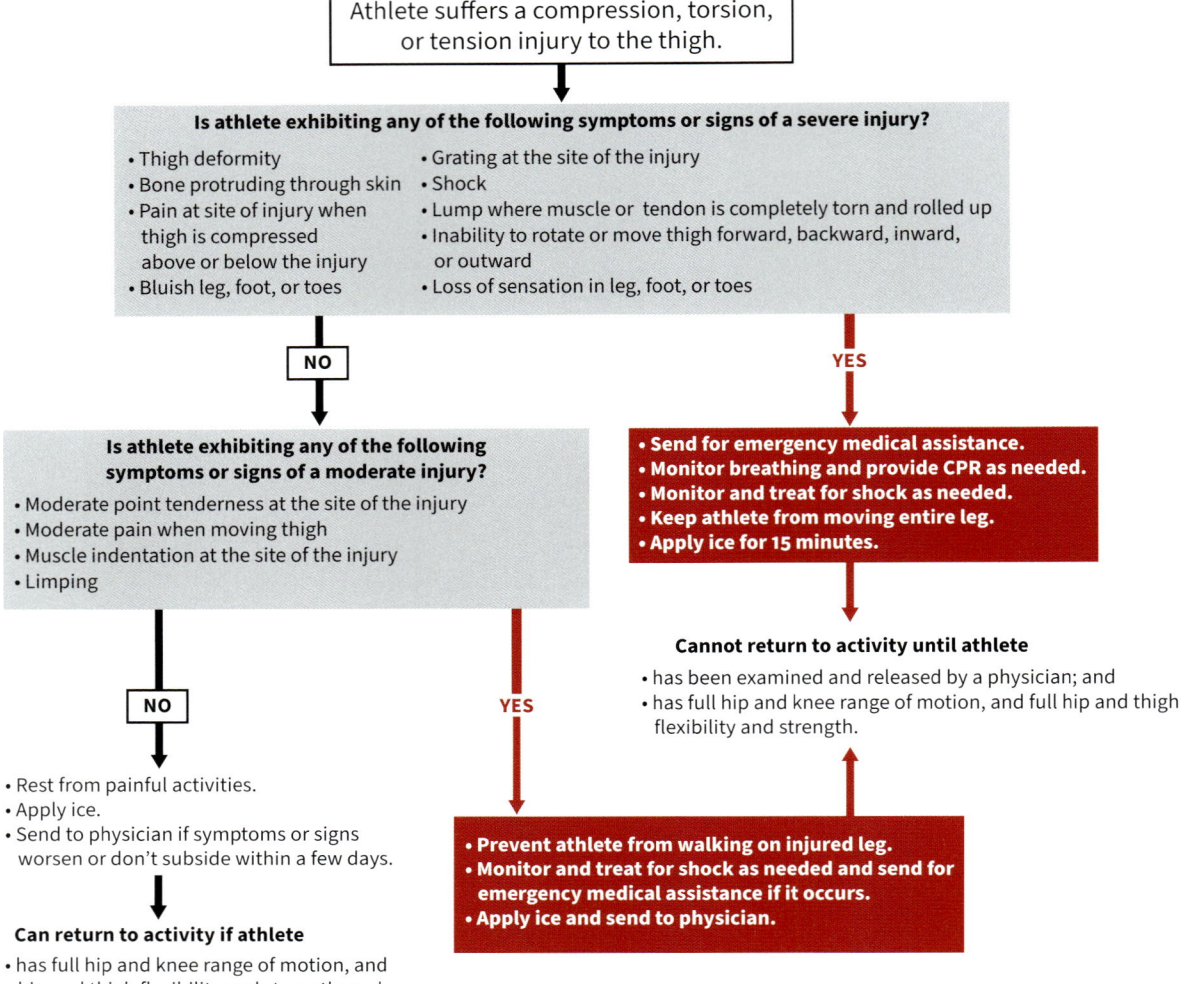

Athlete suffers a compression, torsion, or tension injury to the thigh.

**Is athlete exhibiting any of the following symptoms or signs of a severe injury?**

- Thigh deformity
- Bone protruding through skin
- Pain at site of injury when thigh is compressed above or below the injury
- Bluish leg, foot, or toes
- Grating at the site of the injury
- Shock
- Lump where muscle or tendon is completely torn and rolled up
- Inability to rotate or move thigh forward, backward, inward, or outward
- Loss of sensation in leg, foot, or toes

**NO**

**YES**

- **Send for emergency medical assistance.**
- **Monitor breathing and provide CPR as needed.**
- **Monitor and treat for shock as needed.**
- **Keep athlete from moving entire leg.**
- **Apply ice for 15 minutes.**

**Is athlete exhibiting any of the following symptoms or signs of a moderate injury?**

- Moderate point tenderness at the site of the injury
- Moderate pain when moving thigh
- Muscle indentation at the site of the injury
- Limping

**Cannot return to activity until athlete**

- has been examined and released by a physician; and
- has full hip and knee range of motion, and full hip and thigh flexibility and strength.

**NO**

**YES**

- Rest from painful activities.
- Apply ice.
- Send to physician if symptoms or signs worsen or don't subside within a few days.

- **Prevent athlete from walking on injured leg.**
- **Monitor and treat for shock as needed and send for emergency medical assistance if it occurs.**
- **Apply ice and send to physician.**

**Can return to activity if athlete**

- has full hip and knee range of motion, and hip and thigh flexibility and strength; and
- has been examined and released by a physician (if sent to one).

# ACUTE KNEE INJURY

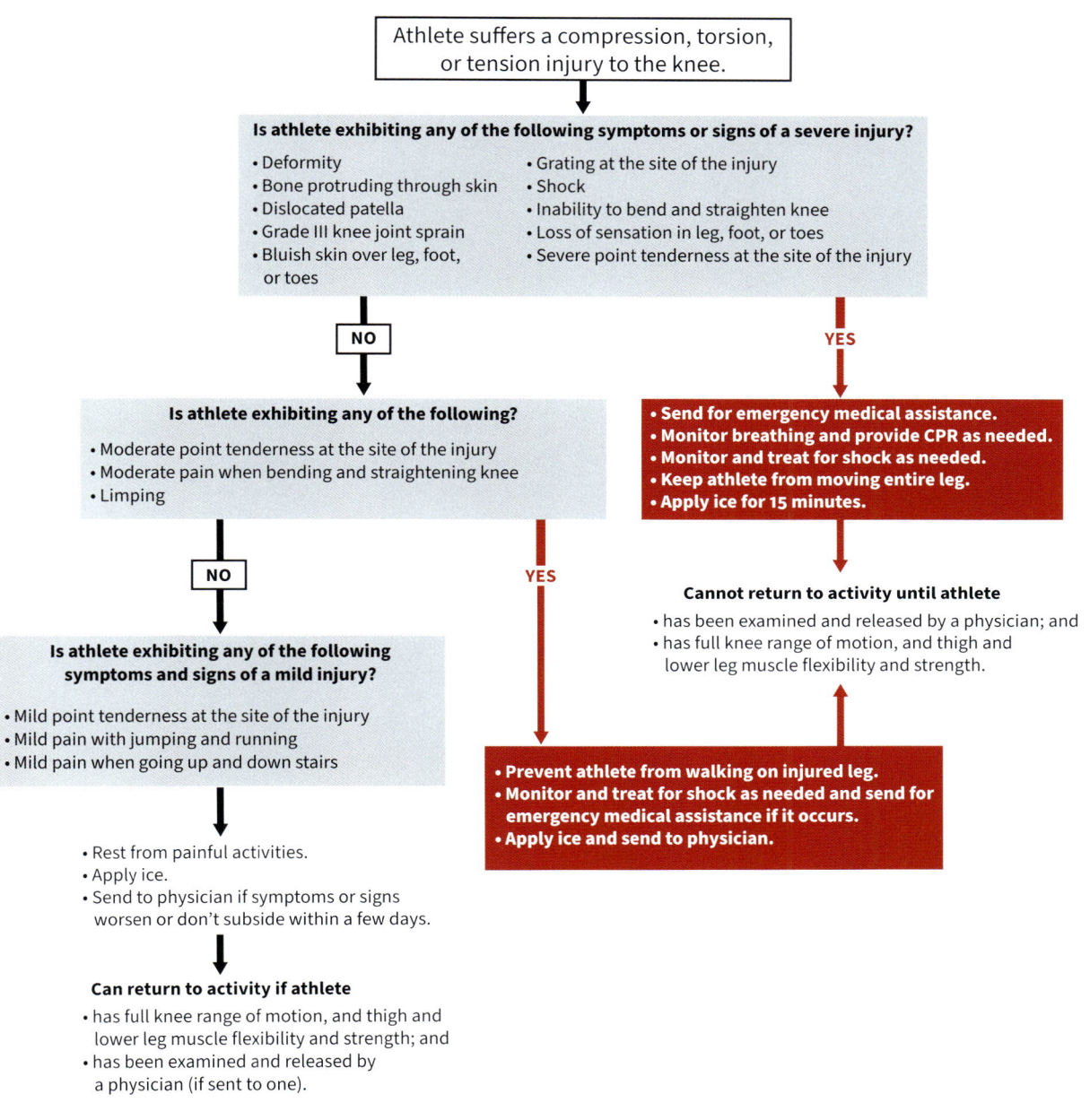

Athlete suffers a compression, torsion, or tension injury to the knee.

**Is athlete exhibiting any of the following symptoms or signs of a severe injury?**

- Deformity
- Bone protruding through skin
- Dislocated patella
- Grade III knee joint sprain
- Bluish skin over leg, foot, or toes
- Grating at the site of the injury
- Shock
- Inability to bend and straighten knee
- Loss of sensation in leg, foot, or toes
- Severe point tenderness at the site of the injury

**NO**

**YES**

**Is athlete exhibiting any of the following?**

- Moderate point tenderness at the site of the injury
- Moderate pain when bending and straightening knee
- Limping

**• Send for emergency medical assistance.**
**• Monitor breathing and provide CPR as needed.**
**• Monitor and treat for shock as needed.**
**• Keep athlete from moving entire leg.**
**• Apply ice for 15 minutes.**

**NO**

**YES**

**Cannot return to activity until athlete**

- has been examined and released by a physician; and
- has full knee range of motion, and thigh and lower leg muscle flexibility and strength.

**Is athlete exhibiting any of the following symptoms and signs of a mild injury?**

- Mild point tenderness at the site of the injury
- Mild pain with jumping and running
- Mild pain when going up and down stairs

**• Prevent athlete from walking on injured leg.**
**• Monitor and treat for shock as needed and send for emergency medical assistance if it occurs.**
**• Apply ice and send to physician.**

- Rest from painful activities.
- Apply ice.
- Send to physician if symptoms or signs worsen or don't subside within a few days.

**Can return to activity if athlete**

- has full knee range of motion, and thigh and lower leg muscle flexibility and strength; and
- has been examined and released by a physician (if sent to one).

# CHRONIC KNEE INJURY

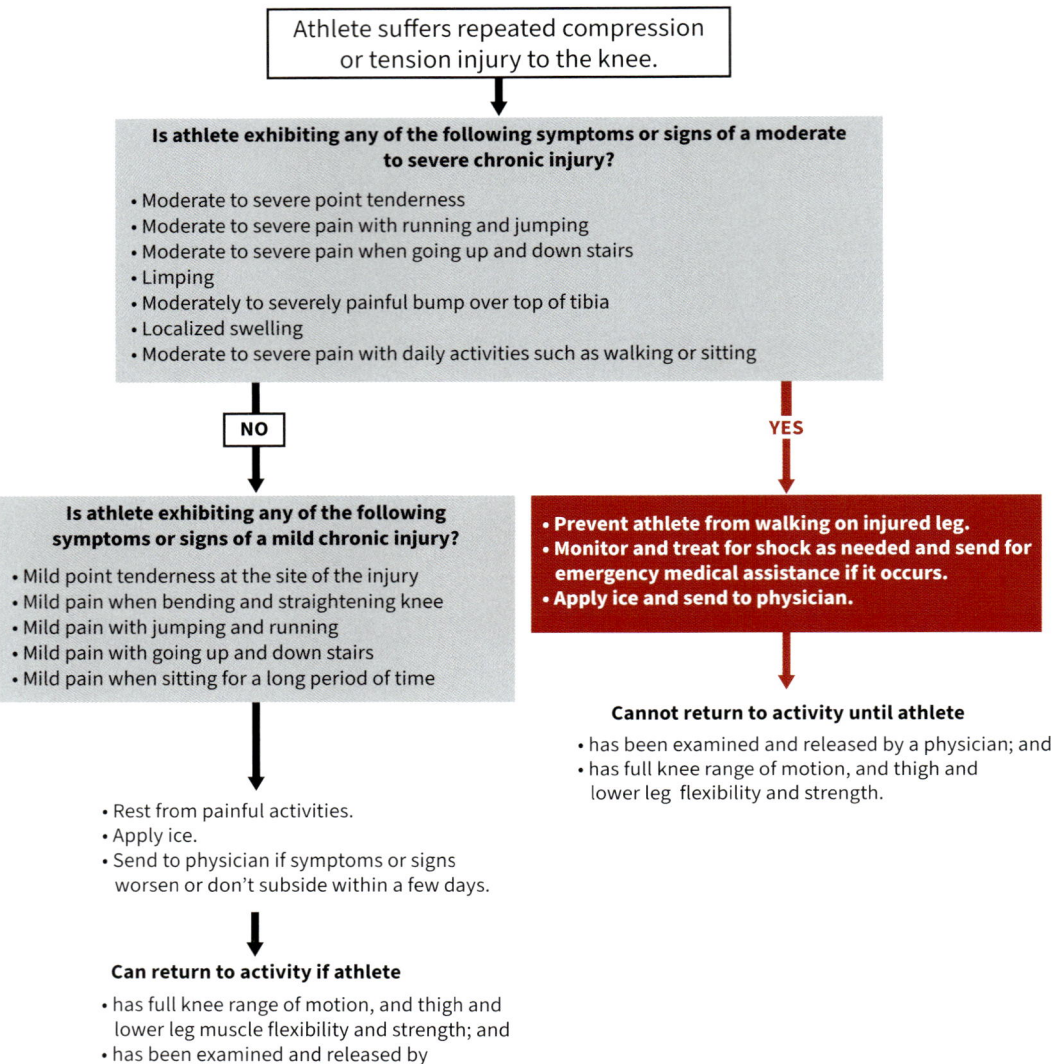

Athlete suffers repeated compression or tension injury to the knee.

**Is athlete exhibiting any of the following symptoms or signs of a moderate to severe chronic injury?**

- Moderate to severe point tenderness
- Moderate to severe pain with running and jumping
- Moderate to severe pain when going up and down stairs
- Limping
- Moderately to severely painful bump over top of tibia
- Localized swelling
- Moderate to severe pain with daily activities such as walking or sitting

**NO**

**YES**

**Is athlete exhibiting any of the following symptoms or signs of a mild chronic injury?**

- Mild point tenderness at the site of the injury
- Mild pain when bending and straightening knee
- Mild pain with jumping and running
- Mild pain with going up and down stairs
- Mild pain when sitting for a long period of time

- **Prevent athlete from walking on injured leg.**
- **Monitor and treat for shock as needed and send for emergency medical assistance if it occurs.**
- **Apply ice and send to physician.**

- Rest from painful activities.
- Apply ice.
- Send to physician if symptoms or signs worsen or don't subside within a few days.

**Cannot return to activity until athlete**

- has been examined and released by a physician; and
- has full knee range of motion, and thigh and lower leg flexibility and strength.

**Can return to activity if athlete**

- has full knee range of motion, and thigh and lower leg muscle flexibility and strength; and
- has been examined and released by a physician (if sent to one).

# ACUTE LEG, FOOT, OR ANKLE INJURY

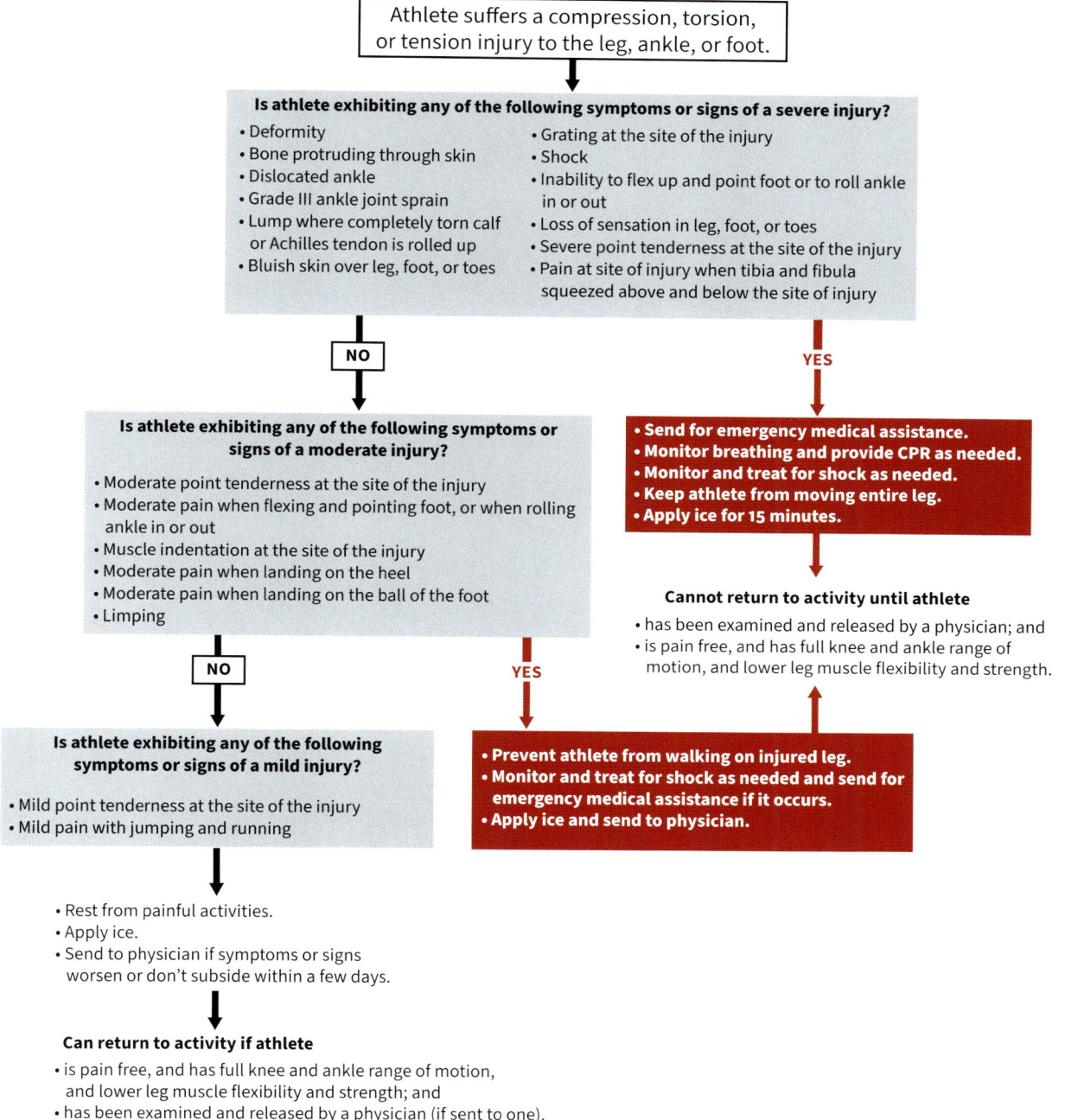

Athlete suffers a compression, torsion, or tension injury to the leg, ankle, or foot.

**Is athlete exhibiting any of the following symptoms or signs of a severe injury?**

- Deformity
- Bone protruding through skin
- Dislocated ankle
- Grade III ankle joint sprain
- Lump where completely torn calf or Achilles tendon is rolled up
- Bluish skin over leg, foot, or toes

- Grating at the site of the injury
- Shock
- Inability to flex up and point foot or to roll ankle in or out
- Loss of sensation in leg, foot, or toes
- Severe point tenderness at the site of the injury
- Pain at site of injury when tibia and fibula squeezed above and below the site of injury

**NO**

**YES**

**Is athlete exhibiting any of the following symptoms or signs of a moderate injury?**

- Moderate point tenderness at the site of the injury
- Moderate pain when flexing and pointing foot, or when rolling ankle in or out
- Muscle indentation at the site of the injury
- Moderate pain when landing on the heel
- Moderate pain when landing on the ball of the foot
- Limping

- **Send for emergency medical assistance.**
- **Monitor breathing and provide CPR as needed.**
- **Monitor and treat for shock as needed.**
- **Keep athlete from moving entire leg.**
- **Apply ice for 15 minutes.**

**Cannot return to activity until athlete**

- has been examined and released by a physician; and
- is pain free, and has full knee and ankle range of motion, and lower leg muscle flexibility and strength.

**NO**

**YES**

**Is athlete exhibiting any of the following symptoms or signs of a mild injury?**

- Mild point tenderness at the site of the injury
- Mild pain with jumping and running

- **Prevent athlete from walking on injured leg.**
- **Monitor and treat for shock as needed and send for emergency medical assistance if it occurs.**
- **Apply ice and send to physician.**

- Rest from painful activities.
- Apply ice.
- Send to physician if symptoms or signs worsen or don't subside within a few days.

**Can return to activity if athlete**

- is pain free, and has full knee and ankle range of motion, and lower leg muscle flexibility and strength; and
- has been examined and released by a physician (if sent to one).

# CHRONIC LEG, FOOT, OR ANKLE INJURY

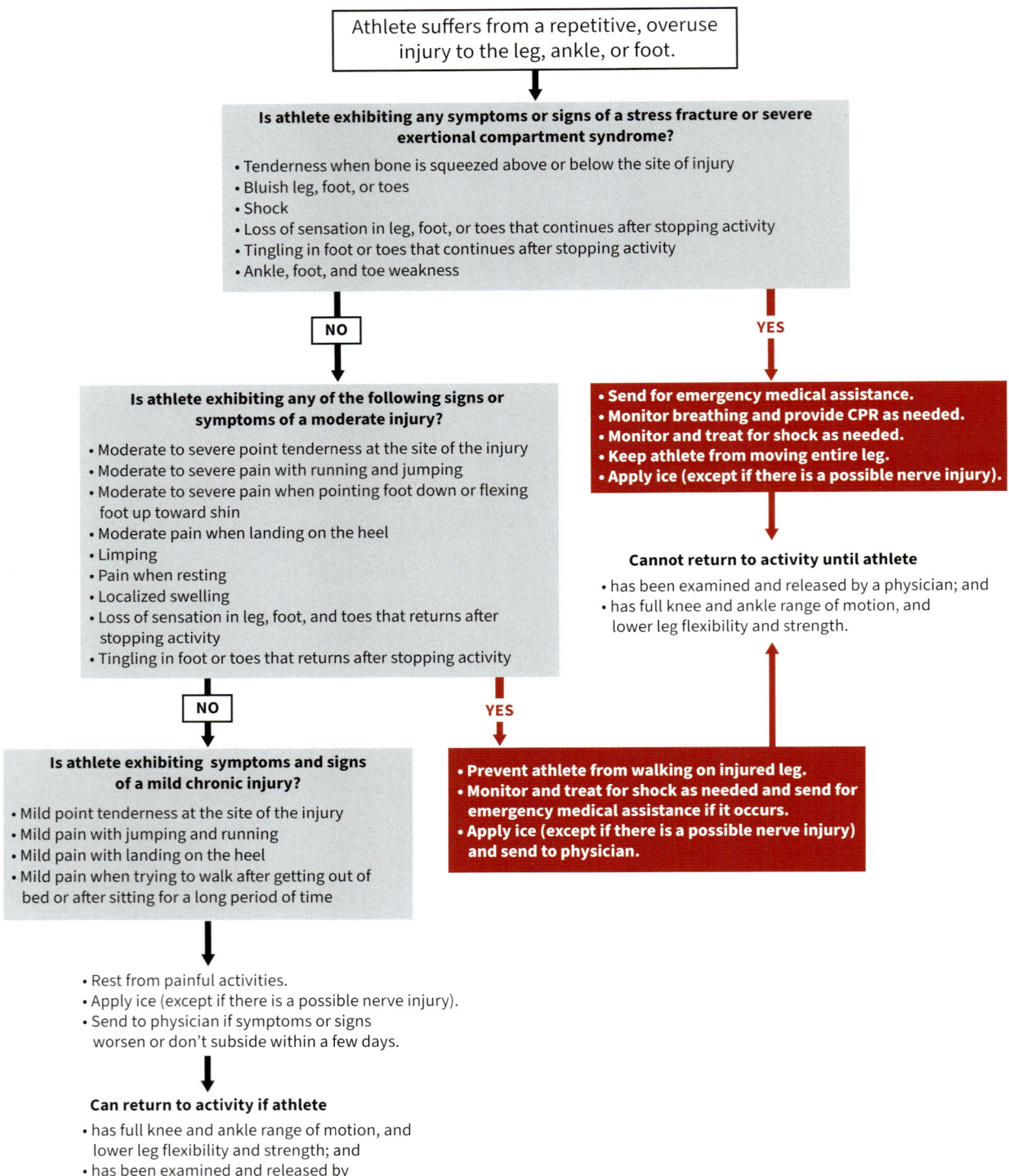

Athlete suffers from a repetitive, overuse injury to the leg, ankle, or foot.

**Is athlete exhibiting any symptoms or signs of a stress fracture or severe exertional compartment syndrome?**
- Tenderness when bone is squeezed above or below the site of injury
- Bluish leg, foot, or toes
- Shock
- Loss of sensation in leg, foot, or toes that continues after stopping activity
- Tingling in foot or toes that continues after stopping activity
- Ankle, foot, and toe weakness

**NO**

**YES**

**Is athlete exhibiting any of the following signs or symptoms of a moderate injury?**
- Moderate to severe point tenderness at the site of the injury
- Moderate to severe pain with running and jumping
- Moderate to severe pain when pointing foot down or flexing foot up toward shin
- Moderate pain when landing on the heel
- Limping
- Pain when resting
- Localized swelling
- Loss of sensation in leg, foot, and toes that returns after stopping activity
- Tingling in foot or toes that returns after stopping activity

- **Send for emergency medical assistance.**
- **Monitor breathing and provide CPR as needed.**
- **Monitor and treat for shock as needed.**
- **Keep athlete from moving entire leg.**
- **Apply ice (except if there is a possible nerve injury).**

**Cannot return to activity until athlete**
- has been examined and released by a physician; and
- has full knee and ankle range of motion, and lower leg flexibility and strength.

**NO**

**YES**

**Is athlete exhibiting symptoms and signs of a mild chronic injury?**
- Mild point tenderness at the site of the injury
- Mild pain with jumping and running
- Mild pain with landing on the heel
- Mild pain when trying to walk after getting out of bed or after sitting for a long period of time

- **Prevent athlete from walking on injured leg.**
- **Monitor and treat for shock as needed and send for emergency medical assistance if it occurs.**
- **Apply ice (except if there is a possible nerve injury) and send to physician.**

- Rest from painful activities.
- Apply ice (except if there is a possible nerve injury).
- Send to physician if symptoms or signs worsen or don't subside within a few days.

**Can return to activity if athlete**
- has full knee and ankle range of motion, and lower leg flexibility and strength; and
- has been examined and released by a physician (if sent to one).

# FACE OR SCALP LACERATION

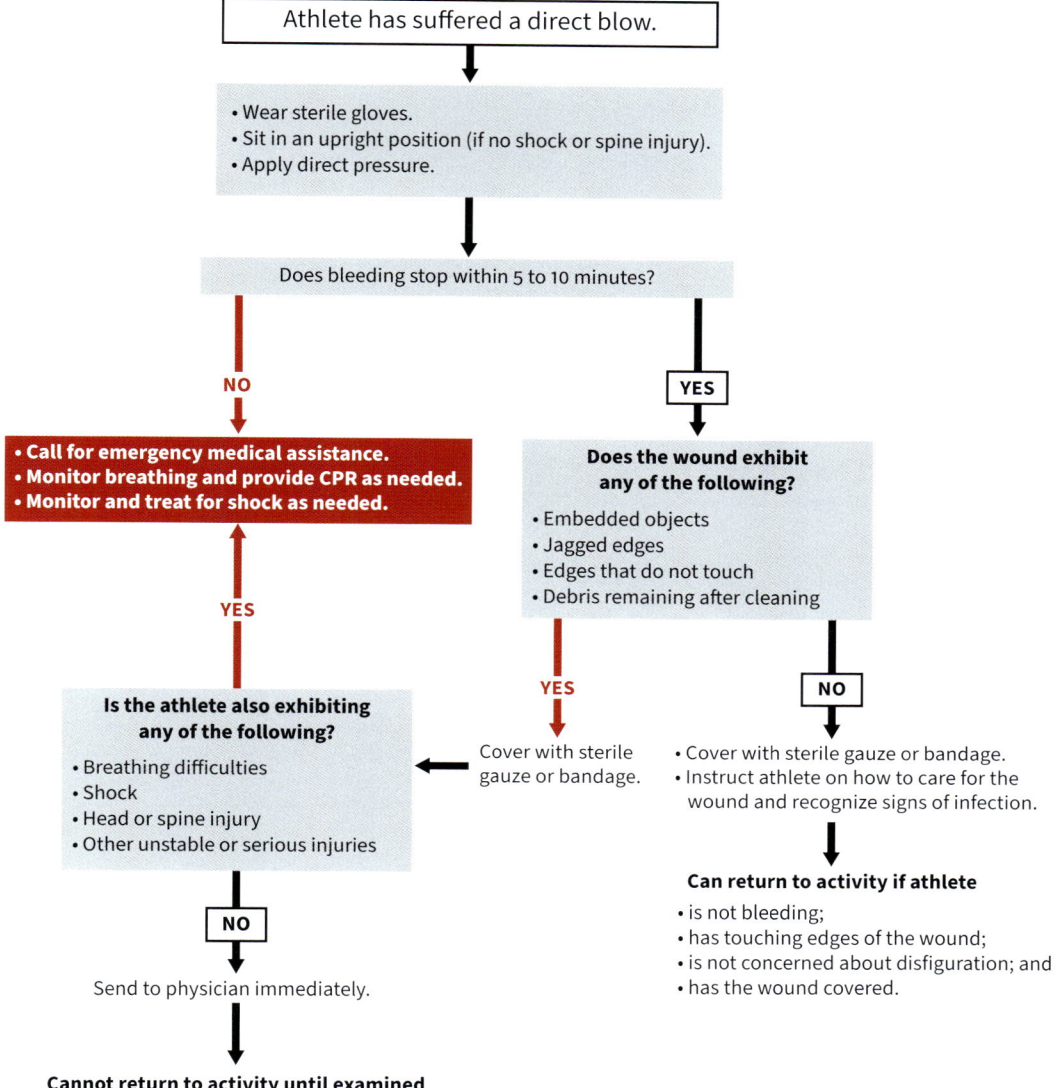

Athlete has suffered a direct blow.

- Wear sterile gloves.
- Sit in an upright position (if no shock or spine injury).
- Apply direct pressure.

Does bleeding stop within 5 to 10 minutes?

**NO**

**YES**

- **Call for emergency medical assistance.**
- **Monitor breathing and provide CPR as needed.**
- **Monitor and treat for shock as needed.**

**Does the wound exhibit any of the following?**

- Embedded objects
- Jagged edges
- Edges that do not touch
- Debris remaining after cleaning

**YES**

**YES**

**NO**

**Is the athlete also exhibiting any of the following?**

- Breathing difficulties
- Shock
- Head or spine injury
- Other unstable or serious injuries

Cover with sterile gauze or bandage.

- Cover with sterile gauze or bandage.
- Instruct athlete on how to care for the wound and recognize signs of infection.

**NO**

**Can return to activity if athlete**

- is not bleeding;
- has touching edges of the wound;
- is not concerned about disfiguration; and
- has the wound covered.

Send to physician immediately.

**Cannot return to activity until examined and released by a physician.**

# DIRECT BLOW TO THE EYE

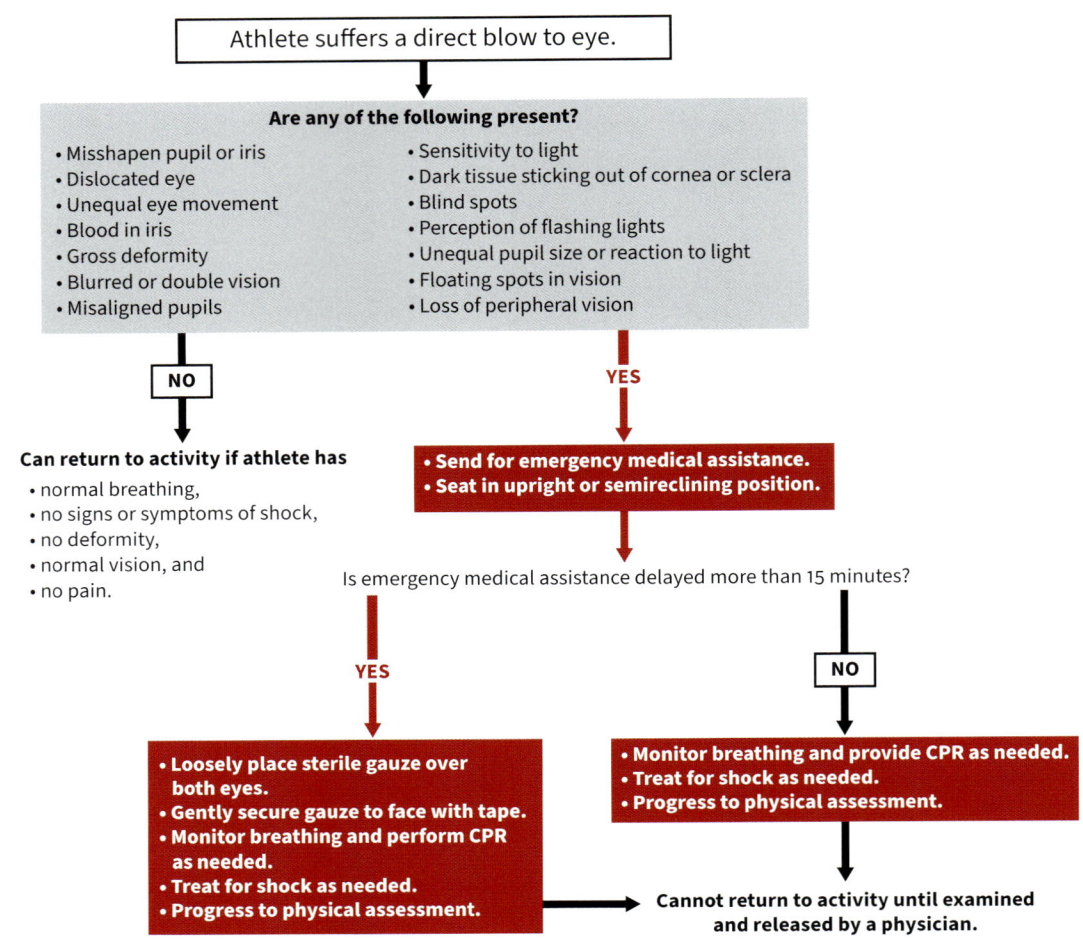

# EYE ABRASION

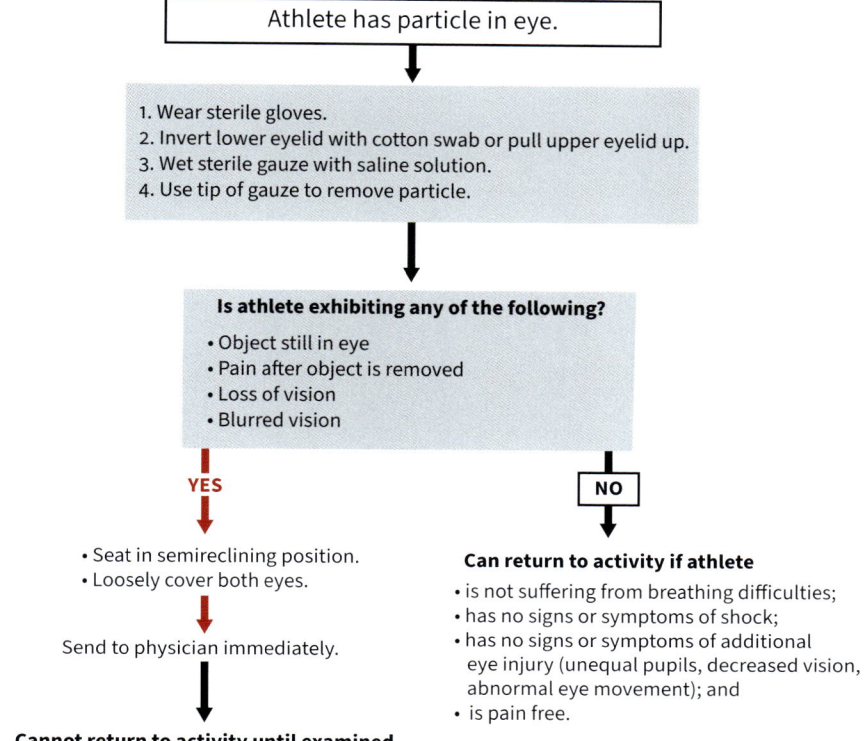

Athlete has particle in eye.

1. Wear sterile gloves.
2. Invert lower eyelid with cotton swab or pull upper eyelid up.
3. Wet sterile gauze with saline solution.
4. Use tip of gauze to remove particle.

**Is athlete exhibiting any of the following?**

- Object still in eye
- Pain after object is removed
- Loss of vision
- Blurred vision

**YES**

- Seat in semireclining position.
- Loosely cover both eyes.

Send to physician immediately.

**Cannot return to activity until examined
and released by a physician.**

**NO**

**Can return to activity if athlete**

- is not suffering from breathing difficulties;
- has no signs or symptoms of shock;
- has no signs or symptoms of additional
  eye injury (unequal pupils, decreased vision,
  abnormal eye movement); and
- is pain free.

# ABRASION

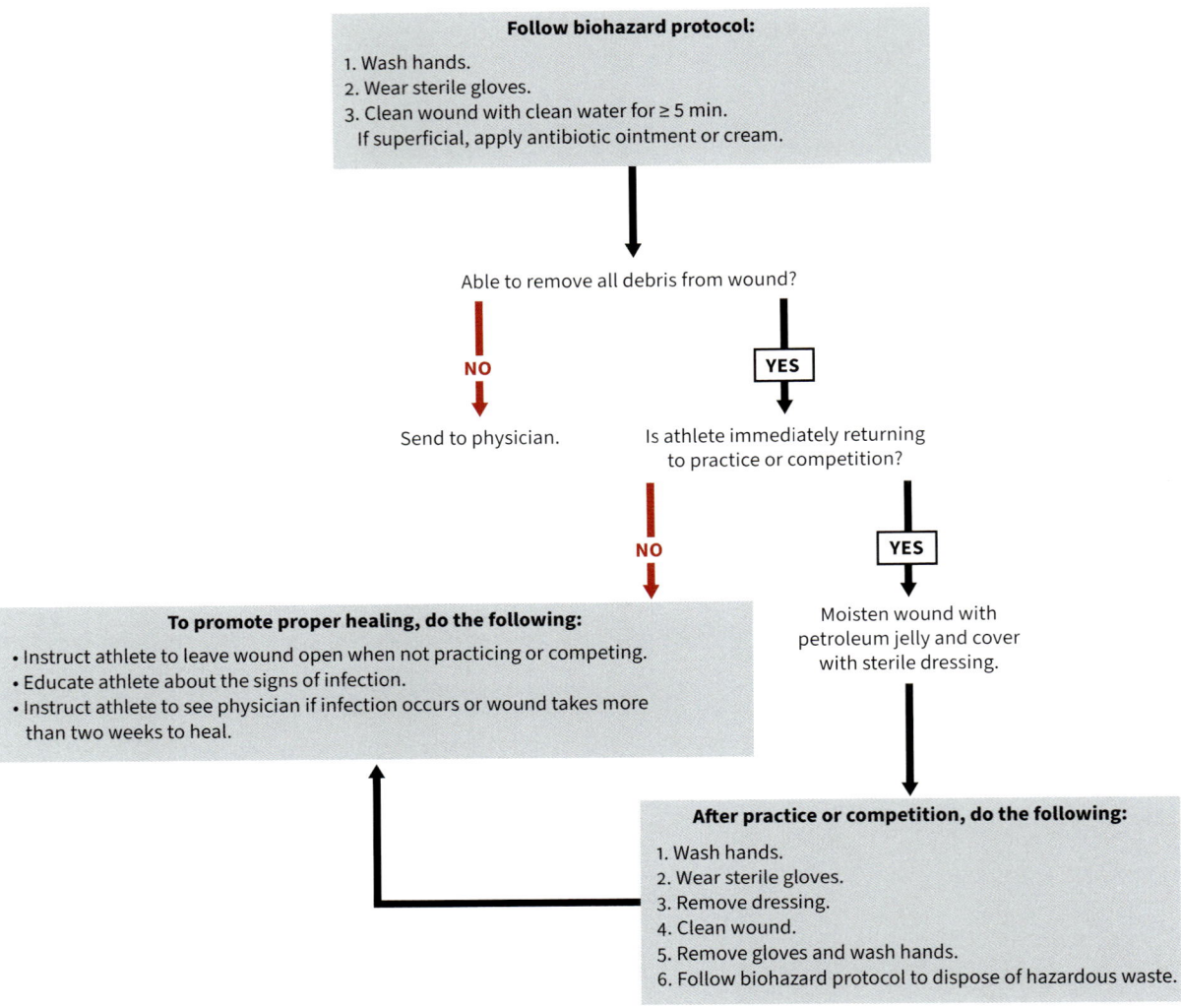

**Follow biohazard protocol:**

1. Wash hands.
2. Wear sterile gloves.
3. Clean wound with clean water for ≥ 5 min.
   If superficial, apply antibiotic ointment or cream.

Able to remove all debris from wound?

**NO**

Send to physician.

**YES**

Is athlete immediately returning to practice or competition?

**NO**

**YES**

**To promote proper healing, do the following:**

• Instruct athlete to leave wound open when not practicing or competing.
• Educate athlete about the signs of infection.
• Instruct athlete to see physician if infection occurs or wound takes more than two weeks to heal.

Moisten wound with petroleum jelly and cover with sterile dressing.

**After practice or competition, do the following:**

1. Wash hands.
2. Wear sterile gloves.
3. Remove dressing.
4. Clean wound.
5. Remove gloves and wash hands.
6. Follow biohazard protocol to dispose of hazardous waste.

# REFERENCES

## Chapter 2

American Safety & Health Institute. 2015. *CPR and AED for the Community and Workplace*. Holiday, FL: American Safety & Health Institute.

Andersen, J.C., R.W. Courson, D.M. Kleiner, and T.A. McLoda. 2002. National Athletic Trainers' Association Position Statement: Emergency Action Planning in Athletics. *Journal of Athletic Training* 37(1): 99-104.

Casa, D.J., K.M. Guskiewicz, S.A. Anderson, R.W. Courson, J.F. Heck, C.C. Jimenez, B.P. McDermott, M.G. Miller, R.L. Sterns, E.E. Swartz, and K.M. Walsh. 2012. National Athletic Trainers' Association Position Statement: Preventing Sudden Death in Sports. *Journal of Athletic Training* 47(1): 96-118.

Clark, N. 2020. *Nancy Clark's Sports Nutrition Guidebook*. 6th ed. Champaign, IL: Human Kinetics.

Conley, K.M., D.J. Bolin, P.J. Carek, J.G. Konin, T.L. Neal, and D. Violette. 2014. National Athletic Trainers' Association Position Statement: Preparticipation Physical Examination and Disqualifying Conditions. *Journal of Athletic Training* 49(1): 102-20.

Ibrahim, W.H. 2007. Recent Advances and Controversies in Adult Cardiopulmonary Resuscitation. *Postgraduate Medical Journal* 83(984): 649-54. https://doi.org/10.1136/pgmj.2007.057133.

Martens, R., and R.S. Vealey. 2024. *Successful Coaching*. 5th ed. Champaign, IL: Human Kinetics.

## Chapter 3

Collins, C., H. Robison, and T. Burus. 2022. Original Sample Summary Report. National High School Sports-Related Injury Surveillance Study, 2021-2022 School Year. https://datalyscenter.org/wp-content/uploads/2023/01/2021-22-High-School-RIO-ORIGINAL-Summary-Report.pdf.

## Chapter 4

American Heart Association. 2020. 2020 American Heart Association Guidelines for Cardiopulmonary Resuscitation and Emergency Cardiovascular Care. https://cpr.heart.org/en/resuscitation-science/cpr-and-ecc-guidelines.

American Heart Association and American Red Cross. 2020. 2020 American Heart Association and American Red Cross Focused Update for First Aid. https://cpr.heart.org/en/resuscitation-science/first-aid-guidelines.

## Chapter 5

American Heart Association. 2020. 2020 American Heart Association Guidelines for Cardiopulmonary Resuscitation and Emergency Cardiovascular Care. https://cpr.heart.org/en/resuscitation-science/cpr-and-ecc-guidelines.

American Heart Association and American Red Cross. 2020. 2020 American Heart Association and American Red Cross Focused Update for First Aid. https://cpr.heart.org/en/resuscitation-science/first-aid-guidelines.

National Safety Council. 2016. *Advanced First Aid, CPR & AED*. Itasca, IL: National Safety Council.

## Chapter 6

Del Rossi, G., M.H. Horodyski, B.P. Conrad, C.P. Di Paola, M.J. Di Paola, and G.R. Rechtine. 2008. The 6-Plus-Person Lift Transfer Technique Compared With Other Methods of Spine Boarding. *Journal of Athletic Training* 43(1): 6-13. http://www.doi.org/10.4085/1062-6050-43.1.6.

Mills, B.M., K.M. Conrick, S. Anderson, J. Bailes, B.P. Boden, D. Conway, J. Ellis, et al. 2020. Consensus Recommendations on the Prehospital Care of the Injured Athlete With a Suspected Catastrophic Cervical Spine Injury. *Journal of Athletic Training* 55(6): 563-72.

Swartz, E.E., B.P. Boden, R.W. Courson, L.C. Decoster, M. Horodyski, S.A. Norkus, R.S. Rehberg, and K.N. Waninger. 2009. National Athletic Trainers' Association Position Statement: Acute Management of the Cervical Spine-Injured Athlete. *Journal of Athletic Training* 44(3): 306-31. http://www.doi.org/10.4085/1062-6050-44.3.306.

## Chapter 7

National Safety Council. 2016. *Advanced First Aid, CPR & AED*. Itasca, IL: National Safety Council.

## Chapter 8

Collins, C., H. Robison, and T. Burus. 2022. Original Sample Summary Report. National High School Sports-Related Injury Surveillance Study, 2021-2022 School Year. https://datalyscenter.org/wp-content/uploads/2023/01/2021-22-High-School-RIO-ORIGINAL-Summary-Report.pdf.

Courson, R., J. Ellis, S. Herring, et al. 2020. Best Practices and Current Care Concepts in Prehospital Care of the Spine-Injured Athlete in American Tackle Football. March 2–3, 2019; Atlanta, GA. *Journal of Athletic Training* 55(6): 545-62.

Kerr, Z., A. Chandran, A. Nedimyer, A. Arakkal, L. Pierpoint, and S. Zuckerman. 2019. Concussion Incidence and Trends in 20 High School Sports. *Pediatrics* 144(5): e20192180. https://publications.aap.org/pediatrics/article/144/5/e20192180/38225/Concussion-Incidence-and-Trends-in-20-High-School.

Marar, M., N.M. McIlvain, S.K Fields, and R.D. Yard. 2012. Epidemiology of Concussions Among United States High School Athletes in 20 Sports. *The American Journal of Sports Medicine* 40: 747-55.

Theye, F., and K.A. Mueller. 2004. "Heads Up": Concussions in High School Sports. *Clinical Medicine & Research* 2(3):165-71. http://www.doi.org/10.3121/cmr.2.3.165.

University of Pittsburgh Medical Center. n.d. Concussion Facts and Statistics. Accessed March 15, 2023. www.upmc.com/services/sports-medicine/services/concussion/about/facts-statistics#:~:text=Between%201.7%20and%203%20million,concussions%20go%20unreported%20or%20undetected.

University of Pittsburgh School of Medicine—Neurological Surgery. n.d. Concussions. Accessed April 16, 2024. https://www.neurosurgery.pitt.edu/centers/brain-and-spine-injury/concussions.

## Chapter 9

Koester, M.C. 2000. Initial Evaluation and Management of Acute Scrotal Pain. *Journal of Athletic Training* 35(1): 76-79.

Rehberg, R., and J.G. Konin. 2018. *Sports Emergency Care: A Team Approach.* 3rd ed. SLACK.

## Chapter 10

American Diabetes Association (ADA). 2023. Treatment and Care of Hypoglycemia (Low Blood Sugar). www.diabetes.org/healthy-living/medication-treatments/blood-glucose-testing-and-control/hypoglycemia.

American Heart Association (AHA). 2020. 2020 American Heart Association Guidelines for Cardiopulmonary Resuscitation and Emergency Cardiovascular Care. Last modified October 21, 2020. https://professional.heart.org/en/science-news/2020-aha-guidelines-for-cpr-and-ecc.

Centers for Disease Control and Prevention (CDC). 2011. National Center for Health Statistics. National Health Interview Survey: 2011 Data Release. https://ftp.cdc.gov/pub/Health_Statistics/NCHS/Dataset_Documentation/NHIS/2011/readme.pdf.

Centers for Disease Control and Prevention (CDC). 2024. CDC Naloxone Fact Sheet: How and When to Use Naloxone for an Opioid Overdose 2024. Last modified April 4, 2024. https://www.cdc.gov/overdose-prevention/media/pdfs/2024/04/Naloxone-Fact-Sheet_FamilyandCaregivers_HowandWhen_4_11_2024.pdf.

Climan, A. 2023. Non-Diabetic Hypoglycemia: Symptoms, Causes, and Treatments. Last modified May 25, 2023. https://www.verywellhealth.com/hypoglycemia-in-non-diabetics-5181737.

Evans, M.W. Jr., H. Ndetan, M. Perko, R. Williams, and C. Walker. 2012. Dietary Supplement Use by Children and Adolescents in the United States to Enhance Sport Performance: Results of the National Health Interview Survey. *The Journal of Primary Prevention* 33: 3-12.

Gargallo-Fernández, M., J.E. San Martín, F. Gómez-Peralta, P. Rozas Moreno, A.M. Martínez, M. Botella-Serrano, C. Tejera Pérez, and J. López Fernández. 2015. Clinical Recommendations for Sport Practice in Diabetic Patients (RECORD Guide). Diabetes Mellitus Working Group of the Spanish Society of Endocrinology and Nutrition (SEEN). *Endocrinology and Nutrition* 62(6): 73-93.

Jimenez, C., M.H. Corcoran, J.T. Crawley, W.G. Hornsby Jr., K.S. Peer, R.D. Philbin, and M.C. Riddell. 2007. National Athletic Trainers' Association Position Statement: Management of the Athlete With Type 1 Diabetes Mellitus. *Journal of Athletic Training* 42(4): 536-45.

Johns Hopkins Medicine. n.d. Health: Absence Seizures. John Hopkins Medicine. Accessed July 31, 2023. www.hopkinsmedicine.org/health/conditions-and-diseases/epilepsy/absence-seizures.

Knapik, J.J., R.A. Steelman, S.S. Hoedebecke, K.G. Austin, E.K. Farina, and H.R. Lieberman. 2016. Prevalence of Dietary Supplement Use by Athletes: Systematic Review and Meta-Analysis. *Sports Medicine* 46(1): 103-23. https://doi.org/10.1007/s40279-015-0387-7.

Lattavo, A., A. Kopperud, and P.D. Rogers. 2007. Creatine and Other Supplements. *Pediatric Clinics of North America* 54: 735-60.

National Institute on Drug Abuse (NIH). 2017. MDMA (Ecstasy) Abuse Research Report. Last modified September 2017. https://nida.nih.gov/publications/research-reports/mdma-ecstasy-abuse/what-are-effects-mdma.

Taylor Hooten Foundation. n.d. *Anabolic Steroids: What Are Anabolic Androgenic Steroids(AAS)?* Accessed July 31, 2023. https://taylorhooton.org/anabolic-steroids.

U.S. Department of Health and Human Services (HHS) and Substance Abuse and Mental Health Services Administration (SAMHSA). 2019. *Tips for Teens: The Truth About Steroids.* Last modified May 2019. https://store.samhsa.gov/sites/default/files/pep19-06.pdf.

## Chapter 11

American Heart Association. 2020. 2020 American Heart Association Guidelines for Cardiopulmonary Resuscitation and Emergency Cardiovascular Care. https://cpr.heart.org/en/resuscitation-science/cpr-and-ecc-guidelines.

American Heart Association and American Red Cross. 2020. 2020 Focused Update for First Aid. https://cpr.heart.org/en/resuscitation-science/first-aid-guidelines.

Casa, D.E., L.E. Armstrong, S.K. Hillman, S.J. Montain, R.V. Reiff, B.S.E. Rich, W.O. Roberts, and J.A. Stone. 2000. National Athletic Trainers' Association Position Statement: Fluid Replacement for Athletes. *Journal of Athletic Training* 35(2): 212-24.

Casa, D.J., and D. Csillan. 2009. Preseason Heat-Acclimatization Guidelines for Secondary School Athletics. *Journal of Athletic Training* 44(3): 332-33.

Casa, D.J., J.K. DeMartini, M.F. Bergeron, D. Csillan, E.R. Eichner, R.M. Lopez, M.S. Ferrara, et al. 2015. National Athletic Trainers' Association Position Statement: Exertional Heat Illnesses. *Journal of Athletic Training* 50(9): 986-1000. https://doi.org/10.4085/1062-6050-50.9.07. Erratum in 2017. *Journal of Athletic Training* 52(4): 401.

Castellani, J.W, A.J. Young, M.B. Ducharme, G.G. Giesbrecht, E. Glickman, and R.E. Sallis. 2006. American College of Sports Medicine Position Stand: Prevention of Cold Injuries During Exercise. *Medicine & Science in Sports & Exercise* 38(11): 2012-29.

Centers for Disease Control and Prevention (CDC). 1998. Hyperthermia and Dehydration-Related Deaths Associated With Intentional Rapid Weight Loss–North Carolina, Wisconsin, and Michigan, November-December 1997. *Morbidity and Mortality Weekly Report* 47(6): 105-08.

Cooper, E., A. Grundstein, A. Rosen, J. Miles, J. Ko, and P. Curry. 2017. An Evaluation of Portable Wet Bulb Globe Temperature Monitor Accuracy. *Journal of Athletic Training* 52(12): 1161-67. https://doi.org/10.4085/1062-6050-52.12.18.

Hopkins, B.E., ed. 2023. *2023-2024 NFHS Wrestling Rule Book.* Indianapolis, IN: National Federation of State High School Associations.

National Federation of State High School Associations (NFHS) and Korey Stringer Institute. 2015. Five Pillars of Exertional Heat Stroke Prevention. Last modified August 31, 2015. www.nfhs.org/articles/five-pillars-of-exertional-heat-stroke-prevention.

National Weather Service (NWS). n.d.-a. What Is the Heat Index? Accessed May 7, 2022. www.weather.gov/ama/heatindex.

National Weather Service (NWS). n.d.-b. Lightning Safety and Outdoor Sports Activities. Accessed May 7, 2022. https://www.weather.gov/safety/lightning-sports.

U.S. Department of Homeland Security. 2021. How Much Do I Need to Drink After Work or Exercise? Last modified September 29, 2021. https://www.dhs.gov/sites/default/files/publications/21_0929_cbp_scale-hydration-chart.pdf.

Walsh, K.M, M.A. Cooper, R. Holle, V.A. Rakov, W.P. Roeder, and M. Ryan. 2013. National Athletic Trainers' Association Position Statement: Lightning Safety for Athletics and Recreation. *Journal of Athletic Training* 48(2): 258-70.

## Chapter 12

American Heart Association. 2020. 2020 American Heart Association Guidelines for Cardiopulmonary Resuscitation and Emergency Cardiovascular Care. https://cpr.heart.org/en/resuscitation-science/cpr-and-ecc-guidelines.

American Heart Association and American Red Cross. 2020. 2020 American Heart Association and American Red Cross Focused Update for First Aid. https://cpr.heart.org/en/resuscitation-science/first-aid-guidelines.

Collins, C., H. Robison, and T. Burus. 2022. Original Sample Summary Report. National High School Sports-Related Injury Surveillance Study, 2021-2022 School Year. https://datalyscenter.org/wp-content/uploads/2023/01/2021-22-High-School-RIO-ORIGINAL-Summary-Report.pdf.

Fleisig, G.S., C.J. Dillman, and J.R. Andrew. 1994. Biomechanics of the Shoulder During Throwing. In *The Athletic Shoulder*, edited by J.E. Andrews and K.E. Wilk. New York: Churchill Livingstone.

Koh, T.J., M.D. Grabiner, and G.G. Weiker. 1992. Technique and Ground Reaction Forces in the Back Handspring. *American Journal of Sports Medicine* 20: 61-66.

Yard, E.E., and R.D. Comstock. 2006. Injuries Sustained by Pediatric Ice Hockey, Lacrosse, and Field Hockey Athletes Presenting to United States Emergency Departments. *Journal of Athletic Training* 41(4): 441-49.

## Chapter 13

American Heart Association. 2020. 2020 American Heart Association Guidelines for Cardiopulmonary Resuscitation and Emergency Cardiovascular Care. https://cpr.heart.org/en/resuscitation-science/cpr-and-ecc-guidelines.

American Heart Association and American Red Cross. 2020. 2020 American Heart Association and American Red Cross Focused Update for First Aid. https://cpr.heart.org/en/resuscitation-science/first-aid-guidelines.

Cavanaugh, P.R., and J.R. Robinson. 1989. A Biomechanical Perspective on Stress Fractures in NBA Players. A Final Report to the National Basketball Association. Research partially supported by and submitted to the NBA.

Collins, C., H. Robison, and T. Burus. 2022. Original Sample Summary Report. National High School Sports-Related Injury Surveillance Study, 2021-2022 School Year. https://datalyscenter.org/wp-content/uploads/2023/01/2021-22-High-School-RIO-ORIGINAL-Summary-Report.pdf.

## Chapter 14

American Heart Association. 2020. 2020 American Heart Association Guidelines for Cardiopulmonary Resuscitation and Emergency Cardiovascular Care. https://cpr.heart.org/en/resuscitation-science/cpr-and-ecc-guidelines.

American Heart Association and American Red Cross. 2020. 2020 American Heart Association and American Red Cross Focused Update for First Aid. https://cpr.heart.org/en/resuscitation-science/first-aid-guidelines.

Collins, C., H. Robison, and T. Burus. 2022. Original Sample Summary Report. National High School Sports-Related Injury Surveillance Study, 2021-2022 School Year. https://datalyscenter.org/wp-content/uploads/2023/01/2021-22-High-School-RIO-ORIGINAL-Summary-Report.pdf.

Knapik, J.J., B.L. Hoedebecke, G.G. Rogers, M.A. Sharp, and S.W. Marshall. 2019. Effectiveness of Mouthguards for the Prevention of Orofacial Injuries and Concussions in Sports: Systematic Review and Meta-Analysis. *Sports Medicine* 49: 1217-32.

Turbert, D., and B. Shelton. 2024. Sports Eye Safety. Last modified January 21, 2024. https://www.aao.org/eye-health/tips-prevention/injuries-sports#:~:text=Nearly%2030%2C000%20sports%2Drelated%20eye,by%20wearing%20appropriate%20protective%20eyewear.

Young, E.J., R. Macias, and L. Stephens. 2015. Common Dental Injury Management in Athletes *Sports Health* 7(3): 250-55.

## Chapter 15

Centers for Disease Control and Prevention (CDC). 2024. Methicillin-Resistant *Staphylococcus aureus* (MRSA) Basics. Last modified April 11, 2024. https://www.cdc.gov/mrsa/about/index.html.

Hopkins, B.E., ed. 2023. *2023-2024 NFHS Wrestling Rule Book*. Indianapolis, IN: National Federation of State High School Associations.

National Athletic Trainers' Association. 2005. Official Statement from the National Athletic Trainers' Association on Community-Acquired MRSA Infections (CA-MRSA). Last modified March 1, 2005. www.nata.org/sites/default/files/mrsa.pdf.

# INDEX

*Note*: The italicized *f* and *t* following page numbers refer to figures and tables, respectively.

# ABOUT THE EDITOR

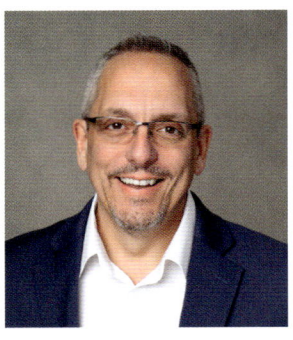

**Robb S. Rehberg, PhD, ATC, NREMT,** has served in many roles in the fields of athletic training, sports medicine, and emergency care. He is currently a professor of sports medicine and athletic training at William Paterson University of New Jersey and a senior medical advisor and director of game day medical operations for the National Football League (NFL). He also served as head athletic trainer at Westwood Regional Junior/Senior High School in Westwood, New Jersey, for 14 years; as a clinical athletic trainer at the Center for Concussion Care at Overlook Medical Center in Summit, New Jersey; and as a high school and youth sport coach.

Rehberg has held several leadership positions, including serving as president of the Athletic Trainers' Society of New Jersey and as a member of the Eastern Athletic Trainers' Association and National Athletic Trainers' Association (NATA) District 2 executive boards. Outside of athletic training, Rehberg has served as the director of first aid and emergency preparedness training and program development for the National Safety Council. His contributions and service to sport safety, athletic training, and sports medicine have been recognized through numerous awards, including induction in the halls of fame of both NATA and the Athletic Trainers' Society of New Jersey.

Rehberg has authored three textbooks in the field of sports medicine and has edited over a dozen first aid, CPR, and emergency preparedness textbooks and related training programs. He has served as an author or coauthor of dozens of publications and presented over 200 lectures on various topics in sports medicine and emergency care. He has also authored several online education programs, including ConcussionWise, a concussion education program that has trained over 2.5 million coaches, parents, and athletes in 53 countries. He served as executive producer for over a dozen first aid, CPR, and emergency preparedness training programs with the National Safety Council.

He is the cofounder of two companies: Sport Safety International, an organization dedicated to the safe participation in sport and physical activity through education, and the Rehberg Konin Group, which is the largest group of athletic training legal experts in the world.

Rehberg earned his bachelor's degree in athletic training with a minor in health science from West Chester University of Pennsylvania, a master of sport science degree from the United States Sports Academy, and a doctor of philosophy degree in health science from Touro University.

# ABOUT THE CONTRIBUTORS

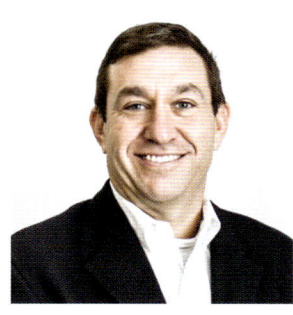

**Michael Prybicien, MA, LAT, ATC, CES, PES,** is a certified and licensed athletic trainer in New Jersey and Pennsylvania and is currently an athletic trainer at Passaic High School in New Jersey, a high school with over 3,100 students and 1,500 student-athletes. He is also an athletic training adjunct faculty member at William Paterson University of New Jersey and an athletic trainer spotter for the NFL.

Prybicien is a graduate of the Pennsylvania State University and holds bachelor's degrees in both health education and exercise and sport science. He earned a master of arts in sport administration teaching, with a concentration in health education, from Kent State University.

Prybicien has received several prestigious awards for his work in the field, including the National Athletic Trainers' Association (NATA) Service Award and Most Distinguished Athletic Trainer Award and the Athletic Trainers' Society of New Jersey (ATSNJ) Distinguished Service Award. Additionally, he has been inducted into both the ATSNJ Hall of Fame and the New Jersey Scholastic State Coaches Association Hall of Fame.

He is active with the NATA, serving on the Secondary School Committee, the ATs Care Committee, and the AT Educationalist Community Board. He has authored numerous online education courses, book chapters, abstract articles, and journal articles in his areas of expertise.

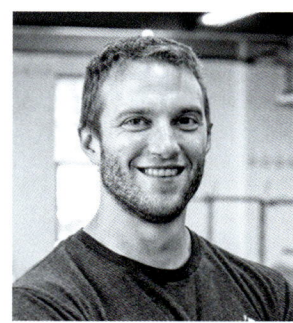

**Ben Chianchiano, MS, ATC, LAT, CSCS,** has a master of science degree in exercise science and physiology from William Paterson University of New Jersey and is a certified strength and conditioning specialist. He has been a strength and conditioning coach at the high school and collegiate levels and has also worked in clinical settings. He is a subject matter expert who works on special projects at Sport Safety International, an organization dedicated to the safe participation in sport and physical activity through education.

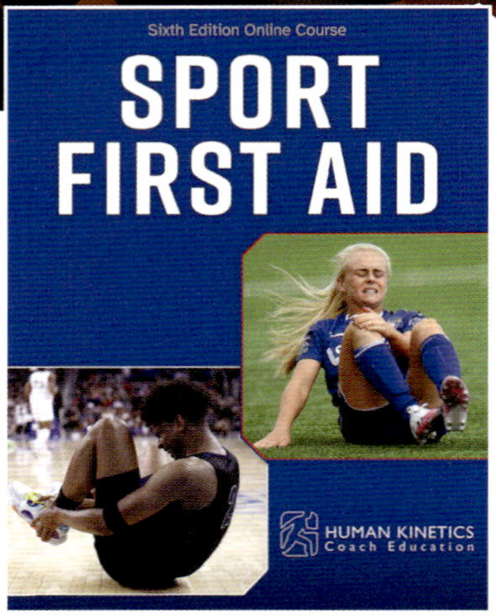

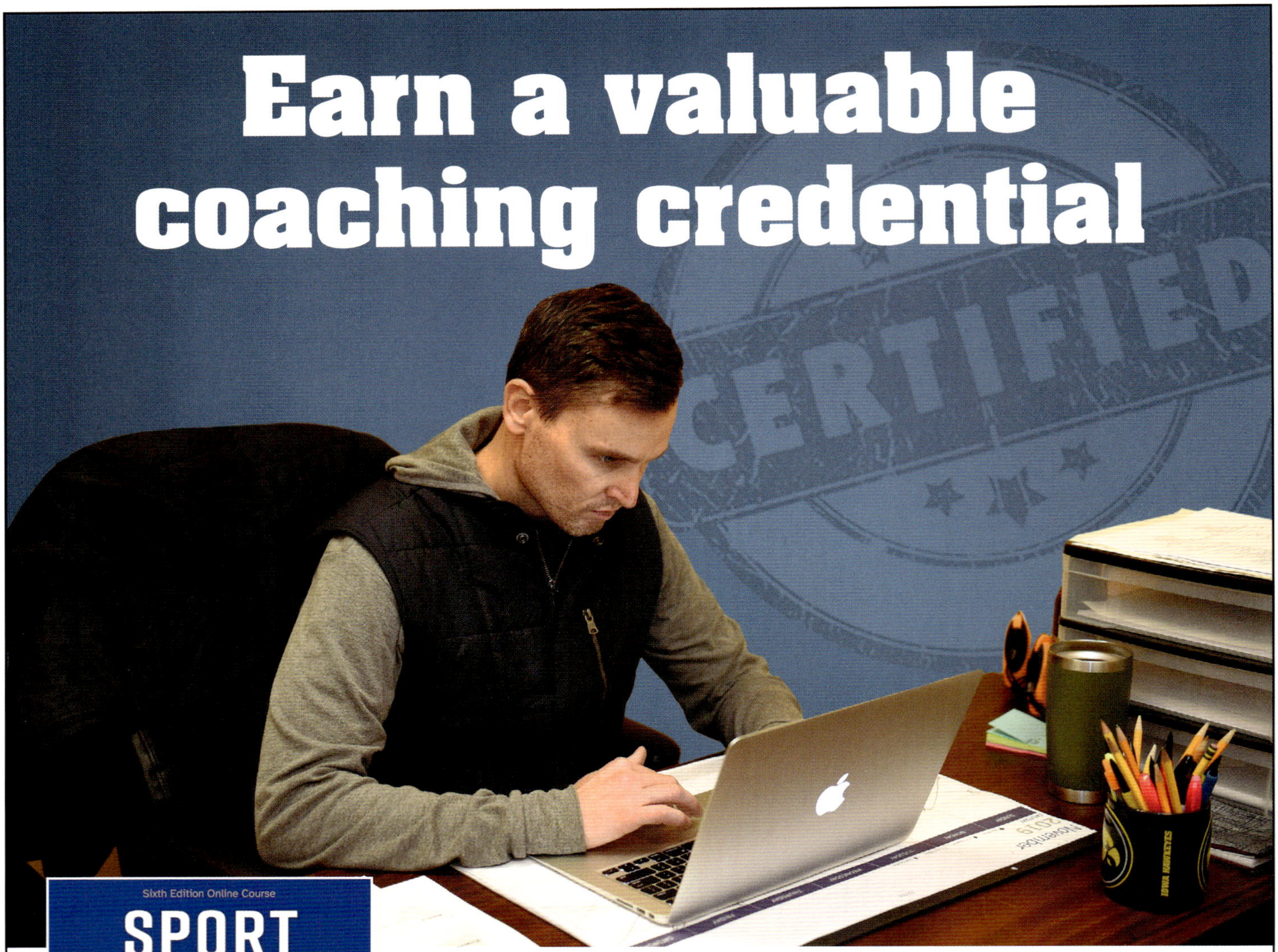

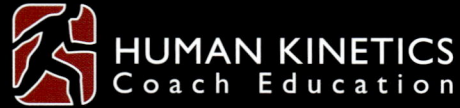